Clinical Focus on
Polycystic Ovary Syndrome

Clinical Focus on
Polycystic Ovary Syndrome

Series Editors

Neharika Malhotra
MD (Gold Medalist) DRM (Germany) FICMCH
Fellow ICOG (Rep Med) ICOG (USG)
Director and Consultant
ART Rainbow IVF and MNMH (P) Ltd
and Ujala Cygnus Rainbow Hospital
Agra, Uttar Pradesh, India
Joint Secretary, FOGSI
Chair, YTP Committee, FOGSI

Jaideep Malhotra
MD FICMCH FICOG FRCOG FRCPI FMAS
Managing Director
ART Rainbow IVF and MNMH (P) Ltd
and Ujala Cygnus Rainbow Hospital
Agra, Uttar Pradesh, India
President, SAFOM/ISPAT
Past President, IMS/ISAR/FOGSI/ASPIRE

Narendra Malhotra
MD FICMCH FICOG FRCOG FICS FMAS FIAP
Managing Director
Global Rainbow Health Care and MNMH (P) Ltd
and Ujala Cygnus Rainbow Hospital
Agra, Uttar Pradesh, India
Professor, Sarajevo School of Science and Technology, Croatia
Past President, FOGSI/IFUMB/ISPAT/ISAR, INSARG
Vice President, WAPM/SAFOG
Director, International IAN Donald School and SAFOG

Editors

Poonam Goyal
MD FICOG FICMCH
HOD, IVF and Infertility Max Hospital; Vaishali
Medical Director and HOD
Department of Obstetrics and Gynecology
Panchsheel Hospital
Delhi, India

Prerna Keshan
MBBS DGO FICOG FICMCH FIAOG
Masters in Cosmetic Gynecology
Consultant OBGYN and Infertility Specialist
Horizon Maternity and Fertility Clinic
Tinsukia, Assam, India

Ruchika Garg
MD FICOG FICMCH MRCOG1 FMAS MAMS
Professor
SN Medical College
Agra, Uttar Pradesh, India

Parul Sinha
MS FICOG
Associate Professor
Department of Obstetrics and Gynecology
All India Institute of Medical Sciences
Raebareli, Uttar Pradesh, India

Foreword
Sonia Malik

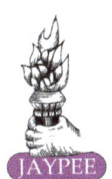

JAYPEE BROTHERS MEDICAL PUBLISHERS
The Health Sciences Publisher
New Delhi | London

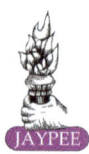

Jaypee Brothers Medical Publishers (P) Ltd

Headquarters

Jaypee Brothers Medical Publishers (P) Ltd
EMCA House, 23/23-B
Ansari Road, Daryaganj
New Delhi 110 002, India
Landline: +91-11-23272143, +91-11-23272703
+91-11-23282021, +91-11-23245672
Email: jaypee@jaypeebrothers.com

Corporate Office

Jaypee Brothers Medical Publishers (P) Ltd
4838/24, Ansari Road, Daryaganj
New Delhi 110 002, India
Phone: +91-11-43574357
Fax: +91-11-43574314
Email: jaypee@jaypeebrothers.com

Overseas Office

JP Medical Ltd
83 Victoria Street, London
SW1H 0HW (UK)
Phone: +44 20 3170 8910
Fax: +44 (0)20 3008 6180
Email: info@jpmedpub.com

Website: www.jaypeebrothers.com
Website: www.jaypeedigital.com

© 2023, Jaypee Brothers Medical Publishers

The views and opinions expressed in this book are solely those of the original contributor(s)/author(s) and do not necessarily represent those of editor(s) or publisher of the book.

All rights reserved. No part of this publication may be reproduced, stored or transmitted in any form or by any means, electronic, mechanical, photocopying, recording or otherwise, without the prior permission in writing of the publishers.

All brand names and product names used in this book are trade names, service marks, trademarks or registered trademarks of their respective owners. The publisher is not associated with any product or vendor mentioned in this book.

Medical knowledge and practice change constantly. This book is designed to provide accurate, authoritative information about the subject matter in question. However, readers are advised to check the most current information available on procedures included and check information from the manufacturer of each product to be administered, to verify the recommended dose, formula, method and duration of administration, adverse effects and contraindications. It is the responsibility of the practitioner to take all appropriate safety precautions. Neither the publisher nor the author(s)/editor(s) assume any liability for any injury and/or damage to persons or property arising from or related to use of material in this book.

This book is sold on the understanding that the publisher is not engaged in providing professional medical services. If such advice or services are required, the services of a competent medical professional should be sought.

Every effort has been made where necessary to contact holders of copyright to obtain permission to reproduce copyright material. If any have been inadvertently overlooked, the publisher will be pleased to make the necessary arrangements at the first opportunity.

Inquiries for bulk sales may be solicited at: jaypee@jaypeebrothers.com

Clinical Focus on Polycystic Ovary Syndrome

First Edition: 2023

ISBN: 978-93-5696-091-6

Dedicated to

Our parents, teachers, and all practicing Obstetricians and Gynecologists.

Contributors

Akanksha Gupta MD
Senior Resident
Department of Obstetrics and Gynecology
All India Institute of Medical Sciences
New Delhi, India

Amrita Singh MS DNB FRM (Diploma ART)
Consultant
Indira IVF Pvt. Limited
Lucknow, Uttar Pradesh, India

Anand Srivastava MD (Respiratory Medicine)
Additional Professor
Department of Respiratory Medicine
King George's Medical University
Lucknow, Uttar Pradesh, India

Aruna Verma MD FICOG
Professor
Obstetrics and Gynecology
Professor
LLRM Medical College
Meerut, Uttar Pradesh, India

Asha Baxi MS FICOG FRCOG
Lead Consultant
Dr Asha Baxi Fertility Center
Motherhood Hospital
Indore, Madhya Pradesh, India

B Aruna Suman MD FICOG
Professor HOD
Department of Obstetrics and Gynecology
Vice Principal
Government Medical College
Jagtial, Telangana, India

Bhavna Mittal DNB FNB MNAMS FICOG
Director and HOD
Shivam IVF and Infertility Center
Delhi, India

Chandana Bhatt MBBS MS DNB (Obs & Gyn) MCh
(Reproductive Medicine and Surgery)
Consultant
Vishvas Fertility and Gynecology Centre
Bengaluru, Karnataka, India

Charmila Ayyavoo MD DGO DFP FICOG PGDCR
Director
Aditi Hospital and
Parvathy Ayyavoo Fertility Centre, Trichy
Consultant, Southern Railway Hospital
Trichy, Tamil Nadu, India
Vice President Elect FOGSI 2024

Deeba Khanam MD (Obs & Gyn)
Assistant Professor
JN Medical College
Aligarh Muslim University
Aligarh, Uttar Pradesh, India

Deepa Chaudhary
MS (Obs & Gyn) FARM FMAS DIP Urogynecology (Germany)
Associate Professor
SMS Medical College
Jaipur, Rajasthan, India

Dhara Singh MS (Gold Medalist) DNB
Assistant Professor
Department of Obstetrics and Gynecology
MGM Medical College and Associated Hospitals
Indore, Madhya Pradesh, India

Dhaval Baxi
DGO DNB MCh (Reproductive Medicine and Surgery)
Consultant
Disha Fertility and Motherhood Hospital
Indore, Madhya Pradesh, India

Dolly Mehra MS FICOG
Consultant
Mehra Nursing Home Ratlam
Past President
Ratlam Obstetrics and Gynecology Society.
Ratlam, Madhya Pradesh, India

Contributors

Gaurav Rajender MBBS DNB MNAMS FIPS
Associate Professor
Department of Psychiatry
SMS Medical College
Jaipur, Rajasthan, India

Jaideep Malhotra
MD FICMCH FICOG FRCOG FRCPI FMAS
Managing Director
ART Rainbow IVF and MNMH (P) Ltd
and Ujala Cygnus Rainbow Hospital
Agra, Uttar Pradesh, India
President, SAFOM/ISPAT
Past President, IMS/ISAR/FOGSI/ASPIRE

K Geetha MD DVL DDVL
Associate Professor Dermatology
All India Institute of Medical Sciences
Raebareli, Uttar Pradesh, India

Kundan Ingale DGO DNB FICOG
Assisted Reproduction
Fertility Specialist
Nirmiti Clinic: A Center for Assisted
Reproduction, Chinchwad
Pune, Maharashtra, India

Mamta MS (Obs & Gyne)
Associate Professor
Institute of Medical Sciences
Banaras Hindu University
Varanasi, Uttar Pradesh, India

Mayuri More MBBS MS FRM
Assistant Professor
DY Patil School of Medicine
Consultant Bloom IVF
Mumbai, Maharashtra, India

Mohita Agarwal MD (Obs & Gyne)
Professor
SN Medical College
Agra, Uttar Pradesh, India

Mousumi Das Ghosh MD FICOG
Consultant
Tata Main Hospital
Manipal Tata Medical college
Jamshedpur, Jharkhand, India

Nandita Palshetkar MD FRCOG FICOG FCPS
Professor in Obstetrics and Gynecology
DY Patil Medical College
Navi Mumbai
Director at NINE BLOOM IVF Centers
Mumbai, Maharashtra, India

Narendra Malhotra
MD FICMCH FICOG FRCOG FICS FMAS FIAP
Managing Director
Global Rainbow Health Care and MNMH (P) Ltd
and Ujala Cygnus Rainbow Hospital
Agra, Uttar Pradesh, India
Professor, Sarajevo School of Science and
Technology, Croatia
Past President, FOGSI/IFUMB/ISPAT/ISAR, INSARG
Vice President, WAPM/SAFOG
Director, International IAN Donald School and
SAFOG

Natasha Vijayendram MD (Dermatology)
Consultant
AA Derma Science—Complete Clinic for Women
Gurugram, Haryana, India

Neerja Bhatla MBBS MD FICOG FAMS (Obs & Gyne)
Professor and Head
Shobha Wenger Distinguished
Professor of Gynae Oncology
All India Institute of Medical Sciences
New Delhi, India

Neha Kapoor MBBS MD FICMCH
Consultant
Kapoor Medical Center
New Delhi, India

Neharika Malhotra MD (Gold Medalist) DRM
(Germany) FICMCH Fellow ICOG (Rep Med) ICOG (USG)
Director and Consultant
ART Rainbow IVF and MNMH (P) Ltd
and Ujala Cygnus Rainbow Hospital
Agra, Uttar Pradesh, India
Joint Secretary, FOGSI
Chair, YTP Committee, FOGSI

Pallaavi Goel MBBS
PG Resident (General Medicine)
Mahatma Gandhi Medical College and Hospital
Jaipur, Rajasthan, India

Parul Sinha MS FICOG
Associate Professor
Department of Obstetrics and Gynecology
All India Institute of Medical Sciences
Raebareli, Uttar Pradesh, India

Poonam Goyal MD FICOG FICMCH
HOD, IVF and Infertility Max Hospital; Vaishali
Medical Director and HOD
Department of Obstetrics and Gynecology
Panchsheel Hospital
Delhi, India

Priti Kumar MD FICOG
Chairperson Safe Motherhood
Committee FOGSI
Professor and Head
Department of Obstetrics and Gynecology
Naraina Medical College and Research Center
Kanpur, Uttar Pradesh, India

Prerna Keshan MBBS DGO FICOG FICMCH FIAOG
Masters in Cosmetic Gynecology
Consultant OBGYN and Infertility Specialist
Horizon Maternity and Fertility Clinic
Tinsukia, Assam, India

Priyankur Roy MBBS MS FIRM FAGE
Consultant Roy's Clinic, Siliguri
Assistant Professor LBKMCH
Saharsa, Bihar, India

Ragini Agrawal
MS FICOG FICMCH Fellow Clinical Gyne Endoscopy, UK
Director Medical Services and
Clinical Director & Head
Cosmetic Gynecology and
Pelvic Reconstructive Surgery
W Pratiksha Hospital
Gurugram, Haryana, India

Ramesh Patodia MD
Chief Executive Officer
CEO at Ambrosia Nutrition Pvt Ltd
Mumbai, Maharashtra, India

Rashmika Gandhi MD
Reproductive Medicine and Endoscopy Fellow
Solo Clinic: A Center of Excellence and Research
Pune, Maharashtra, India

Rohan Palshetkar
MS (Obs and Gyne) FRM BDRME ADRME
Associate Professor
Head of Unit Bloom IVF
Mumbai, Maharashtra, India

Ruchika Garg
MD FICOG FICMCH MRCOG1 FMAS MAMS
Professor
SN Medical College
Agra, Uttar Pradesh, India

S Ashok Kumar
MS MRCOG DRM MIMS FRM
Consultant Fertility and Gynec Endoscopic
Surgeon
Apollo Fertility Center
Chennai, Tamil Nadu, India

Sadhana Gupta
MS (Obs & Gyne) MNAMS FICOG FICMU FICMCH
Vice President FOGSI 2016
Co-Chair SAFOG NCD Committee
Senior Consultant
Department of Obstetrics and Gynecology
Jeevan Jyoti Hospital and Medical Research Center
Gorakhpur, Uttar Pradesh, India

Sangeeta Rai
PhD FICOG FMAS FICMCH
Professor
Department of Obstetrics and Gynecology
Institute of Medical Sciences
Banaras Hindu University
Varanasi, Uttar Pradesh, India

Sarita Kumari
MD DNB MCH (Gynecologic Oncology)
Assistant Professor
National Cancer Institute
All India Institute of Medical Sciences
New Delhi, India

Shaheen Anjum
MS ACME Fellowship in Reproductive Medicine
Professor & In-charge ART Unit
Department of Obstetrics and Gynecology
JN Medical College
Aligarh Muslim University
Aligarh, Uttar Pradesh, India

Contributors

Shama Batra MBBS MD FICOG
Medical Director
HOD
Department of Obstetrics and Gynecology
Patel Hospital
Delhi, India

Shikha Sachan MS (Obs & Gyne)
Associate Professor
Institute of Medical Sciences
Banaras Hindu University
Varanasi, Uttar Pradesh, India

Sonalica Suresh DGO DNB
Specialist
Department of Obstetrics and Gynecology
NMC Hospital
Al-An-Nahda
Dubai, United Arab Emirates

Soniya Dhiman MBBS MD
Assistant Professor
Department of Obstetrics and Gynecology
All India Institute of Medical Sciences
New Delhi, India

Subash Mallya
DGO DNB MNAMS FICOG Diploma in Gyne Endoscopy
HOD
Department of Minimal Access Surgery
Baby Memorial Hospital
Calicut, Kerala, India

Suman Chaudhary MBBS MS (Gyne-Oncology, TATA)
Associate Professor
Department of Obstetrics and Gynecology
SMS Medical College
Jaipur, Rajasthan, India

Sunita Tandulwadkar MD (Obs & Gyn) FICS (Endoscopic Surgery) FICOG, Diploma in Endoscopy (Germany)
Chief and Head of Department
Ruby Hall Clinic, Pune
Chief, IVF Department
DY Patil Medical College
Pune, Maharashtra, India

Swapnil Langde MD
Consultant
Solo Clinic: A Center of Excellence and Research
Pune, Maharashtra, India

Tanushree Pandey Padgaonkar
MBBS MS OBGY FRM DE (Germany)
Director at Samadhan Nursing Home and Hope Fertility Center
Private Practice
Mumbai, Maharashtra, India

Vandana Gupta MBBS MS CCGDM FICOG
Senior Consultant
Department of Obstetrics and Gynecology
Apex Citi Hospital
Lifeline Hospital
New Delhi, India

Vandana Verma MD (Obs & Gyne)
Associate Professor
All India Institute of Medical Sciences
Raebareli, Uttar Pradesh, India

Vidya Thobbi MD FICOG
Professor and Head
Obstetrics and Gynecology
Ameen Medical College
Bijapur, Karnataka, India

Vishwajeet A Burungale MD
Radiodiagnosis
Registrar
Deenanath Mangeshkar Hospital and Research Center
Pune, Maharashtra, India

Foreword

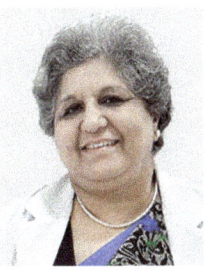

The book "*Clinical Focus on Polycystic Ovary Syndrome*" has been brought out by the stalwarts of Gynecology. It is a wonderful amalgamation of the latest guidelines, algorithms, and practical tips.

The book contains all the latest information required by practitioners. It is indeed extensive work covering every aspect of PCOS-PCOD. All the authors must be congratulated for this book on PCOS. It is a must in all departmental libraries to keep postgraduate students abreast of the latest advances in PCOS. There is a continuous need to be updated in the interest of our patients.

I feel the editors and authors have done a great job by doing justice to all topics. It is recommended for MD/DNB students and practicing consultants and also for those appearing in the MRCOG exam.

I congratulate learned Dr Narendra Malhotra and Dr Jaideep Malhotra for this clinical focus series. It is actually a tedious task to bring out such a needed book. I appreciate the hard work of Dr Poonam Goyal, Dr Neharika Malhotra, and Dr Ruchika Garg. Dr Parul Sinha and Dr Prerna Keshan have also given their valuable inputs. All the editors have worked hard for this to be on your table to update yourself.

My best wishes and good luck to them for the success of the book.

Sonia Malik DGO MD FICOG FIAMS
HOD, NOVA Southend Fertility and IVF
Past President, Indian Fertility Society 2014–16
Past President Indian Menopause Society 2007–08
Member Editorial Board Fertility and Sterility India
Member Editorial Board Journal of Reproductive Health and Medicine
Member, ICMR Task Force on Genital Tuberculosis and PCOS

Preface

The book "*Clinical Focus on Polycystic Ovary Syndrome*" aims at addressing a holistic approach toward understanding and managing this otherwise less understood clinical spectrum. The reason why this book is being launched is the ever-increasing incidence of the syndrome in today's modern world. PCOS has become an endemic of the modern Era. Even with such huge affection of females in the reproductive period and beyond, there is no absolute consensus on the guidelines and strategies of management. There is an ongoing research starting from the pathophysiology to environmental factors as well genetic basis and the in utero causes of this syndrome. While researches help us to understand PCOS better, this book will definitely prove as a clinical and methodical updation of our acumen to understand, diagnose and treat PCOS.

The contributors have taken immense efforts to dissipate a quality information that would prove beneficial for undergraduates, postgraduates and practitioners. We look forward toward a gennext with lesser incidence of this syndrome by understanding it wide and forth and a better tomorrow.

Neharika Malhotra
Jaideep Malhotra
Narendra Malhotra

Acknowledgments

We have the pleasure of introducing "*Clinical Focus on Polycystic Ovary Syndrome*".

We thank the Almighty God for helping us throughout the journey of completing this task.

Our heartfelt gratitude and indebtedness to Dr Sonia Malik for accepting to write the foreword for this book and also for sharing his expertise and pearls of wisdom.

It is with utmost pleasure that we thank Dr Narendra Malhotra and Dr Jaideep Malhotra, our mentors and guide for this clinical series, who lent their considerable clinical and academic prowess. Their enthusiasm and encouragement kept us motivated to accomplish this task.

In constructing a compilation of this breadth, clinicians from several departments and their expertise were needed to add vital, contemporaneous information. We wish to thank all our contributors who responded to our requests with promptness. Our heartfelt thanks to them.

We wish to appreciate the efforts of M/s Jaypee Brothers Medical Publishers(P) Ltd, New Delhi, India for bringing out this book in its final shape with their talent of skillfully and expediently coordinating and overseeing composition. We also thank the publishing team of JP specially Ms Rajni D Chauhan. Without the thoughtful, creative efforts of many, our Focus Series would have been a barren wasteland of words. Their attention to detail and accurate renderings added important academic support to our words.

Our special appreciation and thanks to all our colleagues, friends who supported our idea of bringing out this series and gave us the confidence to finish this book.

Lastly, we offer an enthusiastic thanks to our families and friends. Without their patience, generosity and encouragement, this task would have been impossible. We sincerely thank you for your love and support which kept us going to finish this work of ours

Poonam Goyal
Ruchika Garg
Prerna Keshan
Parul Sinha

Contents

1. PCOS: Introduction and Epidemiology 1
   Poonam Goyal, Dhaval Baxi

2. Pathophysiology in PCOS 4
   Aruna Verma, Mohita Agarwal

3. PCOS its Root in Womb 14
   Charmila Ayyavoo, Priyankur Roy

4. Diagnosis of PCOS 18
   Deeba Khanam, Shaheen Anjum

5. Ultrasound in PCOD 23
   Poonam Goyal, Vishwajeet A Burungale, Pallaavi Goel

6. PCOS in Adolescents 30
   Dhara Singh, B Aruna Suman

7. Metabolic Syndrome and PCOS 44
   Parul Sinha, Amrita Singh

8. Insulin Resistance in PCOS 50
   Aruna Verma, Vandana Verma

9. Hirsutism and Hyperandrogenism in PCOS 56
   K Geetha

10. Psychological Aspects of PCOS 65
    Deepa Chaudhary, Suman Chaudhary, Gaurav Rajender

11. Sleep Apnea and PCOS 73
    Anand Srivastava, Parul Sinha

12. Role of Micronutrients in PCOS 81
    Priti Kumar, Sangeeta Rai

13. Gut Microbiome and PCOS 86
    Ruchika Garg, Soniya Dhiman, Akanksha Gupta

14. Endocrine Disruptors in PCOS 92
    Neha Kapoor, Ruchika Garg, Poonam Goyal

15. Protisol/Nutraceuticals in PCOS 95
    Neharika Malhotra, Narendra Malhotra, Ramesh Patodia

16. **Clinical Spectrum of PCOS** 100
    Vidya Thobbi, Parul Sinha

17. **PCOS in Peri and Post Menopause** 104
    Dolly Mehra

18. **Cancer in PCOS** 112
    Sarita Kumari, Neerja Bhatla

19. **Lifestyle Interventions in PCOS** 116
    Prerna Keshan

20. **Medical Management of PCOS** 121
    Mousumi Das Ghosh

21. **Surgery in PCOS** 128
    Sunita Tandulwadkar, Swapnil Langde, Rashmika Gandhi

22. **Infertility in PCOS** 136
    Kundan Ingale, S Ashok Kumar

23. **Ovulation Induction in PCOS** 142
    Nandita Palshetkar, Tanushree Pandey Padgaonkar, Rohan Palshetkar

24. **Role of Adjuvants in PCOS** 149
    Bhavna Mittal, Chandana Bhatt, Poonam Goyal

25. **ART in PCOS** 154
    Rohan Palshetkar, Nandita Palshetkar, Mayuri More

26. **Pregnancy in PCOS** 161
    Jaideep Malhotra, Parul Sinha, Asha Baxi

27. **Bariatric Surgery in PCOS** 167
    Subash Mallya, Sonalica Suresh

28. **Aesthetics in PCOS** 173
    Ragini Agrawal, Natasha Vijayendram

29. **Sequelae of PCOS** 180
    Shama Batra, Vandana Gupta

30. **PCOS in Indian Scenario** 186
    Sadhana Gupta, Shikha Sachan, Mamta

Annexure 199

Index 217

CHAPTER 1

PCOS: Introduction and Epidemiology

Poonam Goyal, Dhaval Baxi

INTRODUCTION: POLYCYSTIC OVARIAN DISEASE AND POLYCYSTIC OVARY SYNDROME

Polycystic ovary syndrome (PCOS) is a common and perplexing condition affecting metabolic, reproductive, cardiovascular, and psychological health in women. Going back to history, it seems that the existence was noted long back. In ancient times, Hippocrates and Soranus had reported that "Many women have masculine and robust body; they do not menstruate regularly and they don't become pregnant."[1,2] Some other authors suggested that these women have greatest capacity of energy storage to fight the necessary fasting periods.[3,4]

As such in ancient times, the PCOS-related subfertility was good in a way as it was related to low parity and decreased maternal mortality as delivery-related complications were too high in that period, especially in women of reproductive age. Over the years, many gene variants have survived and now we see so much of heterogenicity in phenotypes and genotypes of PCOS.[5]

Previously, the disease was poorly understood; studies point to widespread dissatisfaction and frustration in these women. Studies have found delays with the diagnosis of PCOS. There were gaps in the knowledge of physicians regarding the diagnosis and management of polycystic ovarian disease (PCOD) and PCOS.

But the concept of hyperandrogenism was understood long back in the 18th century and its correlation with truncal fat was established. Later, with time it was proved that it was related to insulin resistance.

Now, in literature there are enough studies to indicate that PCOS is an endocrine disorder, the crux of which is metabolic disorder and insulin resistance being interrelated to each other. There is a vicious circle which is difficult to break. The obesity is android type with accumulation of abdominal fat which is typically male type. This all leads to an increased risk of cardiovascular problems. There is a strong tendency to develop gestational diabetes. Later in life, these women are prone to becoming diabetic.

In a nutshell, it should be considered as a chronic health problem which should be taken care of in all phases of life right from adolescence to postmenopause.

Coming to the terminology used, there is sometimes confusion. Polycystic ovary (PCO) is used as a short form of the polycystic appearance of ovaries on ultrasonography (USG). This does not signify that the patient has the disease; it is just a typical morphology on USG. PCOD is a short form of polycystic ovarian disease and PCOS is polycystic ovarian syndrome. Actually, PCOS has a lot of symptoms common with PCOD—weight gain, infertility, acne, irregular periods, etc. PCOS also includes metabolic syndrome, which increases the risk of heart disease, strokes, and diabetes. It may also cause sleep apnea, which affects the body's ability to breathe while you are sleeping; this means sudden pauses in breathing or inability to breathe while asleep, which in turn leads to a highly disturbed sleep cycle. As no ovulation is taking place, the uterine lining-endometrium—builds up every month, which can also increase chances of endometrial cancer. So, in PCOD it is ovarian–pituitary axis disturbance whereas in PCOS there is endocrine disturbance as well as metabolic disturbance leading to multiple system defects. PCOD is a medical condition where the ovaries release the eggs prematurely, which turn into cysts over time. The ovaries become bigger in size and start to release higher levels of male hormones in the body. This occurs because of unhealthy lifestyle habits, consuming junk food, and being overweight and is reversible with lifestyle interventions. PCOS has genetic onset and is rather refractory to manage.

Polycystic ovary syndrome has different presentations. The findings of study conducted in a university in Hyderabad showed obesity (84.37%), oligomenorrhea (79.68%), infertility (71.87%), and hyperandrogenism (62.49%). According to another study conducted in Islamabad, 75% patients presented with primary infertility, 84.6% with hirsutism, 75% oligomenorrhea, and obesity 86.5%. Amenorrhea, infertility, and hirsutism are main problems.[6,7] If diagnostic criterion is Rotterdam, the incidence is 1.5–2% times more as compared to the National Institutes of Health (NIH) PCOS group. So, the same criterion should be used for comparison.

Polycystic ovary syndrome, thus reflects multiple potential etiologies and has variable clinical manifestations. There is strong evidence that it is a genetic disease. Such evidence includes the familial clustering of cases, greater concordance in monozygotic compared with dizygotic twins, and heritability of endocrine and metabolic features of PCOS. PCOS in adolescents arises as a result of a genetically determined disorder of ovarian function that results in hypersecretion of androgens, possibly during fetal life and also during physiological activation of the hypothalamic–pituitary–ovarian axis in infancy and at the onset of puberty.

Obesity unmasks or amplifies symptoms, and endocrine and metabolic abnormalities. Basic problem is sedentary lifestyle with fast foods, amplified by stress. Obesity is an invitation to various medical disorders. So, to control this, a regular exercise schedule is very crucial—15 minutes daily, adding 5 min/day, and taking it to 150 min/week of aerobic activity. Combining it with right food is very helpful.

The increasing incidence of childhood obesity has resulted in an alarming increase not only in distressing symptoms but also in impaired glucose tolerance and even diabetes among adolescent girls with PCOD and PCOS. In due course, however, identification of the major susceptibility loci is likely to provide key insight into the etiology of the syndrome and improve diagnosis and management.[7] A fall in serum testosterone level in response to insulin-sensitizing therapy with metformin and lifestyle change helps.[8]

Role of gut microbiome is all set to alter the understanding of etiology and management of this disease. Various new drugs, epigenetics, and recent ovulation induction protocols in anovulatory infertile patients will open new horizons in disease prevention and management.

■ CONCLUSION

PCOD and PCOS involve a spiraling cycle of generations of unhealthy body weight and obesity. It is imperative to prevent excessive weight gain and to promote healthy lifestyle during prenatal and postnatal periods. The link between maternal lifestyle and its effects on fetus cannot be underestimated.

It is obvious that humans are not well adaptable to the changing environment as we used to envisage. Many disciplines are required in health care. The future of community health is bright if we not only treat established illnesses but also put great attention on prevention of the disease at its origin.[9]

Better understanding of genetics and epigenetics sets the stage for hopeful outcomes.

■ REFERENCES

1. Hanson AE. Hippocrates: Disease of women 1. Signs (chic). 1975;1(2):567-84.
2. Temkin O, Soranus. Soranus' gynecology. Baltimore: Johns Hopkins University Press; 1991.
3. Chakravarthy MV, Booth FW. Eating, exercise and thrifty genotype: connecting the dots towards an evolutionary understanding of modern chronic disease. J Appl Physiol. 2004; 96:3-10.
4. Neel JV. Diabetes Mellitus a "thrifty" genotype rendered detrimental by "progress"? Am J Hum Genet. 1962;14:353-62.
5. Vague J. La differentiation sexuelle Facteur determinant des forms de l'obesite'. Presse Med. 1947;66:339-40.
6. Hart R. Definitions, prevalence and symptoms of polycystic ovaries. In: Allahabadia GN, Agarwal R (Eds). Polycystic Ovary Syndrome. Kent: Anshan; 2007. pp.15-26.
7. Azziz R, Sanchez L, Knochenhaur ES, Moran C, Lazenby J, Stephens KC, et al. Androgen excess in women: experience with over 1000 consecutive patients. J Clin Endocrinol Metab. 2004;89(2):453-62.
8. Stracquadanio M, Ciotta L. Metabolic Aspects of PCOS. New York: Springer; 2015. pp. 2-3.
9. Shah MB. Obesity and sexuality in women. Obstet Gynecol Clin North Am. 2009;36(2): 347-60.

Pathophysiology in PCOS

Aruna Verma, Mohita Agarwal

INTRODUCTION

Approximately 90% of individuals with polycystic ovary syndrome (PCOS) have abnormal ovarian androgenic effects,[1] and the common denominator of PCOS is ovarian hyperandrogenism. Insulin-resistant hyperinsulinemia is a minor but common complicating factor in pathophysiology. The propensity for luteinizing hormone (LH) excess and obesity appears to accompany underlying ovarian hyperandrogenism and hyperinsulinemia.

So, a unified minimal model of PCOS pathophysiology is given, which incorporated the major features of the syndrome[1] and is as follows:
- Functional ovarian hyperandrogenism (FOH)
- Insulin resistance
- LH excess.

PRIMARY FUNCTIONAL OVARIAN HYPERANDROGENISM

According to ovarian androgenic dynamic testing, approximately 90% of PCOS patients have FOH.[1] Excess circulating androgens act on the skin's pilosebaceous units, causing cutaneous manifestations such as hirsutism and acne. Granulosa cell dysfunction results from an excessive intraovarian androgenic milieu, which manifests as oligo-anovulation and, in some cases, polycystic ovarian morphology (PCOM) **(Figs. 1A and B)**.

Polycystic ovary syndrome is classified into several functional groups, each representing a different source of androgen excess **(Table 1 and Fig. 2)**:
- *Functionally typical PCOS/FOH:* Two-thirds of PCOS/FOH cases are considered "functionally typical" because they show an exaggerated increase in 17-hydroxyprogesterone (17-OHP) in response to LH receptor stimulation achieved clinically with either gonadotropin-releasing hormone agonist (GnRHa) or human chorionic gonadotropin (hCG). The increased 17-OHP response appears to be an indicator of dysregulated cytochrome P450c17 function. Furthermore, these patients have an abnormal response to the dexamethasone androgen-suppression test (DAST): dexamethasone suppresses adrenocortical steroidogenesis but is unable to suppress serum testosterone, indicating an ovarian origin.
- *Functionally atypical PCOS/FOH:* PCOS is classified as "functionally atypical" if the remaining one-third of cases have a normal 17-OHP response to GnRHa or hCG but an abnormal response to DAST. Some patients have isolated primary functional adrenal hyperandrogenism (FAH), as shown by adrenocorticotropic hormone (ACTH) stimulation, or PCOS without FOH or FAH. The majority of the latter group has obesity-related atypical PCOS, while a small percentage has

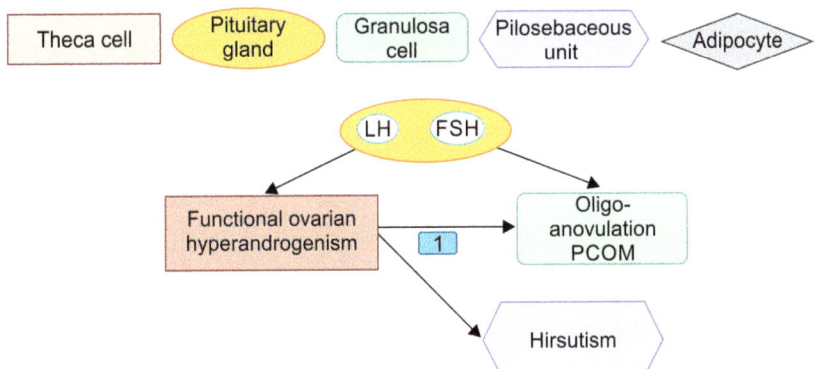

Fig. 1A: Functional ovarian hyperandrogenism in all PCOS.

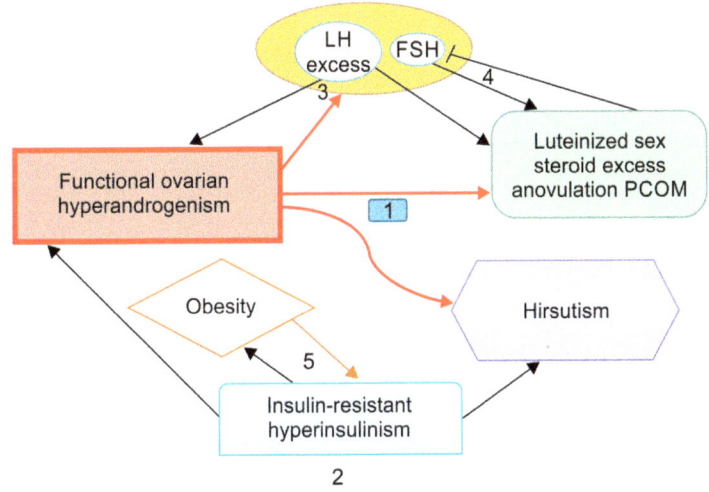

Fig. 1B: Insulin-resistant hyperinsulinism in PCOS.
(FSH: follicle-stimulating hormone; LH: luteinizing hormone; PCOS: polycystic ovary syndrome; PCOM: polycystic ovarian morphology)

idiopathic atypical PCOS **(Table 1 and Fig. 2)**.

The mechanisms for FOH include the following:
- *Dysregulation of theca cell steroidogenesis:* The steroid secretion pattern in PCOS typically indicates generalized overactivity of the whole steroidogenic pathway, from cholesterol to androgens and estrogens, with drastic elevation in 17-OHP stating dysregulation of cytochrome P450c17 activities, which are encoded by the *CYP17A1* gene.[1,2] Cytochrome P450c17 is active in both 17-hydroxylase and 17,20-lyase, the latter being the rate-limiting step in androgen formation.

Androgen production within the ovary is strictly regulated because androgen is a necessary evil in the ovary: androgen serves as the substrate for estrogen formation, and androgen is needed for optimal fertility.[1,3] Excess androgen, on

TABLE 1: Functional classification of polycystic ovary syndrome according to source of androgen excess.

PCOS functional type	Source of androgen	GnRHa test: 17-OHP response	DAST testosterone response	ACTH test: DHEA response	Prevalence among PCOS
Typical PCOS (PCOS-T)	Primary FOH (typical FOH)	High	High in 92.5%	High in 28% (associated FAH)	67%
Atypical PCOS (PCOS-A)	Primary FOH (atypical FOH)	Normal	High	High in 30% (associated FAH)	20%
	Isolated primary FAH (isolated FAH)	Normal	Normal	High	5%
	PCOS without FOH or FAH (atypical PCOS of obesity or idiopathic atypical PCOS)	Normal	Normal	Normal	8%

(ACTH: adrenocorticotropic hormone; DAST: dexamethasone androgen suppression test; DHEA: dehydroepiandrosterone; FAH: functional adrenal hyperandrogenism; FOH: functional ovarian hyperandrogenism; GnRHa: gonadotropin-releasing hormone agonist; 17-OHP: 17-hydroxyprogesterone; PCOS: polycystic ovary syndrome)

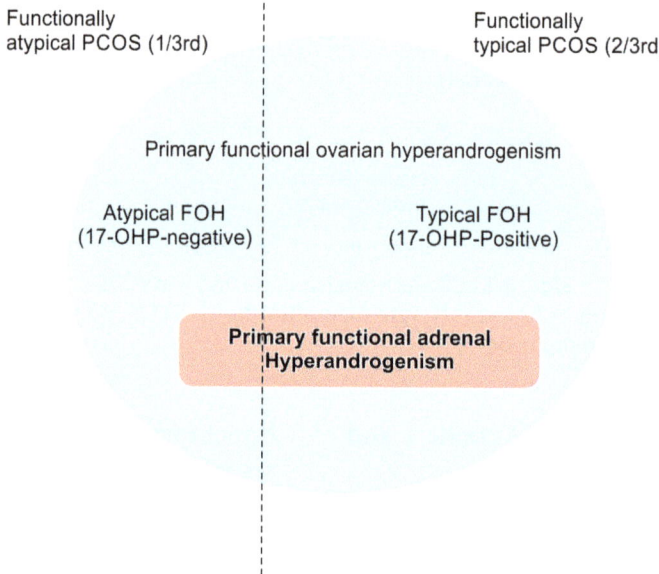

Fig. 2: Atypical PCOS of obesity.
(FOH: functional ovarian hyperandrogenism; 17-OHP: 17-hydroxyprogesterone; PCOS: polycystic ovary syndrome)

the other hand, disrupts the development of ovarian follicles. LH stimulates ovarian theca cells to form androgen and follicle-stimulating hormone (FSH) stimulates granulosa cells to form estrogen during the small antral follicle stage of development.

Intraovarian (paracrine/autocrine) mechanisms, rather than endocrine negative feedback loops, normally coordinate theca cell androgen production with granulosa cell estrogen production. The balance of downregulation and upregulation processes within the ovary modulates the response to LH.

Desensitization of LH receptor-binding sites in the presence of elevated LH levels ("homologous desensitization") and inhibition of P450c17 activities by local androgens and estrogens cause downregulation. Granulosa cell factors that upregulate P450c17 activities, particularly insulin-like growth factors (IGFs) and inhibin, balance out the downregulation.

Extraovarian factors such as insulin and proinflammatory cytokines [e.g., tumor necrosis factor α (TNF-α), transforming growth factor β (TGF-β), interleukin 1 (IL-1) and IL-6, and lipopolysaccharide] produced by specialized monocytic cells of adipose tissue and the gut microbiome can disrupt this synchronized intraovarian regulation. These also increase P450c17 activity, whereas other cytokines (e.g., IL-22) suppress androgenic enzymes.[4,5]

Downregulation of thecal androgen production is completely misguided in PCOS because PCOS ovaries are hyperresponsive to LH stimulation **(Figs. 1A and B)**.[1] Clinical evidence suggested that steroidogenesis dysregulation in PCOS is primarily of ovarian origin.[1]

- *Granulosa cell dysfunction:* Granulosa cells synthesize estrogens from androgens (via aromatase expression) and secrete peptides and growth factors that control follicle and oocyte development.[6] Androgens normally stimulate the transformation of dormant primordial follicles into primary follicles ("recruitment"), the first step in their growth and development into small antral follicles.[7] Androgens then normally synergize with FSH to induce LH receptor expression on granulosa cells, resulting in "luteinization," which allows granulosa cells to produce progesterone in response to LH and initiates the formation of the preovulatory follicle.[1]

Excess intraovarian androgen causes granulosa cell dysfunction in PCOS, which leads to anovulation and PCOM **(Figs. 1A and B)**.[1] High androgen levels promote the growth of an abnormally large number of small follicles which is primarily due to increased granulosa cell proliferation, and responsible for the increased anti-müllerian hormone (AMH) levels in women with PCOS (AMH is a product of the granulosa cells of small growing follicles that normally restrain the growth of primordial follicle). Androgens also contribute to follicular luteinization occurring in the mid- rather than a late follicular phase, which appears to be the basis for the follicular maturation arrest that prevents the emergence of a dominant follicle and prevents ovulation.[8]

Alternatively, granulosa cell dysfunction in PCOS could be the result of an intrinsic defect in the intraovarian (paracrine) regulation of follicle dynamics. Excessive granulosa cell secretion of factors that stimulate androgens, such as inhibin B, may reflect intrinsic granulosa cell dysfunction. Indeed, a subset of women with PCOS has deleterious variants in the genes encoding AMH or its receptor that impairs the restraint of follicular growth and granulosa cell aromatase activity.[8]

INSULIN-RESISTANT HYPERINSULINISM

Insulin resistance is a contributing factor in roughly half of PCOS cases: insulin resistance is disproportionately high for the severity of their obesity [body mass index (BMI)].[1,9] Insulin resistance is thus thought to be intrinsic in these women.

Compensatory hyperinsulinemia is a mechanism by which insulin resistance aggravates PCOS. Excess insulin action in some tissues, most notably the ovary, is paradoxically caused by hyperinsulinemia, which compensates for resistance to insulin's glucose-metabolic effect. This "insulin-resistant hyperinsulinism" is a major extraovarian factor in the pathophysiology of roughly half of all PCOS cases.

Polycystic ovary syndrome with insulin resistance is remarkable because resistance to insulin's metabolic effects is tissue-specific.[1] While skeletal muscle is resistant to insulin action on glucose metabolism due to mitochondrial gene dysfunction,[7] compensatory hyperinsulinemia causes excess insulin action in the ovary, liver, and adipocytes. As a result, signaling pathways that mediate insulin's mitogenic, growth factor-like, protein-anabolic, and lipogenic actions remain insulin sensitive. These insulin actions aggravate steroidogenic dysregulation and contribute to obesity and acanthosis nigricans, which are common PCOS comorbidities.

This insulin-resistant hyperinsulinism is an important aggravating factor in PCOS pathogenesis because it promotes FOH.

Hyperinsulinemia sensitizes the intrinsically dysregulated ovarian theca cells to secrete excess androgen in response to LH[1] (**Fig. 1B**, step 2). It does this by reversing the LH-induced homologous desensitization of LH-binding sites, which then upregulates cytochrome P450c17 activities. Insulin also upregulates testosterone formation by type 5 17-beta-hydroxysteroid dehydrogenase via a transcription factor (*KLF15*) that stimulates adipogenesis.

Insulin excess also synergizes with androgen excess and FSH to prematurely induce LH receptors on granulosa cells, leading to their premature luteinization and follicle maturation arrest.[1]

The severity of insulin resistance correlates with the severity of hyperandrogenism, the severity of anovulatory symptomatology, and the prevalence of PCOM. Any treatment that lowers insulin levels, therefore, improves hyperandrogenism (including in experimental models of PCOS[10]), though the hyperandrogenism of typical PCOS is seldom fully corrected by such treatments alone in most populations.

Associated Pathophysiologic Disturbances

Excess gonadotropin secretion, adiposity, and adrenal androgenic dysfunction are inconsistent features of PCOS that seem related to dysregulation of steroidogenesis and/or insulin-resistant hyperinsulinism.

Gonadotropin Abnormalities

Luteinizing hormone is necessary for the expression of steroidogenic enzymes. Thus, PCOS is gonadotropin-dependent, i.e., functional, a form of ovarian hyperandrogenism. Any treatment that suppresses LH levels (e.g., estrogenic–progestin oral contraceptives) suppresses ovarian hyperandrogenism.[1]

Increased LH, often accompanied by decreased FSH, was the first laboratory abnormality identified in classic PCOS and was historically thought to play a role in its pathogenesis by increasing ovarian androgen production. This discrepancy between adolescents and adults suggests that this resistance only becomes apparent when the high sensitivity to sex-steroid negative feedback of childhood fully wanes with maturity.

Such data suggest that LH excess in PCOS is the result, rather than the cause, of androgen excess. In more severe cases of PCOS, the moderate testosterone excess stimulates LH secretion (**Fig. 1B**, step 3). Additionally, granulosa cells that have been prematurely luteinized, under the influence of both increased testosterone and insulin levels, begin to secrete estrogenic in response to LH as well as to FSH. The negative feedback effect of the resultant estradiol excess can account for the significantly low FSH levels of PCOS (**Fig. 1B**, step 4).

Obesity

Approximately half of patients with PCOS are obese, and at least one-third of non-obese patients with PCOS have increased intraabdominal fat.[1]

The reason for the high prevalence of obesity in PCOS is not entirely clear. The hyperinsulinism of insulin resistance seems to be an important factor. Insulin signaling is of major importance to the size and function of the white adipose tissue depot. It stimulates adipogenesis and lipogenesis while inhibiting lipolysis.[11] Androgens oppose insulin effects on subcutaneous fat stores, instead favoring a myogenic differentiation. However, mild hyperandrogenemia also promotes visceral fat accumulation, which promotes insulin resistance. There also appear to be inherent differences in the subcutaneous abdominal fat cells of normal-weight and obese women with PCOS; normal-weight women can form small adipocytes in subcutaneous fat depots that retain insulin sensitivity.

Obesity aggravates the clinical severity of FOH by increasing insulin resistance (**Fig. 1B**). In PCOS, visceral fat contributes more to insulin resistance than subcutaneous abdominal fat because of its enhanced lipolytic response to catecholamines.[1] Enhanced visceral fat lipolysis is unique to PCOS and not attributable to androgen excess; the free fatty acids and diacylglycerol released from visceral fat appear to promote insulin resistance in the liver and muscle, respectively.

The mechanisms by which obesity causes insulin resistance include a deficiency of insulin-sensitizing adipokines that are secreted by a unique population of adipose tissue–derived, monocytic, regulatory T cells[12] and by an altered intestinal microbiome.[4,5] Inflammatory cytokines not only cause insulin resistance but also aggravate ovarian hyperandrogenism. Hyperandrogenism, in turn, sensitizes circulating mononuclear cells to secrete inflammatory cytokines in response to glucose and saturated fat ingestion,[1] which, in a vicious cycle, aggravates hyperandrogenism and insulin resistance.

Obesity also causes low microbial diversity of the intestinal microbiome, which results in a "leaky gut" and resultant endotoxemia.[13] This "leaky gut" leads to increased serum lipopolysaccharide, IL-1β, and TNF-α levels, which directly stimulate thecal androgen production.[4,13] Dysbiosis is also found in nonobese PCOS, indicating that hyperandrogenism is a causative factor.

In contrast with energy-storing white adipose tissue, women with PCOS have been shown to have less energy-consuming brown adipose tissue. The study of the regulation of brown fat development is in its infancy.[14]

In addition to aggravating PCOS via insulin resistance, obesity seems to be the sole cause of most functionally atypical PCOS (sometimes termed "atypical PCOS of obesity") (*see* **Table 1 and Fig. 2**).[1] Both androgen and estrogen are formed in excess by the adipose tissue of obese women. Obesity also suppresses gonadotropin levels by accelerating their metabolism. Thus, obesity should be suspected as the cause of menstrual irregularity when dehydroepiandrosterone sulfate (DHEAS) and LH are normal in obese PCOS women with marginally elevated testosterone levels.

FUNCTIONAL ADRENAL HYPERANDROGENISM

In 25–50% of cases, primary FOH is accompanied by primary FAH. In another 5% of cases of PCOS, FAH is the only detectable source of androgen excess **(Table 1 and Fig. 2)**.[1] Isolated primary FAH usually occurs in hirsute women without menstrual abnormalities, i.e., without PCOS.

Primary FAH is defined as 17-ketosteroid hyper-responsiveness to ACTH that is otherwise unexplained. This FAH has been postulated to result from a dysregulation of adrenal zona reticularis steroidogenesis that parallels the dysregulation of ovarian theca cell steroidogenesis.[1] This FAH has been associated not only with mild adrenal enlargement in some cases but also with slightly smaller adrenal volumes and a marginal degree of autonomous adrenocortical function in others. Hyperinsulinism seems to aggravate FAH as it does FOH.

External Factors

Genetics

Multiple population-wide genome-wide association studies (GWAS) have revealed numerous pathogenic variants of PCOS. Out of the several culprit genes, *LHCGR*, *THADA*, and *DENND1A* promoter genes are most important.[15] Polymorphism of LH/chorionic gonadotropic receptors (LHCGR) found in theca and mature granulosa cells of the adult ovary drives excess androgen production.[16] Overexpression of *DENND1A* which encodes for DENN proteins drives excess ovarian steroidogenesis.[17] Altered expression of thyroid adenoma-associated gene (*THADA*) modifies insulin secretion and subsequent insulin resistance by interfering with pancreatic beta-cell function.

Epigenetics

Epigenetics studies inheritable alterations in the gene expression and genomes that take place without any changes in DNA sequences. Due to lack of any single gene defect that could explain the various systemic manifestations of PCOS, scientists have been looking for factors that could change the characteristics of gene expression. Environmental factors, specifically increased exposure to in utero androgens, is one of the most important theories in fetal programming for development of PCOS in later life.[18]

Some genes which undergo reprogramming in PCOS are:
- *LHCGR* gene encoding for LH receptor, present on the theca cell surface
- *FST*—encodes for follistatin
- *LMNA*—encodes for Lamin A/C
- *PPARGC1A*—encodes for peroxisome proliferation
- *EPHX1*—encodes for epoxide hydrolase which degrades aromatic compounds.

Changes in the methylation status of these genes are the precursors which encode for the physiologic processes of steroidogenesis, follicular development, inflammatory mediation, insulin regulation, and glucose metabolism. Xu et al. found that serum global methylation was higher in obese PCOS patients than in nonobese PCOS patients. This indicates that obesity may play a role within the disease process itself, not only as a phenotypic expression but also as an epigenetic modifier itself.[19]

Histone epigenetic modifications, via methylation or acetylation, complements the direct methylation changes in DNA. Proper gene expression requires the presence of the correct pattern of both histone epigenetic modifiers and DNA. Hosseini et al. confirmed that increased serum levels of acetylation in histone H3 and methylation of H3K9 were found in PCOS patients, reducing the expression of *CYP19A1*, ultimately reducing cytochrome P450 aromatase activity, thus contributing to the hyperandrogenic phenotype.[20]

Another epigenetic modification influencing gene expression involves the presence of noncoding single-stranded RNA molecules called microRNA (miRNA). Several miRNAs such as mi222 linked with type 2 diabetes mellitus (T2DM) and gestational diabetes mellitus (GDM) and mi93 linked with cellular glucose and lipid metabolism have been associated with disease pathogenesis.

Environmental Toxicants

The United States Environmental Protection Agency (USEPA) defines endocrine-disrupting chemical (EDC) as "an exogenous agent that interferes with the synthesis, secretion, transport, binding, action, or elimination of natural hormones in the body that are responsible for the maintenance of homeostasis, reproduction, development and/or behaviour."[21] EDCs bind to the cellular hormone receptor as hormones' agonists or antagonists. Studies have approved the higher serum concentration of EDCs in PCOS women with prolonged and continuous exposure from prenatal to adolescence. One such EDC is bisphenol A found in polycarbonate plastics, epoxy resins, baby bottles, dental fillings, etc. Its effects are as follows:

- Directly affects oogenesis by interacting with estrogen receptor (ER)
- Overproduction of androgens
- Potent ligand for sex hormone–binding globulin (SHBG) and replaces testosterone; thereby, free testosterone concentration increases.
- Acts as an obesogen
- Can also change glucose homeostasis by directly influencing the pancreatic cells.

Advanced chemical group is advanced glycation end products (AGEs), also called glycotoxins. AGEs are pro-inflammatory molecules[22] which interact with their receptor called RAGE (receptor for AGE) and stimulate pro-inflammatory pathways and oxidative stress. Increased serum concentration of AGEs has been found in patients with PCOS. AGEs interrupt growth of preovulatory follicles and damage follicles by oxidative stress caused by interaction with RAGEs.

Microbiome and Dysbiosis

Rapid human cultural changes and significant dietary modifications have resulted in development of a mismatch between human metabolic genes and bacteria that enhance fat storage. In PCOS women, harboring such microbes increase energy storage, thereby leading to insulin resistance and development of obesity and T2DM. Evidence suggests that microbiome of obese individuals is capable of extracting more energy from the host diet compared with the microbiome of lean individuals. This results from an increase in pro-inflammatory species of bacteria, such as *Escherichia coli*, and a decrease in anti-inflammatory bacteria such as *Faecalibacterium prausnitzii*.[23] Tremellen in 2012[24] proposed that a poor-quality diet and resulting imbalanced microbiome increase intestinal permeability and endotoxin production, with resultant hyperinsulinemia. This unleashes the cascade of increased androgen production and disrupted follicular development. The "first hit" inside the uterus combines with vertical transmission of a dysbiotic microbiome from a mother with PCOS, resulting in dysbiosis in the offspring.

Adult diet high in saturated fatty acids has also been linked to PCOS by producing an inflammatory reaction and reducing insulin sensitivity. Vitamin D deficiency exacerbates PCOS and its associated comorbidities by inducing an inflammatory response. Calcitriol upregulates insulin receptors and also increases insulin sensitivity directly and indirectly. It activates the PPAR delta receptor involved in fatty acid metabolism in adipose tissue and skeletal muscle, directly. Indirectly, it regulates intracellular calcium.

■ REFERENCES

1. Rosenfield RL, Ehrmann DA. The pathogenesis of polycystic ovary syndrome (PCOS): The hypothesis of PCOS as Functional ovarian hyperandrogenism revisited. Endocr Rev. 2016;37:467-520.
2. Ehrmann DA, Barnes RB, Rosenfield RL. Polycystic ovary syndrome as a form of functional ovarian hyperandrogenism due to dysregulation of androgen secretion. Endocr Rev. 1995;16:322-53.
3. Sen A, Hammes SR. Granulosa cell-specific androgen receptors are critical regulators of ovarian development and function. Mol Endocrinol. 2010;24:1393-403.
4. Fox CW, Zhang L, Sohni A, Doblado M, Wilkinson MF, Chang RJ, et al. Inflammatory stimuli trigger increased androgen production and shifts in gene expression in theca-interstitial cells. Endocrinology. 2019;160:2946-58.
5. Qi X, Yun C, Sun L, Xia J, Wu Q, Wang Y, et al. Gut microbiota-bile acid-interleukin-22 axis orchestrates polycystic ovary syndrome. Nat Med. 2019; 25:1225-33.
6. Hsueh AJ, Kawamura K, Cheng Y, Fauser BC. Intraovarian control of early folliculogenesis. Endocr Rev. 2015;36:1-24.
7. Vendola KA, Zhou J, Adesanya OO, Weil SJ, Bondy CA, et al. Androgens stimulate early stages of follicular growth in the primate ovary. J Clin Invest. 1998;101:2622-9.
8. Willis DS, Watson H, Mason HD, Galea R, Brincat M, Franks S. Premature response to luteinizing hormone of granulosa cells from anovulatory women with polycystic ovary syndrome: relevance to mechanism of anovulation. J Clin Endocrinol Metab. 1998;83:3984-91.
9. Kim JY, Tfayli H, Michaliszyn SF, Arslanian S. Impaired lipolysis, diminished fat oxidation, and metabolic inflexibility in obese girls with polycystic ovary syndrome. J Clin Endocrinol Metab. 2018;103:546-54.
10. Yuan X, Hu T, Zhao H, Huang Y, Ye R, Lin J, et al. Brown adipose tissue transplantation ameliorates polycystic ovary syndrome. Proc Natl Acad Sci U S A 2016;113:2708-13.
11. Rosen ED, Spiegelman BM. What we talk about when we talk about fat. Cell. 2014; 156:20-44.
12. Semple RK. EJE PRIZE 2015: How does insulin resistance arise, and how does it cause disease? Human genetic lessons. Eur J Endocrinol. 2016;174:R209-23.
13. Banaszewska B, Siakowska M, Chudzicka-Strugala I, Chang RJ, Pawelczyk L, Zwozdziak B, et al. Elevation of markers of endotoxemia in women with polycystic ovary syndrome. Hum Reprod. 2020;35:2303-11.
14. Hussain MF, Roesler A, Kazak L. Regulation of adipocyte thermogenesis: mechanisms controlling obesity. FEBS J. 2020;287:3370-85.
15. Combs JC, Hill MJ, Decherney AH. Polycystic ovarian syndrome genetics and epigenetics. Clin Obstet Gynecol. 2021;64(1):20-5.
16. Narayan P. Genetic models for the study of luteinizing hormone receptor function. Front Endocrinol (Lausanne). 2015;6:152.
17. McAllister JM, Modi B, Miller BA, Biegler J, Bruggeman R, Legro RS, et al. Overexpression of a DENND1A isoform produces a polycystic ovary syndrome theca

phenotype. Proc Natl Acad Sci USA. 2014; 111(15):E1519-27.
18. Dumesic DA, Hoyos LR, Chazenbalk GD, Naik R, Padmanabhan V, Abbott DH. Mechanisms of intergenerational transmission of polycystic ovary syndrome. Reproduction. 2020;159(1):R1-R13.
19. Xu J, Bao X, Peng Z, Wang L, Du L, Niu W, et al. Comprehensive analysis of genome-wide DNA methylation across human polycystic ovary syndrome ovary granulosa cell. Oncotarget. 2016;7(19):27899-909.
20. Hosseini E, Shahhoseini M, Afsharian P, Karimian L, Ashrafi M, Mehraein F. Role of epigenetic modifications in the aberrant *CYP19A1* gene expression in polycystic ovary syndrome. Arch Med Sci. 2019;15(4): 887-95.
21. Rocha AL, Oliveira FR, Azevedo RC, Silva VA, Peres TM, Candido AL, et al. Recent advances in the understanding and management of polycystic ovary syndrome. F1000Research. 2019;8:565.
22. Sadeghi HM, Adeli I, Calina D, Docea AO, Mousavi T, Daniali M, et al. Polycystic ovary syndrome: A comprehensive review of pathogenesis, management, and drug repurposing. Int J Mol Sci. 2022;23:583.
23. Ridaura VK, Faith JJ, Rey FF, Cheng J, Duncan AE, Kau AL, et al. Gut microbiota from twins discordant for obesity modulate metabolism in mice. Science. 2013;341: 1241214
24. Tremellen K, Pearce K. Dysbiosis of gut microbiota (DOGMA)—a novel theory for the development of polycystic ovarian syndrome. Med Hypotheses. 2012;79:104-12.

PCOS its Root in Womb

Charmila Ayyavoo, Priyankur Roy

INTRODUCTION

Polycystic ovary syndrome (PCOS) is the most common endocrinopathy in women.[1]

It causes a wide range of problems in women in all age groups. It is known to cause reproductive, metabolic, and psychological problems in women.[2]

The prevalence of the disease is around 20% and can vary based on the diagnostic criteria. This high prevalence has made PCOS the target of intensive research regarding the origins of this perplexing disease.[3]

Many theories have been proposed regarding the origins. These theories can be divided to be of genetic origin, epigenetic programming, or intrauterine origin.[4,5]

Developmental origin of health and disease (DoHAD) is the term used to describe a condition where the metabolic and endocrine conditions of the mother can permanently program the functioning of the fetus and modify its susceptibility to disease after birth. The exposure of the fetus can happen at crucial gestational ages of development.

The DoHAD theory originates from the Barker hypothesis. The Barker hypothesis proposes that unfavorable conditions during the development of the fetus can lead to permanent alterations in functioning and metabolism which can predispose to adult diseases.[6] This chapter aims to discuss the different theories proposed for the development of different phenotypes of PCOS due to an exposure of the fetus in utero.

THEORY OF GENETIC ORIGIN OF THE DISEASE

Perturbations of Concerned Genes

The proposed genes involved in the development of PCOS are *FSHB, LHCGR, FSHR, DENND1A, RAB5/SUOX, HMGA2, C9orf3, YAP1, TOX3, RAD50, FBN3,* and *AMH*.[7] These genes are involved in signaling of transforming growth factor beta (TGF-β) and androgens. The proposed genetic theory is that perturbations of these genes in the fetal ovary can lead to PCOS in adulthood.

Transforming growth factor beta can cause stromal cell replication and collagen production in the stroma of the fetal ovary. It is known that increase in ovarian stroma and collagen deposition in the ovary are features of PCOS. There is a likelihood of the fetal ovary developing a tendency for PCOS because of the perturbations in the candidate genes of PCOS. These changes in the genes can cause a signaling of TGF-β and androgens which can lead to an increased exposure of the fetus to androgens and an increased activity of TGF-β. This may lead to the development of PCOS in adulthood.[8]

Intergenerational Transmission

In a study by Risal et al. in 2019, it is reported that there is a 62% risk of transmission of PCOS to their daughters by women conceiving with PCOS.[9] There is also an increased prevalence of PCOS in sisters of women with PCOS.[10] Their parents are found to have a high incidence of metabolic syndrome.[11]

THEORY OF EPIGENETIC PROGRAMMING

There is a proposed theory that PCOS phenotypes can occur when there is an incongruity between primeval genetically programmed mechanisms and contemporary lifestyle. The mechanisms involved are the metabolic and reproductive survival mechanisms. An in utero exposure can lead to the activation of gene variants which can alter the metabolic and endocrine pathways. When this fetus is exposed to specific conditions in the postnatal period, it may predispose to the development of PCOS. The proposed postnatal elements which can modulate the pathways which are epigenetically programmed in these children are diet, unhealthy lifestyle, and endocrine system disrupting chemicals. This modulation can result in the development of the typical features of PCOS.[12]

Theory of Maternal Nutrition and the Development of PCOS in Offspring

When the fetus is undernourished, it will favor the expression of genes involved in energy conservation called the thrifty genotype. This tendency will be useful when there is scarcity of food. But if there is abundance of food, it will lead to metabolic syndrome in adulthood.[13] Similarly, fetal growth restriction is also associated with the development of PCOS symptoms in adult life.[14]

Maternal overnutrition can also lead to changes in the fetus which predispose to adult disease.[15]

THEORY OF INTRAUTERINE ORIGIN

Hyperandrogenism in Utero

If the woman has congenital adrenal hyperplasia, the female offspring has symptoms of PCOS. This is thought to be due to the exposure to high androgens in utero.[16]

Increase in maternal androgens cannot directly cause a programming of the fetus if the placental aromatase activity is normal.[17] Placental aromatase, if working optimally, can prevent the maternal androgens from reaching the fetus. If the placental aromatase activity is abnormal which can be seen in women with PCOS, it can then lead to an increase in exposure of the fetus to maternal androgens in utero.[18]

In animal models, the exposure of high doses of androgens to the mother caused PCOS in the fetuses when they became adults.[10,19-21]

In some animal models, it was noted that there was a higher level of anti-mullerian hormone (AMH) in pregnant animals whose offspring developed PCOS as adults. There is no proof of this theory in humans still.[22]

There is an association of mid-gestation levels of maternal testosterone and high AMH in female offspring in adolescence. This propounds the theory that increase in maternal testosterone can cause changes in ovarian function of female progeny.[23]

All the above studies favor the following mechanism: metabolic changes in the mother cause placental dysfunction of a female fetus which leads to hyperandrogenism and altered follicular development in the ovaries. This also promotes fetal hyperinsulinemia.

Ultimately, the fetus is born with a genetic susceptibility to PCOS.[24]

There is also evidence in some female fetuses that they have been exposed to an increased level of androgens in utero. An elongated anogenital distance is a reliable marker of exposure to mid-gestation androgens of the fetus which can be assessed in the postnatal period. This is seen in female children of PCOS mothers and women with PCOS.[25]

CLINICAL IMPLICATIONS OF THE FETAL ORIGIN OF ADULT DISEASE—POLYCYSTIC OVARY SYNDROME

In the crucial period of human fetal development, if there is a maternal exposure to an altered endocrine and metabolic environment it can change the programming of the female fetus. It can lead to a permanently altered gene expression which makes the fetus vulnerable to childhood and adult diseases. The epigenetic modification leads to fetal genetic susceptibility to PCOS. It is proved that maternal–fetal–placental–infant alterations cause the phenotypic expression of the different types of PCOS in adulthood.

To reduce this intergenerational susceptibility to PCOS, women with PCOS should improve their endocrine and metabolic health before conception. This will help to improve the metabolic and reproductive health of their daughters.[26]

CONCLUSION

All the above theories support the view that PCOS is an inherited disease. The exposure of the female fetus to an adverse maternal endocrine and metabolic environment causes an epigenetic programming of normal gene variants. The genes can be intensified by in utero exposure to androgens. This leads on to a genetic susceptibility to the development of PCOS when there is exposure to unhealthy lifestyle, environmental factors, and endocrine disrupting chemicals.

If the mother follows lifestyle interventions to reduce the adverse endocrine and metabolic profile, there is a potential to diminish the symptoms and prevent the transgenerational transmission of this dreaded disease, PCOS.

REFERENCES

1. Homburg R. Polycystic ovary syndrome—from gynecological curiosity to multisystem endocrinopathy. Hum Reprod. 1996;11:29-39.
2. Teede H, Deeks A, Moran L. Polycystic ovary syndrome: a complex condition with psychological, reproductive and metabolic manifestations that impacts on health across the lifespan. BMC Med. 2010; 8:41.
3. Sirmans SM, Pate KA. Epidemiology, diagnosis, and management of polycystic ovary syndrome. Clin Epidemiol. 2013;6:1-13.
4. Homburg R. Where does polycystic ovary syndrome come from? Ann Transl Med. 2018;6(18).
5. Wang T, Leng J, Li N, Martins de Carvalho A, Huang T, Zheng Y, et al. Genetic predisposition to polycystic ovary syndrome, postpartum weight reduction, and glycemic changes: A longitudinal study in women with prior gestational diabetes. J Clin Endocrinol Metab. 2015;100:E1560-7.
6. Barker F (Ed). Trondhjemite: definition, environment and hypotheses of origin. In Developments in Petrology, vol. 6. Philadelphia: Elsevier; 1979, pp. 1-12.
7. Dumesic DA, Phan JD, Leung KL, Grogan TR, Ding X, Li X, et al. Adipose insulin resistance in normal-weight women with polycystic ovary syndrome. J Clin Endocrinol Metab. 2019;104(6):2171-83
8. Hartanti MD, Rosario R, Hummitzsch K, Bastian NA, Hatzirodos N, Bonner WM, et al. Could perturbed fetal development of

8. the ovary contribute to the development of polycystic ovary syndrome in later life? PLoS One. 2020;15(2):e022935.
9. Risal S, Pei Y, Lu H, Manti M, Fornes R, Pui HP, et al. Prenatal androgen exposure and transgenerational susceptibility to polycystic ovary syndrome. Nature Med. 2019;25(12):1894-904.
10. Dumesic DA, Hoyos LR, Chazenbalk GD, Naik R, Padmanabhan V, Abbott DH. Mechanisms of intergenerational transmission of polycystic ovary syndrome. Reproduction. 2020;159(1):R1-3.
11. Crisosto N, Sir-Petermann T. Family ties: offspring born to women with polycystic ovary syndrome. Curr Opin Endocr Metab Res. 2020;12:119-24.
12. Parker J, O'Brien C, Gersh FL. Developmental origins and transgenerational inheritance of polycystic ovary syndrome. Aust N Z J Obstet Gynaecol. 2021;61(6):922-6.
13. Neel JV, Weder AB, Julius S. Type II diabetes, essential hypertension, and obesity as "syndromes of impaired genetic homeostasis": the "thrifty genotype" hypothesis enters the 21st century. Perspect Biol Med. 1998;42(1):44-74.
14. Davies MJ, March WA, Willson KJ, Giles LC, Moore VM. Birthweight and thinness at birth independently predict symptoms of polycystic ovary syndrome in adulthood. Hum Reprod. 2012; 27:1475-80.
15. Desai M, Beall M, Ross MG. Developmental origins of obesity: programmed adipogenesis. Curr Diabetes Rep. 2013;13(1):27-33.
16. Goodarzi MO, Carmina E, Azziz R. DHEA, DHEAS and PCOS. J Steroid Biochem Mol Biol. 2015;145:213-25.
17. Sloboda DM, Hickey M, Hart R. Reproduction in females: the role of the early life environment. Hum Reprod Update. 2011; 17(2):210-27.
18. Maliqueo M, Lara HE, Sánchez F, Echiburú B, Crisosto N, Sir-Petermann T. Placental steroidogenesis in pregnant women with polycystic ovary syndrome. Eur J Obstet Gynecol Reprod Biol. 2013;166(2):151-5.
19. Padmanabhan V, Veiga-Lopez A. Animal models of the polycystic ovary syndrome phenotype. Steroids. 2013;78:734-40.
20. Walters KA. Androgens in polycystic ovary syndrome: lessons from experimental models. Curr Opin Endocrinol Diabetes Obes. 2016;23:257-63.
21. Filippou P, Homburg R. Is foetal hyperexposure to androgens a cause of PCOS? Hum Reprod Update. 2017;23:421-32.
22. Tata B, Mimouni NEH, Barbotin AL, Malone SA, Loyens A, Pigny P, et al. Elevated prenatal anti-Mullerian hormone reprograms the fetus and induces polycystic ovary syndrome in adulthood. Nat Med. 2018;24:834-46.
23. Hart R, Doherty DA, Norman RJ, Franks S, Dickinson JE, Hickey M, et al. Serum antimullerian hormone (AMH) levels are elevated in adolescent girls with polycystic ovaries and the polycystic ovarian syndrome (PCOS). Fertil Steril. 2010;94(3):1118-21.
24. Dumesic DA, Hoyos LR, Chazenbalk GD, Naik R, Padmanabhan V, Abbott DH. Mechanisms of intergenerational transmission of polycystic ovary syndrome. Reproduction. 2020 Jan 1;159(1):R1-3
25. Hernández-Peñalver AI, Sánchez-Ferrer ML, Mendiola J, Adoamnei E, Prieto-Sánchez MT, Corbalán-Biyang S, et al. Assessment of anogenital distance as a diagnostic tool in polycystic ovary syndrome. Reprod Biomed Online. 2018;37(6):741-9.
26. Willging MM, Abbott DH, Dumesic DA. Intergenerational Implications of PCOS. In Pal L, Seifer DB (Eds). Polycystic Ovary Syndrome. Cham: Springer;2022. pp. 555-76.

CHAPTER 4

Diagnosis of PCOS

Deeba Khanam, Shaheen Anjum

■ INTRODUCTION

Polycystic ovarian syndrome (PCOS) is one of the most common endocrinopathies seen in women of the reproductive age group with a prevalence ranging from 2.2 to 26% globally[1] and 3.7 to 22.5%[2] in the Indian population. Diagnosis and treatment of PCOS remain controversial and challenging as there are significant variations in the components included in the diagnostic criteria, owing to clinical heterogeneity, differences in ethnic characteristics of population, and variation in clinical features at the individual level throughout her life course.

Different criteria evolved over a period of years in order to better diagnose the disorder.

NATIONAL INSTITUTES OF HEALTH CRITERIA (1990)

National Institutes of Health (NIH) criteria included only the presence of clinical and/or biochemical hyperandrogenism and oligo/amenorrhea anovulation[3] for the diagnosis of PCOS but did not include ultrasound features.

■ ROTTERDAM CRITERIA

Rotterdam criteria used polycystic ovarian morphology on ultrasound as a new criterion to be added to the two previous criteria of NIH.[4,5] This is the most widely used criteria for the diagnosis of PCOS; however, as it includes two out of three parameters and may skip hyperandrogenism, it was criticized for including milder phenotypes in diagnosis. The three proposed parameters in *revised Rotterdam criteria include*:

- *Oligomenorrhea* (irregular menstrual periods) or amenorrhea (absence of menstrual periods)
- *Hyperandrogenism* [based on clinical (signs on the body) and/or biochemical signs (hormone levels in the blood)]
- *Polycystic ovaries* (on the ultrasound): The following features on ultrasound
  - Number of immature follicles: 12 or more in each ovary
  - Size of immature follicles: 2–9 mm in diameter
  - Ovarian volume: >10 cm^3. However, international evidence-based guidelines 2018 recommend the threshold of more than 20 follicles per ovary while using endovaginal ultrasound with a band frequency of 8 MHz and volume of >10 cm^3 with a transabdominal ultrasound.[6]

Based on different combinations, four different phenotypes were identified:
1. *Phenotype A (classic PCOS)*
   - Clinical or biochemical evidence of hyperandrogenism
   - Absent or irregular periods
   - Polycystic ovaries on ultrasound

2. *Phenotype B (essential NIH criteria)*
   - Clinical or biochemical evidence of hyperandrogenism
   - Absent or irregular periods
3. *Phenotype C (ovulatory PCOS)*
   - Clinical or biochemical evidence of hyperandrogenism
   - Polycystic ovaries on ultrasound
4. *Phenotype D (nonhyperandrogenic PCOS)*
   - Absent or irregular periods
   - Polycystic ovaries on ultrasound

ANDROGEN EXCESS SOCIETY

The Androgen Excess Society defined PCOS as hyperandrogenism with ovarian dysfunction or polycystic ovaries; thus, androgen excess was considered as a central event in the development and pathogenesis of PCOS, and androgen excess should be present and accompanied by oligomenorrhea or polycystic ovarian morphology (PCOM) or both of them.[7] Exclusion of other androgen excess disorders should be excluded such as nonclassical congenital adrenal hyperplasia (NC-CAH), Cushing's syndrome, androgen-secreting tumors, hyperprolactinemia, thyroid diseases, drug-induced androgen excess, and other causes of oligomenorrhea or anovulation.[8,9]

INTERNATIONAL EVIDENCE-BASED GUIDELINES (2018)

Rotterdam criteria are recommended for the diagnosis of PCOS in adults but emphasize stricter criteria to be employed while labeling irregular cycles and hyperandrogenism and ultrasonographic features as well. Diagnosis of adolescents and menopausal females did not require PCOM as it interferes with the normal physiology, and therefore the guideline provided certain specific recommendations. The guideline also facilitates appropriate diagnosis of PCOS and avoids overdiagnosis, especially in adolescents.

Specific recommendations included in the guidelines:
- Ultrasound is not recommended for diagnosis in those within 8 years of menarche.
- Young women where diagnosis is unclear should be followed up for reassessment.
- Diagnostic features are refined to limit overlap with those without PCOS to improve diagnostic accuracy.

It has been identified that insulin resistance and metabolic syndrome are inherent features of PCOS pathophysiology but their evaluation is not included in the diagnostic criteria as they lack accuracy. Similarly, testing for glucose tolerance is a part of risk stratification in already diagnosed cases of PCOS but is not included in the diagnosis.

Defining the individual characteristics of Rotterdam criteria appropriately is important to make correct diagnosis as specified in the guideline.

Irregular Cycles

Irregular cycles in the first year of menarche are considered normal.

In the first 3 years post menarche, cycle length <21 or >45 days is considered abnormal.

After 3 years post menarche to perimenopause, cycle length <21 or >35 days is considered abnormal.

Post menarche 1 year, cycle length >90 days for any one cycle.

Clinical Hyperandrogenism

A comprehensive history and physical examination should be completed for symptoms and signs of clinical hyperandrogenism, including acne, alopecia, and hirsutism.

Hirsutism

Hirsutism is labeled as growth of terminal hair in a male-like pattern in women. The most common visual assessment tool is the modified Ferriman–Gallwey (mFG) score to assess terminal hairs that would grow > 5 mm in length and are pigmented, and medullated at nine specific areas in the body and a score is provided.[10] The international evidence-based guideline development group after reviewing all available evidence recommends the cutoff of ≥4–6 on mFG; ethnicity and hormonal pill consumption should also be taken into consideration.

Alopecia and Acne

The Ludwig visual score is preferred for assessing the degree and distribution of alopecia. There are no universally accepted visual assessment tools for evaluating acne.[11]

Biochemical Hyperandrogenism

Free testosterone, free androgen index (FAI), or calculated bioavailable testosterone should be used to assess biochemical hyperandrogenism in the diagnosis of PCOS. Liquid chromatography mass spectrometry (LCMS) and extraction/chromatography immunoassays should be used for assessment of total or free testosterone in PCOS rather than radiometrics or enzyme-linked assay as they are less accurate[12] and have cross-reactivity with other androgens. Androstenedione and dehydroepiandrosterone sulfate (DHEAS) could be considered if total or free testosterone is not elevated but is of lesser significance and is commonly used to exclude other causes of hyperandrogenism. Where assessment of biochemical hyperandrogenism is required in a woman on hormonal contraception, drug withdrawal for 3 months is recommended.

The diagnostic utility of LH and the LH:FSH ratio in PCOS is much debated in literature. The Rotterdam consensus criteria proposed that LH had no role in the diagnosis.[13] This is supported by multiple studies[14,15] using consecutive series of women which showed that LH and FSH had practically no diagnostic utility.

Polycystic Ovarian Morphology

Ultrasound should not be used for the diagnosis of PCOS in those <8 years after menarche, due to the high incidence of polycystic ovaries at this stage.

The transvaginal ultrasound approach is preferred in the diagnosis of PCOS.

Using endovaginal ultrasound transducers with a frequency bandwidth of 8 MHz, the threshold for PCOM should be on either ovary, with a number of follicles per ovary ≥20 and/or an ovarian volume ≥10 mL in either ovary.[6] With transabdominal ultrasound, the criteria of ovarian volume should be considered rather than the number of follicles. In patients with irregular menstrual cycles and hyperandrogenism, an ovarian ultrasound is not necessary for PCOS diagnosis; however, ultrasound will identify the complete PCOS phenotype.

Anti-müllerian Hormone Levels

Serum anti-müllerian hormone (AMH) levels are significantly higher in women with PCOS compared with normal ovulatory women and strong correlations exist between circulating AMH levels and antral follicle count on ultrasound in PCOS;[16,17] however, serum AMH levels should not yet be used as an alternative for the detection of PCOM or as a single test for the diagnosis of PCOS.

Evidences suggest that with standardization of serum AMH levels and specific cutoffs, it may be used for the diagnosis of PCOS in future.

Diagnosis of Polycystic Ovarian Syndrome in Adolescents

Evaluation of an adolescent for irregular cycles requires optimum timings in relation to menarche and also should take into consideration psychosocial and cultural factors.

Those who have features of PCOS, but do not meet diagnostic criteria, are considered for reassessment once gynecological maturity is reached, i.e., 8 years post menarche. Those consuming oral contraceptive pills (OCPs) should also be evaluated at the mentioned time while they are being assessed 3 months after the withdrawal of the hormonal pills.

In adolescents, moderate or severe comedonal acne (i.e., 10 or more facial lesions) is common.

There are no studies evaluating alopecia in adolescents. For these reasons, mild acne and alopecia are not recommended as considerations in the diagnostic criteria for adolescents and only severe acne and hirsutism[10] are preferred.

Diagnosis of Polycystic Ovarian Syndrome in Menopause

A natural history of PCOS is not known and whether PCOS resolves and/or persists remains unclear. Menstrual cycles become more regular in PCOS with age as suggested by some studies.[18] It was seen that there was less decrease in ovarian volume and follicle number in women with PCOS. With increasing age, the syndrome evolves from a reproductive disease to a more metabolic disorder.

Diagnosis of PCOS in post menopause could be considered if there is a past diagnosis of PCOS, a long-term history of irregular menstrual cycles and hyperandrogenism and/or PCOM, during the reproductive years.

Less conventional measures of androgen excess such as the FAI and androstenedione and 17-hydroxyprogesterone levels remain higher in menopausal females.[11,12] It has been suggested that PCOM persists into menopause. Postmenopausal women presenting with new-onset, severe or worsening hyperandrogenism require further investigation to rule out androgen-secreting tumors and ovarian hyperthecosis.[19]

Polycystic ovarian syndrome has a complex pathophysiology and its diagnosis requires multiple considerations including, age, ethnicity, and psychosocial and cultural aspects. With more validated research, newer diagnostic modalities may appear and as this population is more prone to developing cardiovascular morbidities and endometrial cancer, its timely diagnosis is essential.

ACKNOWLEDGMENTS

All the contributions in every aspect are acknowledged.

REFERENCES

1. Joshi B, Mukherjee S, Patil A, Purandare A, Chauhan S, Vaidya R. A cross-sectional study of polycystic ovarian syndrome among adolescent and young girls in Mumbai, India. Indian J Endocrinol Metab. 2014;18(3):317-24.
2. Malik S, Jain K, Talwar P, Prasad S, Dhorepatil B, Devi G, et al. Management of polycystic ovary syndrome in India. Fertil Sci Res. 2014;1(1):23-43.
3. Zawadski JK, Dunaif A. Diagnostic criteria for polycystic ovary syndrome: Towards a rational approach. In Dunaif A, Givens JR, Haseltine F (Eds). Polycystic Ovary Syndrome. Boston, MA: Blackwell Scientific; 1992. pp. 377-84.
4. Legro RS, Feingold KR, Anawalt B, Boyce A, Chrousos G, de Herder WW, et al. Evaluation and treatment of polycystic ovary syndrome. Endotext [Internet]. South Dartmouth

(MA): MDText.com, Inc.; 2000. Available from: https://pubmed.ncbi.nlm.nih.gov/25905194/ [Last accessed November, 2022].
5. Kovacs G, Norman R (Eds). Polycystic Ovary Syndrome. Cambridge: Cambridge University Press; 2001.
6. Monash Centre for Health Research and Implementation (MCHRI). (2018). International evidence-based guideline for the assessment and management of polycystic ovary syndrome. [online] Available from: Monash Centre for Health Research and Implementation (MCHRI). International evidence-based guideline for the assessment and management of polycystic ovary syndrome [Last accessed November, 2022].
7. Azziz R, Carmina E, Dewailly D, Diamanti-Kandarakis E, Escobar-Morreale HF, Futterweit W, et al. Positions statement: criteria for defining polycystic ovary syndrome as a predominantly hyper-androgenic syndrome: an Androgen Excess Society guideline. J Clin Endocrinol Metab. 2006;91:4237-45.
8. Spritzer PM. Polycystic ovary syndrome. Arq Bras Endocrinol Metab. 2014;58:182-7.
9. Elting MW, Korsen TJ, Rekers-Mombarg LT, Schoemaker J. Women with polycystic ovary syndrome gain regular menstrual cycles when ageing. Hum Reprod. 2000;15(1):24-8.
10. Lizneva D, Gavrilova-Jordan L, Walker W, Azziz R. Androgen excess: Investigations and management. Best Pract Res Clin Obstet Gynaecol. 2016;37:98-118.
11. Eichenfield LF, Krakowski AC, Piggott C, Del Rosso J, Baldwin H, Fallon Friedlander S et al. Evidence-based recommendations for the diagnosis and treatment of pediatric acne. Pediatrics. 2013;131(Suppl 3):S163-86.
12. Taieb J, Mathian B, Millot F, Patricot MC, Mathieu E, Queyrel N, et al. Testosterone measured by 10 immunoassays and by radio-isotope dilution gas chromatography-mass spectrometry in sera from 116 men, women, and children. Clin Chemi. 2003;49:1381-95.
13. The Rotterdam ESHRE/ASRM-Sponsored PCOS Consensus Workshop Group. Revised 2003 consensus on diagnostic criteria and long-term health risks related to polycystic ovary syndrome (PCOS). Fertil Steril. 2004;81(1):19-25.
14. Balen AH, Michelmore K. What is polycystic ovary syndrome? Are national views important? Human Reprod. 2002;17;2219-27.
15. Cho LW, Jayagopal V, Kilpatrick ES, Holding S, Atkin SL. The LH/FSH ratio has little use in diagnosing polycystic ovarian syndrome. Ann Clin Biochem. 2006;43:217-9.
16. Vulpoi C, Lecomte C, Guilloteau D, Lecomte P. Ageing and reproduction: is polycystic ovary syndrome an exception? Ann Endocrinol (Paris). 2007;68(1):45-50.
17. Minooee S, Ramezani Tehrani F, Rahmati M, Mansournia MA, Azizi F. Prediction of age at menopause in women with polycystic ovary syndrome. Climacteric. 2018;21:29-34.
18. Alsamarai S, Adams JM, Murphy MK, Post MD, Hayden DL, Hall JE, et al. Criteria for polycystic ovarian morphology in polycystic ovary syndrome as a function of age. J Clin Endocrinol Metab. 2009;94:4961-70.
19. Schmidt J, Brännström M, Landin-Wilhelmsen K, Dahlgren E. Reproductive hormone levels and anthropometry in post-menopausal women with polycystic ovary syndrome (PCOS): a 21-year follow-up study of women diagnosed with PCOS around 50 years ago and their age-matched controls. J Clin Endocrinol Metab. 2011;96(7):2178-85.

CHAPTER 5

Ultrasound in PCOD

Poonam Goyal, Vishwajeet A Burungale, Pallaavi Goel

■ INTRODUCTION

Ovarian imaging is very important in the evaluation of patients suspected to have polycystic ovary syndrome (PCOS). The report of radiological imaging has to be very precise and essentially include ovarian volumes and antral follicle counts, along with other relevant findings (e.g., the presence of a dominant follicle or corpus luteum). Morphologically, the typical feature of polycystic ovaries is an apparent failure in selecting a dominant follicle and the accumulation of antral follicles 2–8 mm in size. It is assumed that this appearance reflects an androgen-induced arrest in antral follicle development.[1]

■ EVOLUTION OF CRITERIA

Several attempts were made to form a consensus as to the definition of PCOS. At the first international conference on PCOS, held at the National Institute of Health (NIH) in 1990, there was little agreement on the standard diagnostic criteria for PCOS. The lack of clinical trial evidence at that time led to the making of the following criteria based on majority expert opinion:
- Clinical or biochemical evidence of hyperandrogenism
- Chronic anovulation
- Exclusion of other disorders.[2]

These criteria prompted a number of large-scale clinical trials, which in turn led to an awareness that PCOS likely had clinical manifestations broader than those defined by the 1990 NIH criteria.[3] In acknowledgment of the heterogeneous nature of the syndrome, the Rotterdam European Society of Human Reproduction and Embryology (ESHRE)/American Society for Reproductive Medicine (ASRM)-sponsored PCOS consensus workshop group sought for a comprehensive definition for PCOS. This assembly added the ultrasonographic (USG) finding of polycystic ovaries to the diagnostic criteria.[2]

These 2003 criteria required at least two of the subsequent three conditions to be fulfilled for the diagnosis of PCOS **(Fig. 1)**:
1. Oligo- or anovulation
2. Clinical or biochemical signs of hyperandrogenism
3. Polycystic ovaries.

The Androgen Excess and PCOS Society issued its own criteria in 2009, describing their work as a modification of the original 1990 NIH criteria.[4] These criteria highlight the role of hyperandrogenism and include the presence of polycystic ovaries at USG. These criteria precisely define patients with PCOS as having both.
- Hyperandrogenism (hirsutism or hyperandrogenemia)
- Ovarian dysfunction (oligo- or anovulation or polycystic ovaries).[4]

What establishes the best definition of PCOS is still a matter of dispute. The

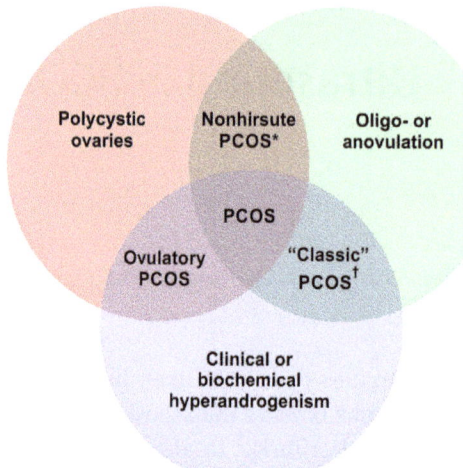

Fig. 1: Venn diagram illustrates the Rotterdam criteria for polycystic ovary syndrome (PCOS). The diagnosis of PCOS requires two of the three criteria to be met, after the exclusion of other diagnoses. These criteria created two new phenotypes for PCOS, in addition to the patient group identified by the original National Institutes of Health (NIH) criteria.
*Controversial subgroup later excluded by the 2009 Androgen Excess and PCOS Society criteria
†Subgroup defined by 1990 NIH criteria.

Androgen Excess and PCOS Society criteria, even though the most recent, should not essentially be interpreted as being the most correct. Nevertheless, the two most recent sets of consensus criteria have established the USG finding of polycystic ovaries as part of the diagnostic criteria for PCOS.

Thus, a correct ultrasound is crucial to arrive at diagnosis.

■ ULTRASONOGRAPHY FINDINGS

The aim of imaging in PCOS is to correctly identify and document the presence of polycystic ovaries. However, because PCOS is a syndrome, the presence of polycystic ovaries alone is insufficient for diagnosis. The clinical implication of incidentally discovered polycystic ovaries is still unidentified, and women with this finding should not be considered to have PCOS unless and until further workup is completed.[4-6]

The updated diagnostic criteria at the time of review are based on a 2018 international consensus guideline. According to its definition, polycystic ovaries are present when:
- One or both ovaries demonstrate 20 or more follicles measuring 2-9 mm in diameter or
- The ovarian volume exceeds 10 cm.^{3}

Only one ovary meeting either of these criteria is sufficient to establish the presence of polycystic ovaries.[7]

Ovarian Volume

The enquiry of what constitutes an abnormally large ovarian volume has been the topic of substantial investigation.[8-13] This literature compares ovarian volumes in healthy women with those in women with PCOS. A volume of 10 cm^3 was designated as the threshold volume for a polycystic ovary.[8]

There are several formulas available for the calculation of ovarian volume, and data regarding the degree of association between some of these formulas and true three-dimensional (3D) USG volume measurements have been considered.[14] Investigators decided that ovarian volume should be calculated on the basis of the simplified formula for a prolate ellipsoid (0.5 × length × width × thickness of the ovary) **(Figs. 2A to D)**.[10,11,15-17] The ellipsoid defined with this formula is not prolate, since a prolate ellipsoid is defined mathematically as the shape created by rotating an ellipse around its long axis. Because the mathematic definition of a prolate ellipsoid requires that two of its three axes be equal, it is more accurate to refer to this formula as the simplified formula for an ellipsoid.

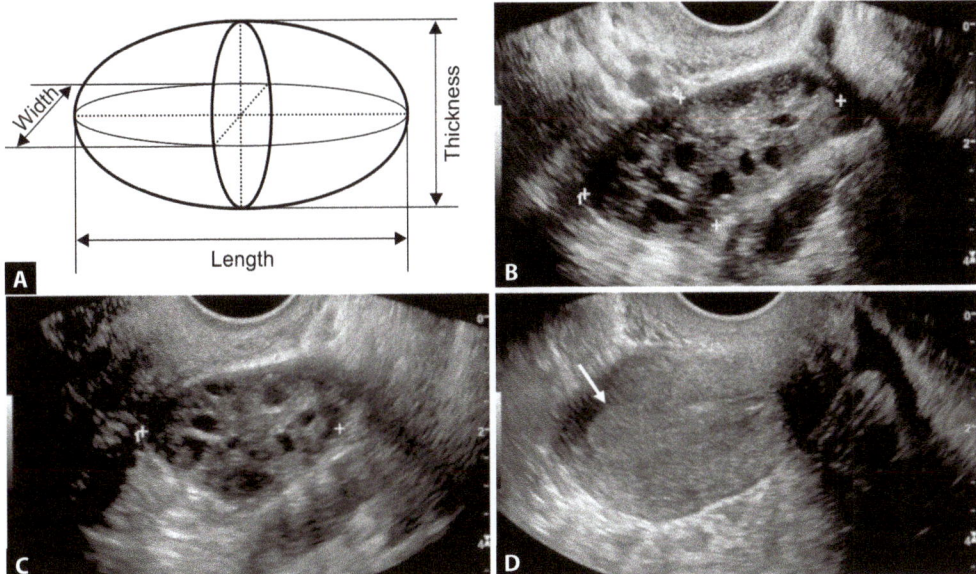

Figs. 2A to D: (A) Drawing illustrates how the calculation of ovarian volume is modeled on the volume of an ellipsoid. Mathematically, the volume of an ellipsoid is calculated using the formula $p/6 \times$ length $\times$ width $\times$ thickness. For the purposes of calculating ovarian volume in the evaluation of polycystic ovaries, the simplified formula $0.5 \times$ length $\times$ width $\times$ thickness is used. (B) Sagittal and (C) transverse ultrasound (US) images of a polycystic left ovary demonstrate axes of measurement corresponding to the three diameters of an ellipsoid. In this example, the length and width are measured in the longitudinal plane. Placement of the US probe in the orthogonal plane provides the third diameter of the ellipsoid. (D) Sagittal US image through the uterus demonstrates a thickened and echogenic endometrium.

Number of Follicles

The threshold for the number of follicles was based on performance data (receiving operator characteristic curves) assessing the ability of different thresholds for the number and size of follicles to help differentiate between healthy control subjects and PCOS patients. These 2003 data suggested that 12 or more follicles 2-9 mm in size per ovary is the best threshold for the diagnosis of PCOS.[17] The main technical requirement for the assessment of the number of follicles is that the number of antral follicles present throughout the entire volume of the ovary be counted.

As the time passed, more and more sensitive and good resolution machines with 3D and sonography-based automated volume count (SonoAVC) functions came into use and it was realized that visibility and pickup rate of follicles became better and if cutoff used is 12, then many patients need unnecessary investigations. The final consensus is to take cutoff of 20 FNPO (follicle number per ovary).

Polycystic Ovaries in Patients without Polycystic Ovary Syndrome

Women who are undergoing investigation for other gynecological complaints may be found to have polycystic ovaries on USG. Data suggests that 23% of women of reproductive age will have findings consistent with polycystic ovaries.[18] However, only 5-10% of these women will have classic symptoms of PCOS such as infertility, amenorrhea, signs of hirsutism, or obesity.[19]

The disparities in ovarian volume and antral follicle counts by age have been studied. The general trend of follicle count relative to age is biphasic, representing a 4.8% annual decline before 37 years of age and a more rapid 11.7% annual decline afterward.[20] However, significant variation in follicle count is seen in particular age groups. In one study, antral follicle counts varied from 7 to 22 during the early follicular phase of the menstrual cycle (day 2, 3, or 4) in women <30 years of age.[20]

The inconsistency in ovarian volume by age has also been studied. One large study measured the mean ovarian volume in 13,963 women undergoing screening for ovarian cancer using the nonsimplified formula for an ellipsoid (0.523 × length × width × thickness).[21] By defining abnormal ovarian volume as two standard deviations above the mean (the same convention as that used by the Rotterdam consensus group), the authors resolute the upper limit of the normal range to be 20 cm³ for premenopausal women and 10 cm³ for postmenopausal women.[21] However, such data in healthy patients are not directly comparable to data regarding ovarian volume in PCOS patients, since ovaries with dominant follicles or corpus luteal cysts were included in the "normal" data. Ideally, volume is measured on day 2 of cycle and it should be avoided if any corpus luteal cyst or dominant follicle is present.

In adolescent girls, ovaries are multicystic in nature as follicles are of >9 mm in size and stroma is also normal.

Stromal Echogenicity and Volume

One of the initial labeled characteristics of a polycystic ovary is an increase in stromal echogenicity.[9] While there have been many efforts to compare the qualitative indexes of stromal echogenicity with PCOS,[10,22] the intrinsic echogenicity of the ovarian stroma is the same in PCOS than in the normal ovary; the subjective impression of increased stromal echogenicity is primarily due to the increase in stromal volume.[23] It has been verified that increased stromal volume associates positively with serum androgen levels.[24] Yet, no standardized method exists for determining stromal volume. Since the overall ovarian volume correlates well with stromal volume in polycystic ovaries[24,25] and is more easily measured in clinical practice, the determination of the overall ovarian volume is a dependable surrogate for ovarian stromal assessment.

Vascularity of stroma is also to be considered, as patients with highly vascular stroma tend to hyper-respond in ovarian stimulation in assisted reproductive technology (ART) leading to ovarian hyperstimulation syndrome (OHSS).

IMAGING AND REPORTING CONSIDERATIONS

- USG:
  - Regularly menstruating women should go through scanning during the early follicular phase (days 3-5).
  - Oligo- or amenorrheic women may be scanned at random or between days 3 and 5 after progesterone-induced bleeding.
  - A history of oral contraceptive use should be obtained, since oral contraceptives cause a decrease in ovarian size, thereby decreasing the sensitivity of USG evaluation.
  - The presence of dominant follicle (defined as a follicle whose longitudinal, transverse, and anteroposterior diameters average is >10 mm) or corpus luteum may increase the ovarian

volume above the 10 cm³ threshold. Such a finding should bring about repeat scanning during the next menstrual cycle.[7]
- Assessment for PCOS in postmenopausal women require specific considerations. It is seen that polycystic ovaries in postmenopausal women tend to have greater volume (6.4 vs. 3.7 cm³) and demonstrate more follicles (9.0 vs. 1.7) than normal postmenopausal ovaries.[26]
- In adolescents females, bilateral ovarian volumes >10 cm³ correlate with the presence of PCOS in patients between 12 and 20 years of age.[27] There is trouble in distinguishing a polycystic ovary from what has traditionally been referred to as a multicystic or multifollicular ovary, defined as an ovary in which there are six or more follicles, usually 4–10 mm in diameter, with normal stromal echogenicity and described as the common appearance of ovaries in adolescents.[24]
- *Transvaginal USG:*
  - It is ideal because it provides good visualization of the internal structure of ovary, particularly in obese patients.
  - The data suggests that polycystic ovaries may not be detected at transabdominal USG in up to 30% of women with PCOS.[28]
- *Transabdominal USG:*
  - It can be compulsory in cases like women who have never been sexually active or if she refuses transvaginal examination.
  - Special care should be taken so that the urinary bladder is sufficiently filled.
  - Overfilled bladder can compress ovary and it can affect the correct estimation of ovarian volume.[7]
- *Magnetic resonance imaging (MRI):*
  - The use of MRI is generally not warranted in the evaluation of polycystic ovaries because of its high cost and the characteristically adequate visualization of the ovaries at transvaginal USG.
  - MRI may be useful in cases in which transvaginal USG cannot be performed and transabdominal USG does not offer adequate visualization.
  - The characteristic T2-weighted MRI appearance of a polycystic ovary is defined as consisting of abundant hypointense central stroma with small peripheral T2-hyperintense cysts.[29] However, the literature on MRI in PCOS is scanty, and no consensus has been reached as to an MRI definition for a polycystic ovary.
- *Computed tomography (CT):*
  - CT is not used in the evaluation of patients with possible PCOS, particularly since the internal ovarian structure is far better depicted at USG or MRI. Polycystic ovaries may sometimes be seen in such patients when they undergo CT for other reasons.

CONCLUSION

Ovarian imaging is important in the evaluation of patients with suspected PCOS. The imaging report should be precise and should include ovarian volumes and antral follicle counts, in addition to relevant findings such as the presence of a dominant follicle or corpus luteum. Therefore, to contribute to workup, radiologists must have a working knowledge of the clinical and imaging criteria for PCOS.

REFERENCES

1. Franks S, Stark J, Hardy K. Follicle dynamics and anovulation in polycystic ovary syndrome. Hum Reprod Update. 2008;14(4):367-78.
2. Rotterdam ESHRE/ASRM-Sponsored PCOS Consensus Workshop Group. Revised 2003 consensus on diagnostic criteria and long-term health risks related to polycystic ovary syndrome. Fertil Steril. 2004;81(1):19-25.
3. Carmina E, Lobo RA. Polycystic ovaries in hirsute women with normal menses. Am J Med. 2001;111(8):602-6.
4. Azziz R, Carmina E, Dewailly D, Futterweit W, Janssen OE, Legro RS, et al. The Androgen Excess and PCOS Society criteria for the polycystic ovary syndrome: the complete task force report. Fertil Steril. 2009;91(2):456-88.
5. Dewailly D. Definition and significance of polycystic ovaries. Baillieres Clin Obstet Gynaecol. 1997;11(2):349-68.
6. ACOG Committee on Practice Bulletins: Gynecology. ACOG Practice Bulletin No. 108: polycystic ovary syndrome. Obstet Gynecol. 2009;114(4):936-49.
7. Balen AH, Laven JS, Tan SL, Dewailly D. Ultrasound assessment of the polycystic ovary: international consensus definitions. Hum Reprod Update. 2003;9(6):505-14.
8. Jonard S, Robert Y, Dewailly D. Revisiting the ovarian volume as a diagnostic criterion for polycystic ovaries. Hum Reprod. 2005;20(10):2893-8.
9. Adams J, Franks S, Polson DW, Mason HD, Abdulwahid N, Tucker M, et al. Multifollicular ovaries: clinical and endocrine features and response to pulsatile gonadotropin releasing hormone. Lancet. 1985;2(8469-70):1375-9.
10. Pache TD, Wladimiroff JW, Hop WC, Fauser BC. How to discriminate between normal and polycystic ovaries: transvaginal US study. Radiology. 1992;183(2):421-3.
11. Fulghesu AM, Ciampelli M, Belosi C, Apa R, Pavone V, Lanzone A. A new ultrasound criterion for the diagnosis of polycystic ovary syndrome: the ovarian stroma/total area ratio. Fertil Steril. 2001;76(2):326-31.
12. Atiomo WU, Pearson S, Shaw S, Prentice A, Dubbins P. Ultrasound criteria in the diagnosis of polycystic ovary syndrome (PCOS). Ultrasound Med Biol. 2000;26(6):977-80.
13. van Santbrink EJ, Hop WC, Fauser BC. Classification of normogonadotropic infertility: polycystic ovaries diagnosed by ultrasound versus endocrine characteristics of polycystic ovary syndrome. Fertil Steril. 1997;67(3):452-8.
14. Nardo LG, Buckett WM, Khullar V. Determination of the best-fitting ultrasound formulaic method for ovarian volume measurement in women with polycystic ovary syndrome. Fertil Steril. 2003;79(3):632-3.
15. Swanson M, Sauerbrei EE, Cooperberg PL. Medical implications of ultrasonically detected polycystic ovaries. J Clin Ultrasound. 1981;9(5):219-22.
16. Hann LE, Hall DA, McArdle CR, Seibel M. Polycystic ovarian disease: sonographic spectrum. Radiology. 1984;150(2):531-4.
17. Saxton DW, Farquhar CM, Rae T, Beard RW, Anderson MC, Wadsworth J. Accuracy of ultrasound measurements of female pelvic organs. Br J Obstet Gynaecol. 1990;97(8):695-9.
18. Polson DW, Adams J, Wadsworth J, Franks S. Polycystic ovaries: a common finding in normal women. Lancet. 1988;1(8590):870-2.
19. Lakhani K, Seifalian AM, Atiomo WU, Hardiman P. Polycystic ovaries. Br J Radiol. 2002;75(889):9-16.
20. Scheffer GJ, Broekmans FJ, Dorland M, Habbema JD, Looman CW, te Velde ER. Antral follicle counts by transvaginal ultrasonography are related to age in women with proven natural fertility. Fertil Steril. 1999;72(5):845-51.
21. Pavlik EJ, DePriest PD, Gallion HH, Ueland FR, Reedy MB, Kryscio RJ, et al. Ovarian volume related to age. Gynecol Oncol. 2000;77(3):410-2.
22. Al-Took S, Watkin K, Tulandi T, Tan SL. Ovarian stromal echogenicity in women with clomiphene citrate-sensitive and

clomiphene citrate–resistant polycystic ovary syndrome. Fertil Steril. 1999;71(5):952-4.
23. Buckett WM, Bouzayen R, Watkin KL, Tulandi T, Tan SL. Ovarian stromal echogenicity in women with normal and polycystic ovaries. Hum Reprod. 1999;14(3):618-21.
24. Kyei-Mensah AA, Lin Tan S, Zaidi J, Jacobs HS. Relationship of ovarian stromal volume to serum androgen concentrations in patients with polycystic ovary syndrome. Hum Reprod. 1998;13(6):1437-41.
25. Franks S, Adams J, Mason H, Polson D. Ovulatory disorders in women with polycystic ovary syndrome. Clin Obstet Gynaecol. 1985;12(3):605-32.
26. Birdsall MA, Farquhar CM. Polycystic ovaries in pre and post-menopausal women. Clin Endocrinol (Oxf). 1996;44(3):269-76.
27. Herter LD, Magalháes JA, Spritzer PM. Relevance of the determination of ovarian volume in adolescent girls with menstrual disorders. J Clin Ultrasound. 1996;24(5):243-8.
28. Fox R, Corrigan E, Thomas PA, Hull MG. The diagnosis of polycystic ovaries in women with oligo-amenorrhoea: predictive power of endocrine tests. Clin Endocrinol (Oxf). 1991;34(2):127-31.
29. Mitchell DG, Gefter WB, Spritzer CE, Blasco L, Nulson J, Livolsi V, et al. Polycystic ovaries: MR imaging. Radiology. 1986;160(2):425-49.

CHAPTER 6

PCOS in Adolescents

Dhara Singh, B Aruna Suman

■ INTRODUCTION

Polycystic ovary syndrome (PCOS) occurs on average in about 10% of women in the reproductive age group and is the cause of over 70% hyperandrogenism. Multiple factors, including hereditary and nonhereditary; intrauterine and extrauterine; environmental factors; disparity in insulin resistance; and steroidogenesis modification, may influence this disease/syndrome. Menstrual irregularity and/or elevated androgen levels have been observed in adolescent women with PCOS, and infertility is encountered later in life, emphasizing the importance of early PCOS diagnosis in adolescence. Adolescent PCOS diagnosis may provide an opportunity to raise awareness of this lifelong condition and provide prospective interventions such as healthy lifestyle counseling, comorbidity testing, or medications to treat clinical manifestations. The diagnosis of PCOS in adolescents, however, can be difficult due to the overlap of normal pubertal physiological changes that occur at the same time. Furthermore, the diagnosis and management of PCOS in adolescence are constantly evolving.[1]

Adolescence is roughly defined as the time between the ages of 10 and 19 years.[2] Adolescent PCOS diagnosis is difficult because PCOS features overlap with normal pubertal development and ovulation, and cycles in adolescents do not match those of reproductive-aged women. Adolescents are prone to obesity, insulin resistance, hyperinsulinemia, and androgen excess. Therefore, the two key phenotypes of PCOS in adolescence are metabolically healthy and metabolically unhealthy.[5]

■ INCIDENCE AND PREVALENCE

In a study of 12–19-year-old females, 18% of individuals had PCOS, and urban populations had a larger proportion of PCOS than their rural counterparts.[3] PCOS is typically detected in adolescents at a rate of 15–26%.

■ ETIOLOGY

Polycystic ovary syndrome is a multifaceted disease. Increased prevalence of the following components is seen among PCOS patients—hyperandrogenemia, type 2 diabetes mellitus (T2DM) in first-degree relatives of women with PCOS. The mode of heritance of PCOS remains unclear. Dominant and/or multigenic modes of transmission are possible. Fibrillin-3 (FBN3), insulin (INS), insulin receptor (INSR), insulin receptor substrate 1 (IRS1), transcription factor 7-like 2 (TCF7L2), calpain 10 (CAPN10), fat and obesity associated gene (FTO), and sex hormone-binding globulin (SHBG) are the genes involved in PCOS **(Fig. 1)**.[4]

Environmental toxins, endocrine-disrupting chemicals (EDCs), and high carbohydrate

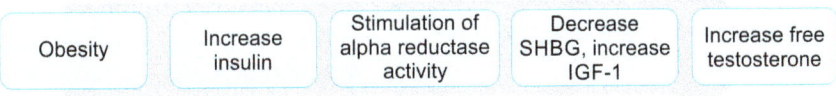

Fig. 1: Etiopathogenesis of polycystic ovary syndrome.
(IGF-1: insulin-like growth factor 1; SHBG: sex hormone-binding globulin)

intake aggravate PCOS, generalized obesity, and body fat distribution.[5]

Polycystic ovary syndrome patients have a significantly higher positive family history of diabetes, breast cancer, endometrial cancer, heart attack, and thrombosis.

CLINICAL FEATURES OF ADOLESCENT POLYCYSTIC OVARY SYNDROME

- The main clinical features of PCOS in adolescence are hyperinsulinemia and hyperandrogenemia.
- Skin disorders/cutaneous manifestations affect nearly 90% of PCOS patients.
- The main pathophysiological feature of PCOS is abnormal steroidogenesis regulation.
- Excessive androgen secretion in PCOS causes hirsutism, acne, seborrhea 1 and AGA, AN, and other symptoms **(Fig. 2)**.[6]

Menstrual Irregularities

Natural changes in antral follicle count occur during the pubertal and menopausal transitions, and up to 70% of adolescents meet the original criteria for polycystic ovarian morphology (PCOM) **(Table 1)**.[7,8] With increasing age, there is a natural progression toward more ovulatory cycles.[9] Girls with PCOS typically have a late onset of menarche. The later menarche occurs, the longer it takes to have regular menstruation.

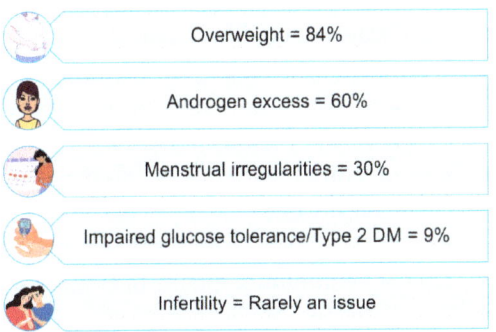

Fig. 2: Clinical features of adolescent polycystic ovary syndrome. (DM: diabetes mellitus)

TABLE 1: Criteria for menstrual irregularities among adolescent.[8]

Menstrual interval persistently >1 to <3 years post menarche: <21 or >45 days	Consecutive menstrual intervals >90 days are rare and require further investigation regardless of years after menarche	Primary amenorrhea by age 15 or >3 years post thelarche (breast development)

Irregular menstrual cycles are defined as:
- Normal in the first year post menarche as part of the pubertal transition
- >1 to <3 years post menarche: <21 or >45 days.
- >3 years post menarche to perimenopause: <21 or >35 days or <8 cycles per year
- >1 year post menarche >90 days for any one cycle
- Primary amenorrhea by age 15 or >3 years post thelarche (breast development)

- When irregular menstrual cycles are present a diagnosis of PCOS should be considered and assessed according to the guidelines.

Hirsutism

For symptoms and indicators of clinical hyperandrogenism in teenagers, such as severe acne and hirsutism, a thorough medical history should be taken.[8]

- Hirsutism, which is an excellent indicator of hyperandrogenism, is the most frequent skin manifestation observed in 60% of women with PCOS,[10] followed by acne and alopecia.
- Excessive facial and/or body hair are the typical symptoms of hirsutism **(Fig. 3B)**.
- The Ferriman-Gallwey score is used to assess hirsutism, and a score of 8 or higher is considered diagnostic.
- Using the Ferriman-Gallwey scoring system, the examiner scored the subjects on a scale of 0–4 for terminal hair growth on 11 different body areas **(Fig. 3A)**.

Alopecia

- Female or male patterns (such as the Christmas tree pattern) impact adolescent PCOS girls' fronto-temporo-occipital scalps **(Figs. 4A and B)**.[11]
- Studies examining alopecia in teens are few.

Acne and Seborrhea

The pilosebaceous unit is a target of androgen stimulation and is sensitive to local enzymes as well as androgen receptors.[6]

Moderate or severe comedonal acne (i.e., 10 or more facial lesions) in early puberty or moderate inflammatory acne through the perimenarcheal years is uncommon (5% prevalence) **(Figs. 5 and 6) (Tables 2 and 3)**.

Acanthosis Nigricans

- It is a marker of insulin resistance and is noticed in 5–10% of PCOS patients and 50% of obese patients with PCOS.[12] Skin hyperpigmentation and diffuse velvety thickening.[13]
- Usually observed on the back of the neck, axillae, beneath the breasts, and in exposed areas (elbows, knuckles) **(Figs. 7 and 8)**.

Obesity

- About 50% of girls with PCOS exhibit obesity.
- Waist circumference >88 cm is a marker of central/visceral obesity. Body weight is the main factor affecting the quality of life.
- Typical obesity of PCOS is described as having a "apple" or "centripetal" type of fat distribution—the center of the body, as opposed to the thighs and hips **(Fig. 9)**.

Ideally, waist circumference, height, and weight should be measured, and body mass index (BMI) should be computed taking into account the following factors:

- In addition to specifying ethnic and teenage ranges, BMI classifications and waist circumference measurements should adhere to World Health Organization recommendations.
- Asians and other high-risk ethnic groups should be taken into account, and monitoring of waist circumference is advised.[8]

Psychological Symptoms

Health professionals should be aware that adults with PCOS have a high prevalence of moderate to severe anxiety and depressive symptoms, with an even higher prevalence in adolescents.[8]

At the time of diagnosis, all adolescents should be routinely screened for anxiety and depressive symptoms. If the screening for these symptoms and/or other aspects of emotional well-being is positive, further

PCOS in Adolescents

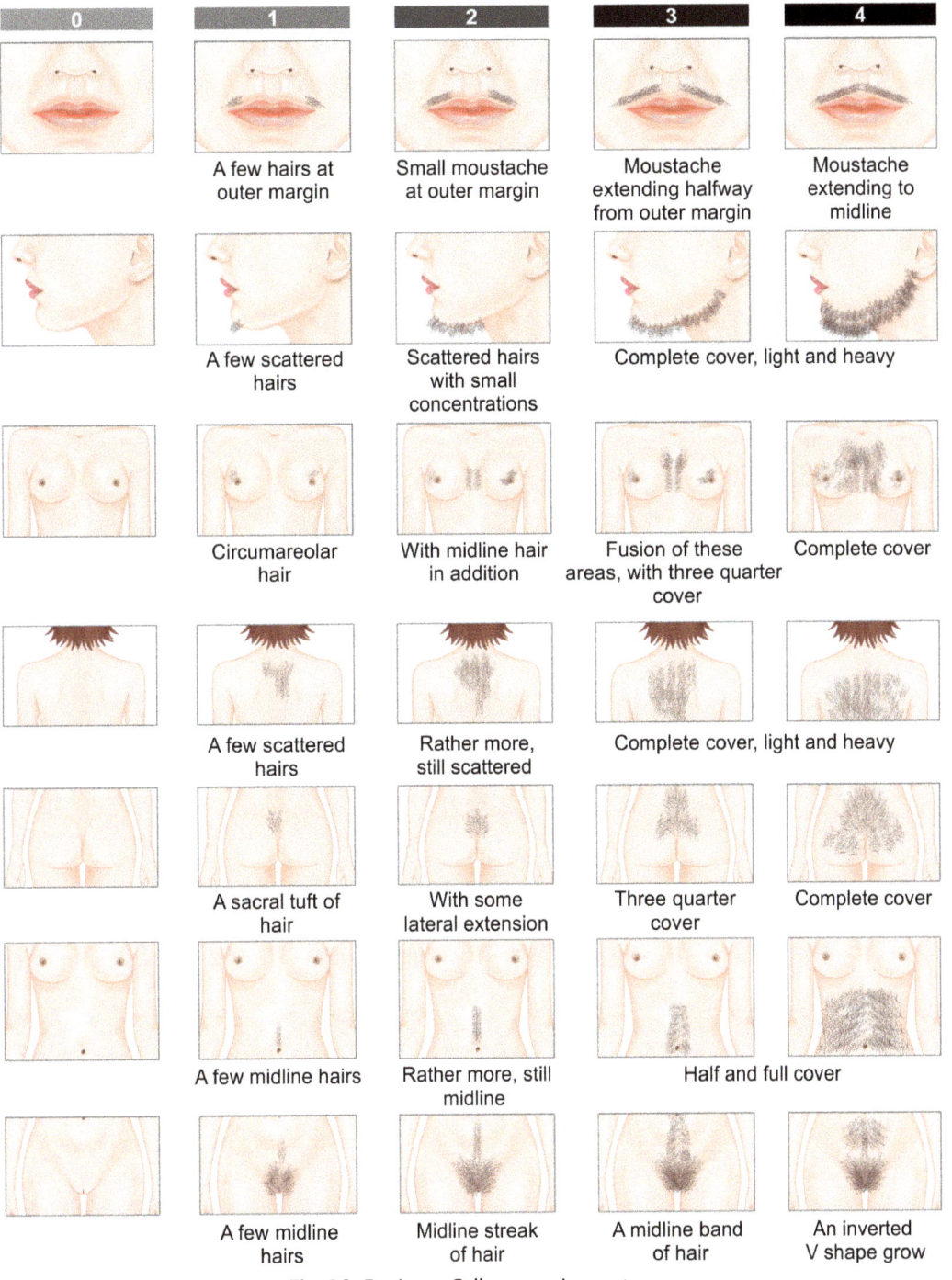

Fig. 3A: Ferriman-Gallwey scoring system.

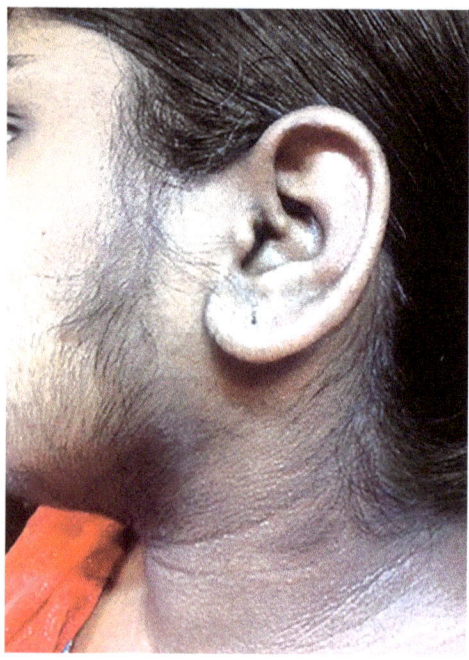

Fig. 3B: Excessive facial hair: A typical symptoms of hirsutism.

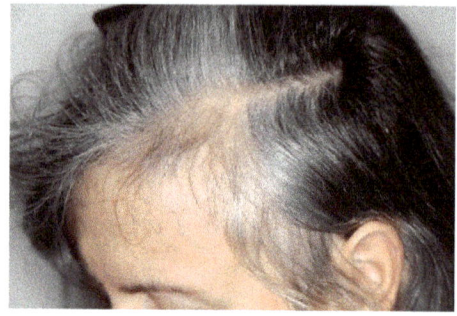

Fig. 4A: Frontotemporal alopecia.

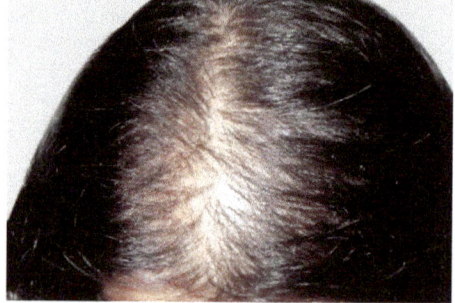

Fig. 4B: Christmas tree pattern of alopecia.

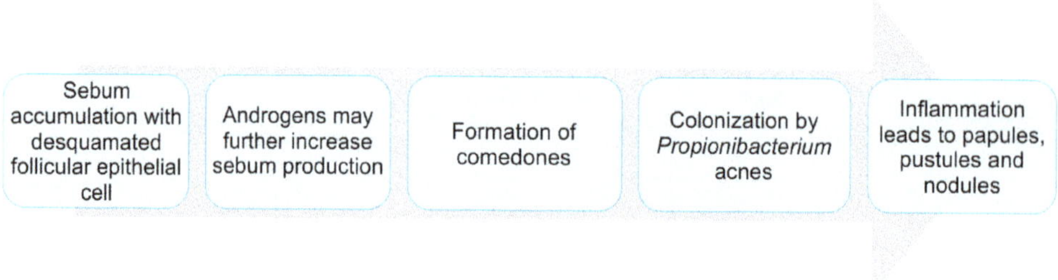

Sebum accumulation with desquamated follicular epithelial cell → Androgens may further increase sebum production → Formation of comedones → Colonization by *Propionibacterium acnes* → Inflammation leads to papules, pustules and nodules

Fig. 5: Formation of Comedonal acne.

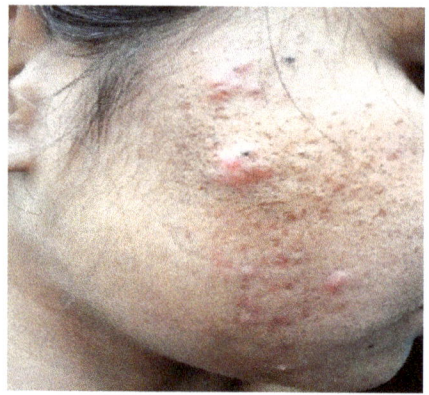

Fig. 6: Sebum accumulation in Comedonal acne.

evaluation and/or referral for evaluation and treatment should take place.[8]
- The high prevalence of eating disorders and disordered eating has been described, and screening can be done using regional guidelines or the stepped approach outlined below. Questions for initial screening may include:
  • Does your weight affect the way you feel about yourself?
  • Are you satisfied with your eating patterns?

TABLE 2: Grading of acne severity: Recommendation of Indian Acne Association.

- Mild acne (Grade 1)
- Predominance of comedones

  - Comedones <30
  - Papules <10
  - No scarring

- Moderate acne (Grade 2)
- Predominance of papules

  - Comedones any number
  - Papules >10
  - Nodules <3
  - With or without scarring

- Severe acne (Grade 3)
- Many nodules

  - Comedones any number
  - Papules any number
  - Nodules/cysts >3
  - With scarring

TABLE 3: Acne distribution by age group: Recommendation of Indian Acne Association.

Age group	Location of lesions	Type of lesions	Sex
Neonates	Cheeks, chin, eyelids, forehead	Papules and pustules, no comedones	Both male and female
Infants	Full face	Comedones, papules, nodules, scars	Male
Preadolescent	Forehead, upper cheeks, nose	Predominantly comedonal, occasional papules	Both
Adolescent	Full face, seborrheic area of torso	All types of lesions	Both
Adults	Chin, upper lip, jaws	Papules, excoriated papules	Both

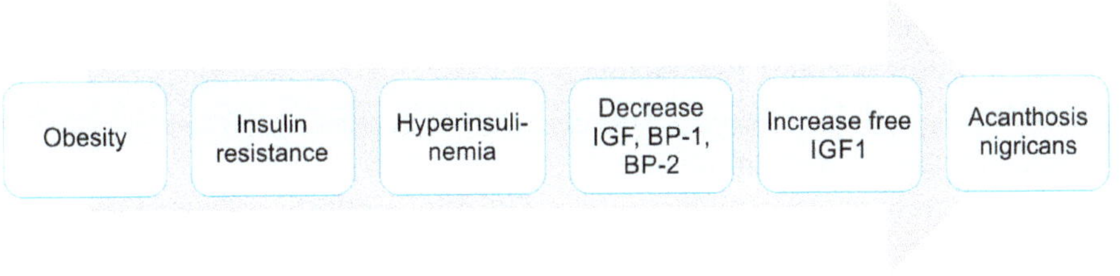

Obesity → Insulin resistance → Hyperinsulinemia → Decrease IGF, BP-1, BP-2 → Increase free IGF1 → Acanthosis nigricans

Fig. 7: Formation of Acanthosis nigricans.
(BP: binding protein; IGF: insulin-like growth factor)

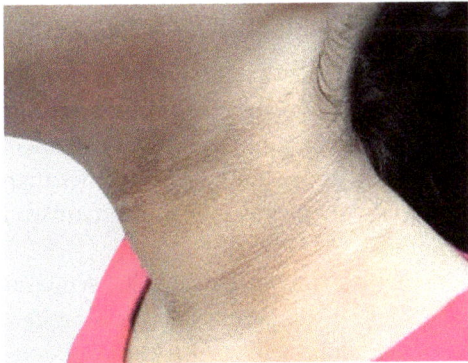

Fig. 8: Appearance of Acanthosis nigricans.

- Acne, hirsutism, and obesity have all been linked to decreased self-esteem, which can be screened for using regional guidelines or a stepped approach. Initial inquiries could include:
  - Do you worry a lot about the way you look and wish you could think about it less?
  - On a typical day, do you spend more than 1 h/day worrying about your appearance?

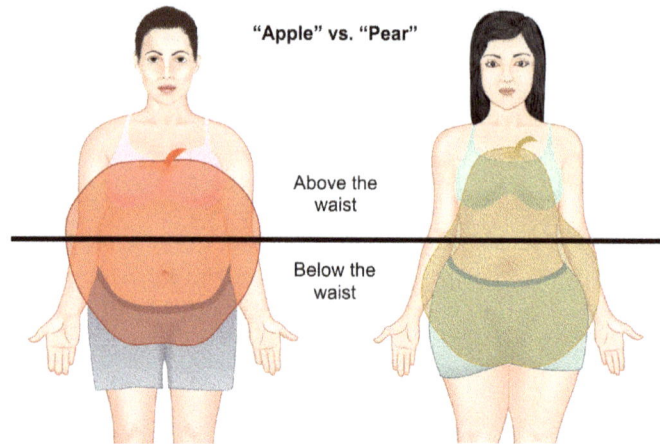

Fig. 9: Apple vs pear shape of fat distribution in obesity.

- What specific concerns do you have about your appearance?
- What effect does it have on your life?
- Does it make it hard to do your work or be with your friends and family?
■ Elevated levels of anxiety and depression—routine screening for everyone at diagnosis and then depending on clinical judgment, taking into account risk factors, comorbidities, and life events. Initial questions OR suggested screening depending on area criteria could include: In the past 2 weeks, how frequently have you had the following issues:
  - Feeling down, depressed or hopeless?
  - Little interest or pleasure in doing things?
  - Feeling nervous, anxious or on edge?
  - Not being able to stop or control worrying?

Factors including obesity, infertility, and hirsutism need consideration along with use of hormonal medications in PCOS, which may independently exacerbate depressive and anxiety symptoms and other aspects of emotional wellbeing
■ Behavioral problem

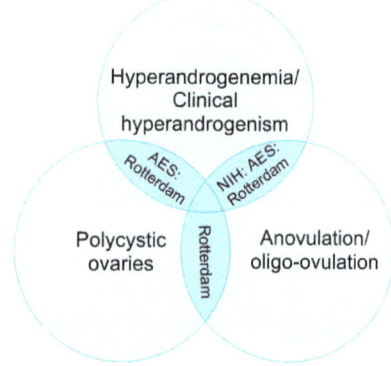

Fig. 10: Diagnostic criteria of polycystic ovary syndrome.
(AES: Androgen Excess Society; NIH: National Institutes of Health)

DIAGNOSTIC CRITERIA OF POLYCYSTIC OVARY SYNDROME

■ A detailed history and physical examination should be done to look for symptoms and signs of clinical hyperandrogenism, such as acne, alopecia, and hirsutism, along with severe acne and hirsutism in adolescents **(Fig. 10)**.[8]
  - For adolescents having PCOS symptoms but who do not meet diagnostic criteria, an "increased risk" may be considered, and assessment may be advised at or

before complete reproductive maturity, typically occurs 8 years after menarche. This includes those who had PCOS symptoms before to using the combined oral contraceptive pill (COCP), people with persistent symptoms, and people who had significant weight increase during adolescence.[8]
- *There were no studies on alopecia in adolescents. Mild acne and alopecia are not recommended as diagnostic criteria for adolescents for these reasons.*[8]

Diagnostic Criteria for Metabolic Syndrome in Adolescent Girls[14,15]

- The International Diabetes Federation (IDF) Census group criteria for diagnosis of metabolic syndrome among girls 10–16 years are shown in **Figure 11**.
- For girls older than 16 years, the IDF adult criteria can be used **(Fig. 12)**.

Precautions during Diagnosis of PCOS in Adolescence[8]

- Aim is to facilitate timely diagnosis while preventing overdiagnosis and unnecessary treatment in otherwise healthy normal pubertal girls (Level C).
- It should be kept in mind that the overlap between normal pubertal development and characteristic features of PCOS confound an accurate diagnosis of PCOS in adolescence (Level A).
- Other disorders associated with irregular menses or hyperandrogenism must be excluded (Level A).
- Presence of clinical features of androgen excess such as hirsutism and biochemical hyperandrogenism in absence of oligomenorrhea of more than 2 years is not diagnosed in PCOS but considered to be at risk for PCOS.

Diagnostic Recommendations for PCOS in Adolescence[8]

- To avoid misdiagnosing physiological pubertal changes as PCOS, deferred diagnostic labeling accompanied by frequent longitudinal reevaluations of these girls who are considered to be "at risk for PCOS" is beneficial and prudent during adolescence (Level C)
- Despite no definitive diagnosis or approved therapy for PCOS in adolescence, treat the symptoms to decrease the risk for subsequent associated comorbidities (Level B).
- Although obesity, insulin resistance, and hyperinsulinemia are common findings in adolescents with hyperandrogenism

Blood glucose >100 mg/dL or >5.6 mmol/L	HDL-cholesterol <40 mg/dL or <1.03 mmol/L	Triglycerides >150 mg/dL or >1.7 mmol/L	Obesity >90th percentile or adult cutoff if lower	Blood pressure >130/85 mm Hg [Systolic/Diastolic]

Fig. 11: International Diabetes Federation Census group criteria for diagnosis of metabolic syndrome in girls of age 14–16 year. (HDL: high-density lipoprotein)

Blood glucose >100 mg/dL or >5.6 mmol/L	HDL-cholesterol <50 mg/dL or <1.29 mmol/L	Triglycerides >150 mg/dL or 1.7 mmol/L	Obesity >80 cm [Ethnicity variability]	Blood pressure >130/85 mm Hg [Systolic/Diastolic]

Fig. 12: International Diabetes Federation Census group criteria for diagnosis of metabolic syndrome in girls older than 16 year. (HDL: high-density lipoprotein)

they are not considered for diagnosis in this group (Level A).
- The objective assessment of cutaneous manifestations such as hirsutism, acne, and androgenic alopecia, Indian specific grading should be performed with appropriate scales and possibility of other etiologies should be excluded (Grade B, EL 3).
- Anti-Müllerian hormone (AMH) is not considered as a biomarker for diagnosis of PCOS in adolescence.

INVESTIGATION IN POLYCYSTIC OVARY SYNDROME[16]

Androgen measures are useful to detect biochemical hyperandrogenism where PCOS is suspected, these are likely to be most useful in diagnosis of PCOS in adolescents and women who demonstrate minimal to no features of clinical hyperandrogenism (e.g., hirsutism) **(Box 1)**.[8]

BOX 1: Investigation in polycystic ovary syndrome.
- Ultrasonography—antral follicle count, ovarian volume
- Androgens, DHEAS, total testosterone, free testosterone, FAI—elevated
- 17-OH progesterone—decreased
- SHBG—decreased
- Serum prolactin—elevated
- Serum cortisol—elevated
- Serum FSH—normal or decreased
- LH—elevated
- LH/FSH ratio—elevated
- AMH—elevated
- OGTT, IR, and lipid profile—deranged
- TSH—elevated

(AMH: anti-Müllerian hormone; DHEAS: dehydroepiandrosterone sulfate; FAI: free androgen index; FSH: follicle-stimulating hormone; IR: insulin resistance; LH: luteinizing hormone; OGTT: oral glucose tolerance test; SHBG: sex hormone-binding globulin; TSH: thyroid-stimulating hormone)

MANAGEMENT OF PCOS IN ADOLESCENT

Treatment of PCOS includes treating the symptoms and treatment of insulin resistance.

Psychological Support[17]

Adolescent PCOS is treated using an integrated, personalized, all-encompassing, scientifically devised, multifaceted strategy **(Fig. 13)**.

Consideration should be given to seeking both individual and group psychological counseling.

Lifestyle[17]

Diet and exercise are important and must be recommended early in management of PCOS.

Weight loss of only 5% of total body weight is associated with:
- Decreased insulin and luteinizing hormone (LH) levels, increased SHBG, and decreased free E2

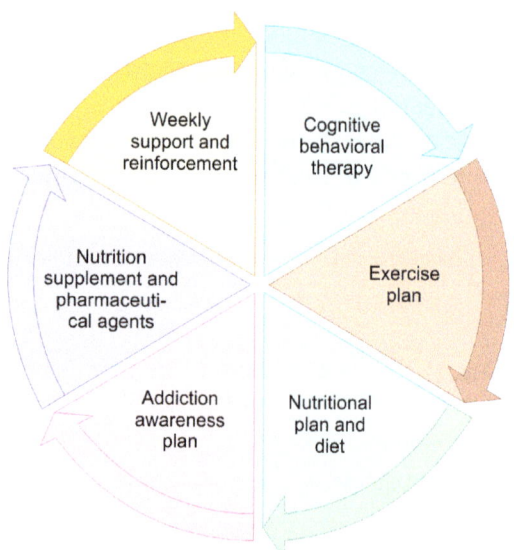

Fig. 13: Multifaceted strategy for treatment of adolescent polycystic ovary syndrome.

- Improved menstrual function
- Reduced hirsutism and acne
- Lower testosterone levels
- Improved cardiovascular risk factors including blood pressure.

In adolescents with PCOS, a multidisciplinary model of care with a dietitian, health psychologist, gynecologist, and endocrinologist demonstrated that a "behavioral intervention" enhanced weight loss when combined with dietary consultation, compared to receiving neither or dietary advice only.[8]

Diet[17]

- Low-calorie diet of 1,000–1,200 Kcal/day with low glycemic index
- Diet rich in fiber and high plant protein
- A calorie restriction of 500 Kcal/day can reduce body weight by 10% in 6 month.

Exercise[17]

Adolescents should engage in physical activity of a moderate to vigorous level for at least 60 minutes each day, including activities that build bone and muscle at least three times per week.[8,18]

Lowers the risk of the metabolic syndrome by 22%.

Treatment for Hyperandrogenic Features[11]

Box 2 shows the treatment for hyperandrogenic features.

Treatment for Menstrual Irregularities[11]

- Treatment is necessary for reducing chronic anovulatory cycles which increase the risk of developing endometrial hyperplasia; endometrial hyperplasia is associated with endometrial carcinoma.

BOX 2: Treatment for hyperandrogenic features.

Hirsutism
Antiandrogens (At least 6 months of therapy for therapeutic response):
- Spironolactone—100–200 mg/day
- Flutamide—250 mg/day. Side effect—hepatotoxicity
- Finasteride—5 mg/day
- Cyproterone acetate (CPA)—25–50 mg/day on day 5–14 of cycle or along with ethinylestradiol (EE)
- Combined oral contraceptive (COC) pills—cyproterone acetate (2 mg), drospirenone (3 mg), desogestrel (150 µg)

Dermatological:
- Permanent method—electrolysis, photoepilation
- Temporary method—waxing, shaving, plucking, bleaching
- Topical method—1% eflornithine hydrochloride

Acne
Pharmacological:
- Combined OCPs
- Antiandrogens
- Insulin-sensitizing agent

Topical:
- Salicylic acid
- Benzoyl peroxide
- Topical antibiotics
- Topical retinoids

Alopecia
- COC with androgen blocker (first line)
- Topical minoxidil 2–5%.

(OCP: oral contraceptive pill)

- Combined OCPs forms the first-line treatment for menstrual irregularities.
- Progestin is the critical ingredient in COCs that inhibits endometrial proliferation; it prevents the hyperplasia that results from unopposed estrogen action.
- Progesterone, either synthetic progesterone or dydrogesterone, is administered in the second half of the cycle.
- The dose of ethinylestradiol varies from 20 to 35 µg and progestins with minimum androgenic property.

- Cyclical micronized progesterone (100–200 mg/day) or medroxyprogesterone acetate (10 mg/day) for 10–14 days can also be given.
- *RCOG guideline:* In oligomenorrhea or amenorrhea, withdrawal bleeding should be induced every 3–4 months with cyclical progestogens for at least 12 days or COC for endometrial protection.[19]
- *Guidelines for prescribing COCP in adolescent:*
  - The COCP alone should be considered in adolescents with a clear diagnosis of PCOS for management of clinical hyperandrogenism and/or irregular menstrual cycles.
  - The COCP could be considered in adolescents who are deemed "at risk" but not yet diagnosed with PCOS, for management of clinical hyperandrogenism and irregular menstrual cycles.
  - When prescribing COCPs in adults and adolescents with PCOS:
    - Various COCP preparations have similar efficacy in treating hirsutism
    - The lowest effective estrogen doses (such as 20–30 μg of ethinylestradiol or equivalent) and natural estrogen preparations need consideration, balancing efficacy, metabolic risk profile, side effects, cost, and availability.
    - The relative and absolute contraindications and side effects of COCPs need to be considered and be the subject of individualized discussion.
    - PCOS-specific risk factors such as high BMI, hyperlipidemia, and hypertension need to be considered.
  - In combination with the COCP, metformin could be considered in adolescents with PCOS and BMI ≥25 kg/m^2 where COCP and lifestyle changes do not achieve desired goals.

Adjuvants[20,21]

- *Metformin:* Metformin, in additional to lifestyle, could be considered in adolescents with a clear diagnosis of PCOS or with symptoms of PCOS before the diagnosis is made.[8] For women with PCOS with menstrual irregularity who cannot take or do not tolerate hormonal contraceptives metformin may be used as second-line therapy.
- *Myoinositol:* Use of myoinositol in PCOS was associated with controlling of metabolic parameters, glucose, C-peptide, insulin, HOMA-IR, slight decrease in androgens, and weight reduction. Myoinositol can prevent developing of serious metabolic disturbances in adolescents with PCOS in future. It regularizes menstrual cycle with spontaneous ovulation, and improves ovarian response.[22]
- *D-chiro-inositol:* It reduces insulin resistance, improves glucose metabolism, lipid profile, and reduces risk of cardiovascular and metabolic complications. Dose is 2–4 g/day.[23]
- *Vitamin D:* Though controversial, vitamin D2 or D3 taken at a dose of 1,000–2,000 U/d or 50,000 U/week shown beneficial effect on insulin resistance, hyperandrogenism, follicular maturation, menstrual regularity, and ovulation.
- *L-methylfolate:* Its dose is 1–5 mg/day for 3 months. It reduces cardiovascular risk factor by increasing DNA synthesis and reducing homocysteine level.
- *Antioxidants:* N-acetyl cysteine, melatonin, L-carnitine

BOX 3: Approach towards PCOS in Adolescents.

Identify etiology
- Detailed history
- Pattern of menstrual cycle
- BMI, visceral fat distribution

Investigations
- Androgens, DHEAS, total testosterone, free testosterone, FAI, 17-OH progesterone, SHBG-decreasd, serum prolactin, serum cortisol, serum FSH, LH, LH/FSH ratio, AMH, OGTT, IR and lipid profile, TSH

USG
- Follicle number per ovary >12 to >25, ovary volume >10 cc

Lifestyle
- Weight loss of only 5% of total body weight is associated with increase insulin and LH level, increase SHBG, decrease free E2, improved menstrual function, reduce hirsutism, acne, lower testosterone level

Diet
- Low calorie diet of 1,000-1,200 Kcal/day with low glycemic index
- Diet rich in fiber and high plant protein

Exercise
- 150 minutes of moderate intensity exercise per week or 75 minutes of vigorous exercise
- Aerobic exercise of 3–4 times/week for 20–30 min burns 100–200 Kcal and 40% improvement in insulin sensitivity in 48 hours.[9]

Pharmacotherapy
- Antiandrogens, combined OCPs, progestins
- Adjuvants—Metformin, inositols (myoinositol, D-chiro inositol), vitamin D, l-methylfolate, antioxidants

(AMH: anti-Müllerian hormone; DHEAS: dehydroepiandrosterone sulfate; FAI: free androgen index; FSH: follicle-stimulating hormone; IR: insulin resistance; LH: luteinizing hormone; OGTT: oral glucose tolerance test; SHBG: sex hormone-binding globulin; TSH: thyroid-stimulating hormone)

CONCLUSION

- Polycystic ovary syndrome is extremely common in adolescents.[24]
- It can manifest as late menarche/primary amenorrhea, or as early menarche/oligomenorrhea with irregular bleeding.
- Obesity in adolescent PCOS is associated with:
  - Insulin resistance leading to functional hyperandrogenism, increase in ovarian and uterine volume and PCOM, and clinical manifestation in those with genetic or developmental predisposition.
- The clinical features of PCOS in adolescence overlap with those of normal puberty, making diagnosis difficult.
- The diagnostic criteria which apply to adults do not apply to adolescent girls.

- Adolescent PCOS may be characterized by hyperandrogenemia and hyperinsulinemia.
- In adolescents who are overweight or obese (BMI >25 kg/m^2 or 23 kg/m^2 in Asians), general guidelines recommend testing for prediabetes and DM.

▪ REFERENCES

1. Fauser JM, Tarlatzis BC, Rebar RW, Legro RS, Balen AH, Lobo R, et al. Consensus on women's health aspects of 3rd polycystic ovary syndrome (PCOS): The Amsterdam ESHRE/ASRM-Sponsored 3 PCOS Consensus Workshop Group. Fertil Steril. 2012;97(1):28-38.e25.
2. Adolescent Health Committee. Age limits and adolescents. Paediatr Child Health. 2003;8(9):577.
3. Malik S, Shah D, Sheth R, Talwar P, Prasad S, Dhorepatil B, et al. PCOS guideline: Management of polycystic ovary syndrome in India. Fertil Sci Res. 2014;1(1):23-43.
4. Kosova G, Urbanek M. Genetics of the polycystic ovary syndrome. Mol Cell Endocrinol. 2013;373(0):29-38.
5. Merkin SS, Phy JL, Sites CK, Yang D. Environmental determinants of polycystic ovary syndrome. Fertil Steril. 2016;106 (1): 16-24.
6. Gowri BV, Chandravathi PL, Sindhu PS, Naidu KS. Correlation of Skin Changes with Hormonal Changes in Polycystic Ovarian Syndrome: A Cross-sectional Study Clinical Study. Indian J Dermatol. 2015;60(4):419.
7. Rosenfield RL. The diagnosis of polycystic ovary syndrome in adolescents. Paediatrics. 2015;136:1154.
8. Teede HJ, Misso ML, Costello MF, Dokras A, Laven J, Moran L, et al. Recommendations from the International evidence-based guideline for the assessment and management of polycystic ovary syndrome. Fertil Steril. 2018;110(3):364-79.
9. Wiksten-Almstromer M, Hirschberg AL, Hagenfeldt K. Prospective follow-up of menstrual disorders in adolescence and prognostic factors. Acta Obstet Gynecol Scand. 2008;87:1162-8.
10. Marques AR, Silva C, Colmonero S, Andrade P. Diabetes Mellitus and Polycystic Ovary Syndrome: Beyond A Dermatological Problem. Diabetes Case Rep. 2016;1:113.
11. Shaw N, Rosenfield RL. Definition, clinical features and differential diagnosis of polycystic ovary syndrome in adolescents. [online] Available from: https://www.uptodate.com/contents/definition-clinical-features-and-differential-diagnosis-of-polycystic-ovary-syndromein-adolescents?source=search_result&search=PCOS&selectedTitle=4~150 [Last accessed November, 2022].
12. Maderal AD. Acanthosis nigricans. [online] Available from: https://www.uptodate.com/contents/acanthosis-nigricans?search=Acanthosis%20nigricans&source=search_result&selectedTitle=1~51&usage_type=default&display_rank=1 [Last accessed November, 2022].
13. Pannil M. Polycystic Ovary Syndrome: An Overview. Advanced Practice Nursing eJournal. 2002;2(3).
14. Rotterdam ESHRE/ASRM-Sponsored PCOS Consensus Workshop Group. Revised 2003 consensus on diagnostic criteria and long-term health risks related to polycystic ovary syndrome. Fertil Steril. 2004;81(1):19-25.
15. International Diabetes Federation Consensus group. (2007). The IDF consensus definition of metabolic syndrome in children and adolescents. Pediatric Diabetes. [online] Available from: https://www.idf.org/e-library/consensus-statements/61-idf-consensus-definition-of-metabolic-syndrome-in-children-and-adolescents.html [Last accessed November, 2022].
16. Shaw N, Rosenfield RL. Diagnostic evaluation of polycystic ovary syndrome in adolescents. [online] Available from: https://www.uptodate.com/contents/diagnostic-evaluation-of-polycystic-ovary-syndrome-in-adolescents [Last accessed November, 2022].
17. Lass N, Kleber M, Winkel K, Wunsch R, Reinehr T. Effect of lifestyle intervention on features of polycystic ovarian syndrome, metabolic syndrome, and intima-media thickness in obese adolescent girls. J Clin Endocrinol Metab. 2011;96(11):3533-40.

18. US Department of Health and Human Services. Physical Activity Guidelines. [online] Available from: https://health.gov/our-work/nutrition-physical-activity/physical-activity-guidelines [Last accessed November, 2022].
19. RCOG. Long-term Consequences of Polycystic Ovary Syndrome (Green-top Guideline No. 33). [online] Available from: https://www.rcog.org.uk/guidance/browse-all-guidance/green-top-guidelines/long-term-consequences-of-polycystic-ovary-syndrome-green-top-guideline-no-33 [Last accessed November, 2022].
20. Legro RS, Arslanian SA, Ehrmann DA, Hoeger KM, Murad MH, Pasquali R, et al. Diagnosis and Treatment of Polycystic Ovary Syndrome: An Endocrine Society Clinical Practice Guideline. J Clin Endocrinol Metab. 2013;98(12):4565-92.
21. Pkhaladze L, Barbakadze L, Kvashilava N. Myo-Inositol in the Treatment of Teenagers Affected by PCOS. Int J Endocrinol. 2016; 2016:1473612.
22. Unfer V, Facchinetti F, Orrù B, Giordani B, Nestle J. Myo-inositol effects in women with PCOS: a meta-analysis of randomized controlled trials. Endocr Connect. 2017;6(8): 647-58.
23. Morley LC, Tang T, Yasmin E, Norman RJ, Balen AH. Insulin-sensitising drugs (metformin, rosiglitazone, pioglitazone, D-chiro-inositol) for women with polycystic ovary syndrome, oligo amenorrhoea and subfertility. Cochrane Database Syst Rev. 2017;11(11):CD003053.
24. Jeffrey CR, Coffler MS. Polycystic ovary syndrome: early detection in the adolescent. Clin Obstet Gynecol. 2007;50:178-87.

CHAPTER 7

Metabolic Syndrome and PCOS

Parul Sinha, Amrita Singh

■ INTRODUCTION

Metabolic syndrome includes central obesity, hypertension, dyslipidemia, and insulin resistance. This syndrome needs to be studied on two major factors, one is cardiovascular risks and the other is endocrinological factors like insulin resistance.

Polycystic ovary syndrome (PCOS) is one of the syndromes which affects around 10–18% of the population and around 33% of PCOS patients suffer from metabolic syndrome and its sequelae.[1] Majority of the times, PCOS management is focused on infertility, hirsutism, and menstrual disturbances but as the disease burden of heart disease and diabetes increases, detecting metabolic syndrome early will help in better management of disease burden.

PATHOPHYSIOLOGY OF METABOLIC SYNDROME IN POLYCYSTIC OVARY SYNDROME

Insulin Resistance–Atherogenic Dyslipidemia–Obesity–Hypertension

- PCOS is a low-grade chronic inflammatory process which mediates insulin resistance.
- Besides this, high glycemic diet and obesity further increase production of proinflammatory cytokines which might accelerate atherogenesis.[2]
- Metabolic and mitogenic pathways are being regulated by insulin; hence, insulin resistance is one of the causes of metabolic inertia in PCOS.
- Insulin resistance leads to increased shunting of free fatty acids from adipose tissue to liver leading to increased production of triglycerides consequently developing atherogenic dyslipidemia.
- Insulin sensitivity in theca cells develops hyperandrogenemia which increases the sensitivity toward central obesity.
- This central obesity is linked with increased sympathetic outflow based on increased sensitivity of renin-angiotensin-aldosterone system (RAAS) because of insulin resistance and increased free fatty acids. This potentiates hypertension.

■ CONSEQUENCES

- *Cardiovascular disease (CVD):*
  - Risk of coronary heart disease and stroke get doubled in the patients of PCOS; according to one of the meta-analyses, despite adjusting for body mass index (BMI), there was 55% increase in risk.[3]
  - Risk factors for CVD in PCOS are obesity, lack of physical activity, dyslipidemia, impaired glucose tolerance (IGT) test, and hypertension.

- PCOS women should undergo regular monitoring of height, weight, and BMI.
- Annual or more frequent blood pressure checkup or as per global risk of CVD.
- PCOS women regardless of age should have their fasting lipid profile monitored according to derangement and global risk of CVD.

▪ *Diabetes:*
- PCOS women with normoglycemia have 16% increased risk for developing IGT per year and those with IGT have 2% increased risk of developing type II diabetes and over 6 years this risk could be 54%.[4]
- There is a threefold increased risk of developing gestational diabetes in PCOS women.
- Glycemic status should be assessed at the baseline evaluation by fasting glucose or glycated hemoglobin (HbA1c); otherwise, oral glucose tolerance test (OGTT) with 75 g glucose should be done in high-risk ethnicity, BMI > 25 kg/m^2, past history of IGT or gestational diabetes, or family history of diabetes.
- All PCOS women planning pregnancy should be offered OGTT; if not done, it should be done at the first visit of conception.

▪ *Cancers:*
- Hyperketonemia leads to endometrial hyperplasia and subsequently increased risk of developing endometrial cancer.
- Metabolic syndrome associated with PCOS is having increased risk for breast and colon cancers.[5]
- Optimal method of screening and prevention of endometrial hyperplasia is still not established.
- Pragmatic approach would be to offer combined oral contraceptives (COCs) and progestin in women with cycles longer than 90 days.

▪ *Obstructive sleep apnea (OSA):*
- There is 30-fold increased risk of OSA in PCOS patients. Key factor is insulin resistance independent of BMI and testosterone levels.
- A simple questionnaire known as Berlin tool is offered and if screened positive, patients should be referred to specialist.

▪ *Psychological problems:*
- PCOS patients are more prone to eating disorders, depression, and relationship dysfunction.
- Similarly, metabolic syndrome is also associated with a higher incidence of depression.
- Emotional well-being can be assessed by PCOS quality of life questionnaire (PCOSQ) or modified PCOSQ to highlight the features causing the distress, treatment outcomes, and subjective concerns.
- Anxiety and depression should be routinely screened in all PCOS adolescents at diagnosis and further evaluated by suitable qualified health professionals following regional guidelines if screened positive.
- Psychosexual dysfunction can be assessed by Female Sexual Function Index.
- All PCOS patients should be offered psychotherapy or pharmacological treatment if needed.

▪ *Nonalcoholic fatty liver disease (NAFLD) and PCOS:*
- NAFLD and PCOS have often been found together in patients because of insulin resistance and

hyperandrogenism leading to chronic liver disease varying from steatosis to cirrhosis; hence, it is a big concern for PCOS patients.
- Most patients are either asymptomatic at diagnosis or present with non-specific features of fatigue, upper quadrant discomfort, and malaise.
- Hepatomegaly might be the only finding.
- Laboratory diagnosis is commonly done on the basis of liver function test after excluding alcohol consumption and other secondary causes. Other tests include cytokeratin 18, fatty liver index, etc., apart from imaging.
- Rising incidence of NAFLD in PCOS since its first diagnosis in 2005 sets an alarm to screen liver enzyme derangements at the baseline.

■ DIAGNOSTIC CRITERIA

Defining criteria for metabolic syndrome vary according to the shift in pathogenesis (**Table 1**). Multiple definitions have been proposed according to different bodies which are mentioned in **Table 2**.

Screening

Screening parameters for metabolic syndrome are given in **Table 3**.

Management

- Primary intervention for metabolic syndrome requires adopting lifestyle changes that may prevent or slow progression to adverse events in high-risk individuals.
- In those who do not respond adequately to lifestyle modifications, secondary interventions can be considered, including drug therapy and bariatric surgery.

Lifestyle Modifications

- Exercise and dietary habits need to be modified for better outcome.

TABLE 1: Diagnostic criteria for metabolic syndrome.

Measure	Categorical cutoff points
1. Elevated waist circumference	≥88 cm[6,7] ≥80 cm[8,9]
2. Elevated triglycerides	≥150 mg/dL (1.7 mmol/L), or receiving drug treatment
3. Reduced HDL-C levels	<50 mg/dL (1.3 mmol/L), or receiving drug treatment
4. Elevated BP	Systolic BP ≥130 mm Hg or diastolic BP ≥85 mm Hg, or treatment of previously diagnosed hypertension
5. Elevated fasting glucose levels	≥100 mg/dL (5.6 mmol/L)[7-9] ≥110 mg/dL (6.1 mmol/L)[6] or receiving drug treatment

(BP: blood pressure; HDL-C: high-density lipoprotein-cholesterol)

TABLE 2: International organizations and groups involved in defining metabolic syndrome.

Based on insulin resistance	Based on central obesity
• World Health Organization (WHO) criteria, 1998 • European Group for the Study of Insulin Resistance (EGIR), 1999 • American Association of Clinical Endocrinology (AACE), 2003	• National Cholesterol Education Program: Adult Treatment Panel III (NCEP:ATP III) criteria, 2001[6] • American Heart Association/ National Heart, Lung, and Blood Institute (AHA/NHLBI) criteria, 2005[7] • International Diabetes Federation (IDF) criteria, 2005[8] • Joint Interim Statement (JIS), incorporating IDF and AHA/NHLBI definitions, 2009[9]

TABLE 3: Recommendations for metabolic syndrome risk factor screening in women with polycystic ovary syndrome.[10]

Screening parameters	Frequency of assessment
Cigarette smoking	At every visit, obtain history of recent smoking habits, if any, or cessation
Obesity (weight, BMI, waist circumference)	At every visit
Blood pressure	• For women with a BMI <25 kg/m^2: Annually • For women with a BMI ≥25 kg/m^2: At every visit
Complete lipid profile	• For women with a normal profile: Every 2 years • For women with an abnormal profile or excess weight: Annually
Oral glucose tolerance test (75 g)	• All women: Every 2 years • Women with risk factors [age >40 years, ethnicity, physical inactivity, smoking, waist circumference (>80 cm), BMI ≥25 kg/m^2, hypertension, previous gestational diabetes mellitus, family history of diabetes mellitus]: Annually

(BMI: body mass index)

- Weight reduction of 5–10% is associated with improved clinical outcomes.[11,12]
- Regular exercise of 150 min/week which should include 90 minutes of moderate aerobic activity is recommended for better cardiometabolic outcomes.[11]
- **Figure 1** illustrates the main components of a diet plan with quantities calculated for a 1,500-calorie diet.[13]

■ MEDICAL MANAGEMENT

Medical management includes insulin-sensitizing agents like inositol and metformin. Anti-obesity agents like orlistat and statins improve dyslipidemia.

Insulin-sensitizing Agents

- *Metformin:*
  - Metformin improves insulin sensitivity in women with PCOS and also decreases fasting insulin levels, but this benefit was restricted to nonobese women with PCOS (BMI <30 kg/m^2).[14,15]
  - There is no strong evidence to use metformin merely for treating insulin resistance associated with PCOS, and it is not recommended by any international organization for use in normoglycemic females.
- *Inositols:*
  - Inositols are compounds with insulin-mimetic properties, particularly the isomers myoinositol (MI) and d-chiro-inositol (DCI).
  - MI and DCI are involved in downstream signaling pathways following the activation of insulin receptors and are considered mediators of insulin action.[16]
  - Preliminary data suggests that supplementing with inositol can be considered for improving a patient's metabolic profile, but more studies are required before its use can be standardized.

Anti-Obesity Agents

- *Orlistat:*
  - Orlistat, rimonabant, and sibutramine are used in the pharmacotherapy of obesity in PCOS.
  - Sibutramine and rimonabant have been withdrawn over safety concerns.
  - Orlistat induces significant and sustainable weight loss in patients with PCOS; hence, based on available evidence, it can be considered for the treatment of overweight and obese

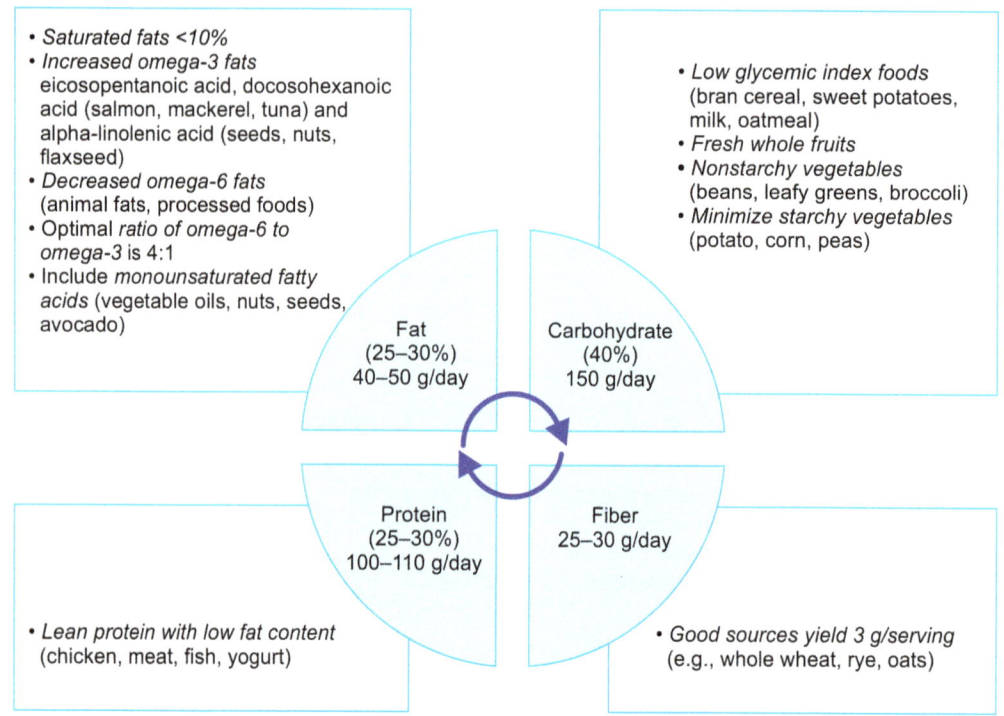

Fig. 1: Components of a healthy diet for women with polycystic ovary syndrome (PCOS).

women with PCOS for whom lifestyle modifications are insufficient.[17]

- Patients take 60–360 mg of orlistat per day, divided between two and three doses.
- *Liraglutide:* Glucagon-like peptide receptor (GLP-1R) agonists, including exenatide and liraglutide, are approved anti-obesity agents. The use of liraglutide for obesity in PCOS-related metabolic syndrome remains limited.

Despite multiple options for the pharmacological correction of metabolic derangements in women with PCOS, no drug is currently recommended as a standard line of management. The apparent benefits of medical therapy must be weighed against the risk of potential adverse effects of prolonged treatment.

CONCLUSION

As is evident from this article, metabolic syndrome is a neglected entity. Multiple mechanisms have been proposed for its occurrence in PCOS. Screening modalities must be developed to enable early diagnosis and institute aggressive measures for secondary prevention. The only universally accepted intervention is lifestyle modification. Metformin may be considered in women with IGT, although there is no established duration of treatment. The use of newer drugs such as inositol and liraglutide require further validation, while the use of statins should be limited only to women with dyslipidemia.

REFERENCES

1. March WA, Moore VM, Willson KJ, Phillips DIW, Norman RJ, Davies MJ. The prevalence of polycystic ovary syndrome

1. in a community sample assessed under contrasting diagnostic criteria. Hum Reprod. 2010;25(2):544-51.
2. Aubuchon M, Bickhaus JA, Gonzalez F. Obesity, metabolic dysfunction and inflammation in polycystic ovary syndrome. In: Lubna P (Ed). Polycystic Ovary Syndrome. New York: Springer; 2014. Pp. 117-44.
3. De Groot PCM, Dekkers OM, Romijn JA, Dieben SWM, Helmerhorst FM. PCOS, coronary heart disease, stroke and the influence of obesity: a systematic review and meta-analysis. Hum Reprod Update. 2011;17(4):495-500.
4. Legro RS, Gnatuk CL, Kunselman AR, Dunaif A. Changes in glucose tolerance over time in women with polycystic ovary syndrome: a controlled study. J Clin Endocrinol Metab. 2005;90(6):3236-42.
5. Chittenden BG, Fullerton G, Maheshwari A, Bhattacharya S. Polycystic ovary syndrome and the risk of gynaecological cancer: a systematic review. Reprod Biomed Online. 2009;19(3):398-405.
6. Expert Panel on Detection Evaluation, and Treatment of High Blood Cholesterol in Adults, Executive Summary of the Third Report of the National Cholesterol Education Program (NCEP) Expert Panel on Detection, Evaluation, and Treatment of High Blood Cholesterol in Adults (Adult Treatment Panel III). JAMA. 2001;285(19):2486-97.
7. Grundy SM, Cleeman JI, Daniels SR, Donato KA, Eckel RH, Franklin BA, et al. American Heart Association; National Heart, Lung, and Blood Institute. Diagnosis and management of the metabolic syndrome: an American Heart Association/National Heart, Lung, and Blood Institute Scientific Statement. Circulation. 2005;112(17):2735-52.
8. Alberti KGMM, Zimmet P, Shaw J. Metabolic syndrome-a new world-wide definition. A Consensus Statement from the International Diabetes Federation. Diabet Med J Br Diabet Assoc. 2006;23:469-80.
9. Alberti KGMM, Eckel RH, Grundy SM, Zimmet PZ, Cleeman JI, Donato KA, et al. Harmonizing the metabolic syndrome: a joint interim statement of the International Diabetes Federation Task Force on Epidemiology and Prevention; National Heart, Lung, and Blood Institute; American Heart Association; World Heart Federation; International Atherosclerosis Society; and International Association for the Study of Obesity. Circulation. 2009;120(16):1640-5.
10. Royal College of Obstetricians and Gynaecologists (2007). Long-term consequences of polycystic ovarian syndrome. [online] Available from: https://www.rcog.org.uk/guidance/browse-all-guidance/green-top-guidelines/long-term-consequences-of-polycystic-ovary-syndrome-green-top-guideline-no-33/ [Last accessed November 2022].
11. Teede HJ, Misso ML, Deeks AA, Moran LJ, Stuckey BGA, Wong JLA, et al. Assessment and management of polycystic ovary syndrome: summary of an evidence-based guideline. Med J Aust. 2011;195(6):S65-112.
12. Alberti KGM, Zimmet P, Shaw J, IDF Epidemiology Task Force Consensus Group. The metabolic syndrome—a new worldwide definition. Lancet. 2005;366(9491):1059-62.
13. Douglas CC, Gower BA, Darnell BE, Ovalle F, Oster RA, Azziz R. Role of lifestyle and diet in the management of polycystic ovarian syndrome. Fertil Steril. 2006;85(3);679-88.
14. Moghetti P, Castello R, Negri C, Tosi F, Perrone F, Caputo M, et al. Metformin effects on clinical features, endocrine and metabolic profiles, and insulin sensitivity in polycystic ovary syndrome: a randomized, double-blind, placebo-controlled 6-month trial, followed by open, long-term clinical evaluation. J Clin Endocrinol Metab. 2000; 85(1):139-46.
15. Tang T, Lord JM, Norman RJ, Yasmin E, Balen AH. Insulin-sensitizing drugs (metformin, rosiglitazone, pioglitazone, D-chiro-inositol) for women with polycystic ovary syndrome, oligo amenorrhoea and subfertility. Cochrane Database Syst Rev. 2012;(5):CD003053.
16. Croze ML, Soulage CO. Potential role and therapeutic interests of myo-inositol in metabolic diseases. Biochimie. 2013;95(10): 1811-27.
17. Panidis D, Tziomalos K, Papadakis E, Vosnakis C, Chatzis P, Katsikis I. Lifestyle intervention and anti-obesity therapies in the polycystic ovary syndrome: impact on metabolism and fertility. Endocrine. 2013;44(3):583-90.

CHAPTER 8

Insulin Resistance in PCOS

Aruna Verma, Vandana Verma

BACKGROUND AND HISTORICAL PERSPECTIVE

The association between abnormalities of glucose metabolism and hyperandrogenism was first described in 1921 by Achard and Thiers as "the diabetes of bearded women (diabetes des femmes a barbe)."[1]

In 1947, Kierland et al. reported the frequent occurrence of acanthosis nigricans, a skin lesion, in women with hyperandrogenism and diabetes mellitus (DM).[2]

In 1976, Kahn et al. described a distinct disorder affecting adolescent girls, designated by them as type A syndrome, characterized by features of virilization, extreme insulin resistance (IR) with DM, and striking acanthosis nigricans in affected females.[3]

In 1980, Burghen et al. observed a significant correlation between basal plasma insulin levels, androstenedione, and testosterone level and also between the levels of insulin and testosterone after giving oral glucose load which suggested the importance of IR and hyperinsulinemia in the pathogenesis of polycystic ovary syndrome (PCOS).[4]

POLYCYSTIC OVARY SYNDROME METABOLIC PHENOTYPES

The metabolic phenotypes of polycystic ovary syndrome are given in the previous chapters of book (*Chapter 4*), here we are explaining about insulin Resistance in them.

Insulin Resistance

Insulin regulates glucose metabolism by stimulating glucose uptake in target tissues such as adipocytes and skeletal and cardiac muscles. It also suppresses glucose production and lipolysis in the liver.[5] When there is less than the normal effect of endogenous- or exogenous-administered insulin on target organs, it is called IR.

Insulin resistance is a common feature in PCOS, especially in obese women as compared to lean women. The women classified with National Institute of Health (NIH) criteria have more marked metabolic dysfunction compared to Rotterdam phenotypes.[5]

The overall prevalence of IR in PCOS women is approximately 50–75% and is more commonly seen in obese PCOS (70–80%) as compared to lean and thin PCOS (20–25%).[6] Up to 35% patients of PCOS show impaired glucose tolerance (IGT) whereas type 2 DM (T2DM) was observed in 7–10% of women with PCOS.

Increased levels of fasting insulin are biochemical evidence of IR; however, it may not be always elevated in PCOS women.

Postprandial abnormalities of glucose metabolism are more common in women with PCOS rather than fasting abnormalities. Therefore, 2 hours post-glucose challenge values are of value in diagnosing IGT and type 2 DM in PCOS.[6] Defects in the insulin-stimulated glucose uptake, especially in glycogen synthesis, are found in PCOS whereas glucose oxidation and the ability to suppress lipid oxidation are less affected in these patients.[5]

The cause of IR is not clear in PCOS; however, more than one mechanism may be involved. Insulin acts on cells by its receptor which is a tetramer of alpha and beta dimers via two different pathways—phosphatidylinositol 3-kinase (PI3K) pathway, which regulates metabolic effects, and the mitogen-activated protein kinase (MAPK) pathway, which regulates mitogenic activity. Conformational change occurs in the receptor after binding with insulin, resulting in tyrosine phosphorylation of the receptor which binds and activates PI3K and Akt, an effector that plays a role in glucose metabolism. Akt stimulation activates the translocation of glucose transporter 4 (GLUT 4) from the intracellular compartment to plasma membrane. Another effector molecule inhibits gluconeogenesis and glycogenolysis while increasing lipid synthesis and decreasing lipid metabolism. It is suggested from the studies on fibroblast, skeletal muscles, and adipocytes that in PCOS, IR is due to defects in the early postreceptor pathway. The number and affinity of receptors do not change in PCOS. In PCOS, there is increased phosphorylation of serine and a decrease in insulin-stimulated phosphorylation of tyrosine. Serine phosphorylation prevents the receptor binding to PI3K, which inhibits the inhibiting insulin signaling. In PCOS, the increased phosphorylation of serine is due to increased intracellular metabolite free fatty acid, which results in IR. By induction of serine phosphorylation of P450c17, there is increased 17β-lyase activity on increased circulating free fatty acid, which leads to increased production of androgens.

Figures 1 and 2 explain how the insulin actions can be selectively inhibited and enhanced at the same time through different signaling pathways—PI3K and MAPK.

Other Metabolic Actions of Insulin in Polycystic Ovary Syndrome

Despite peripheral IR, insulin sensitivity remains normal or may be even increased in women with PCOS. Increased level of insulin in circulation stimulates hyperandrogenism.

Hyperandrogenism can be caused by either stimulation of androgen production by theca cells of the ovaries or by a decrease in sex hormone-binding globulin (SHBG) production in liver cells. In women with PCOS, physiological insulin levels can stimulate androgen secretion from theca cells of the ovary. Insulin also stimulates the action of the luteinizing hormone (LH), increasing androgen production **(Flowchart 1)**.[6]

Not much data is available to see the effect of insulin on lipid metabolism in PCOS patients but according to some studies, there is no significant difference in lipid uptake and oxidation in controls or PCOS myotubes.[6]

Insulin resistance and hyperinsulinemia are associated with a decreased level of high-density lipoprotein cholesterol and elevated triglyceride levels.

Altered catecholamine regulation in lipolysis has been reported in PCOS.

A difference was observed in the sensitivity of catecholamine-stimulated lipolysis in adipocytes of subcutaneous and visceral fat (respectively decreased and increased sensitivity) of lean women with PCOS.[5] Because of increased portal-free fatty acid delivery to the liver, increased catecholamine-stimulated lipolysis may result in hepatic IR.

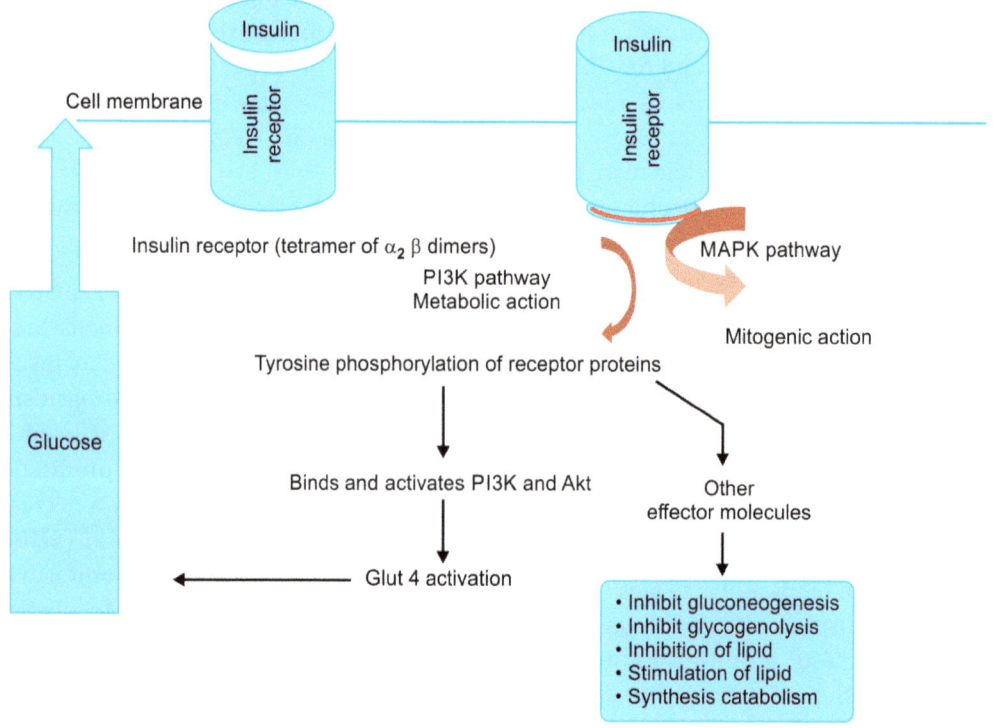

Fig. 1: Mechanism of insulin action in normal individual. (GLUT 4: glucose transporter 4; PI3K: phosphatidylinositol 3-kinase; MAPK: mitogen-activated protein kinase)

Mitogenic Action of Insulin in Polycystic Ovary Syndrome

The mitogenic action of insulin on cell growth and differentiation can be regulated by the MAPK -extracellular signal-regulated kinase (ERK) 1/2 pathway which is independent of the metabolic actions of insulin.[5] This selective IR has been studied in skin fibroblasts and myotubes of PCOS and controls.[5] Selective defect of insulin actions on PCOS granulosa cells has also been found, suggesting ovarian IR, and is associated with enhanced insulin-like growth factor 1 (IGF-1) mitogenic potential.[5]

Thus, the primary defect in insulin action is a postbinding defect affecting primarily adipocytes and skeletal muscle.

Insulin Secretion and Clearance in Polycystic Ovary Syndrome

Hyperinsulinemia and IR are common in patients with PCOS.[5,6] Women with PCOS have higher levels of fasting as well as glucose-stimulated insulin levels. Women with PCOS have less insulin sensitivity than healthy women. Abnormalities in glucose metabolism occur when beta cells are not able to secrete a sufficient amount of insulin.

Insulin response to oral glucose load gives a good understanding of insulin response, sensitivity, and dynamics. In normal individuals after ingestion of 75 g of glucose, peak insulin levels reach after 30 minutes which subsequently decline over 2 hours on the oral glucose tolerance test whereas in

Insulin Resistance in PCOS

In PCOS Individual:

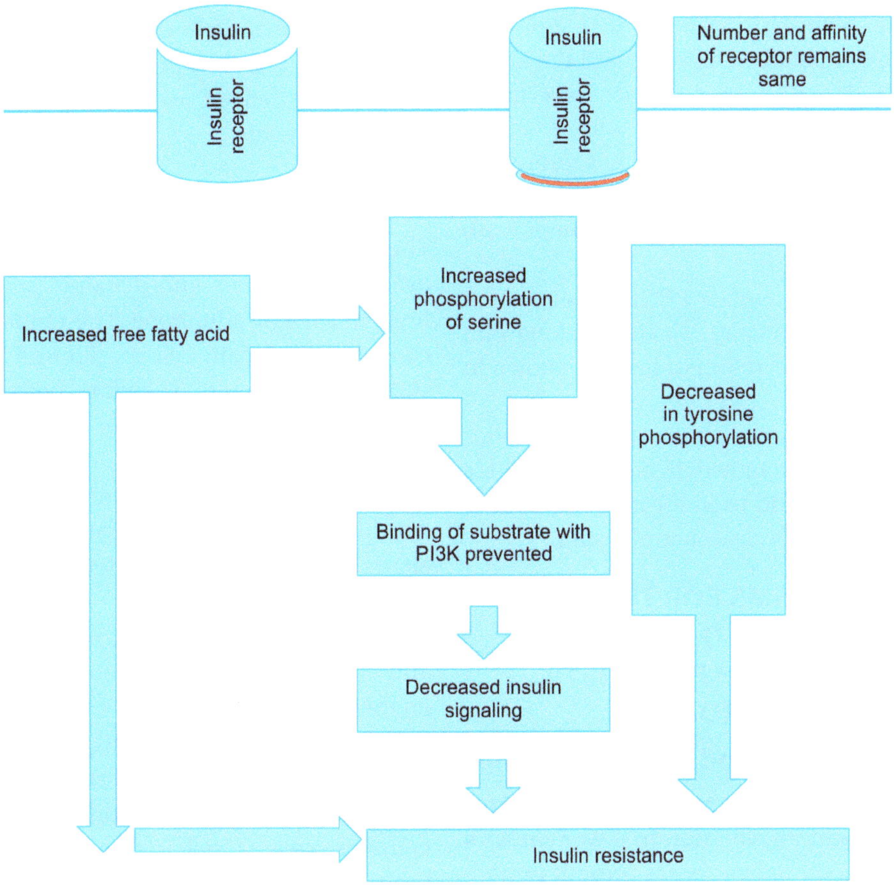

Fig. 2: Mechanism of insulin action in PCOS individual.
(PI3K: phosphatidylinositol 3-kinase)

Flowchart 1: Insulin resistance producing and enhancing factors. (SHBG: sex hormone binding globulin)

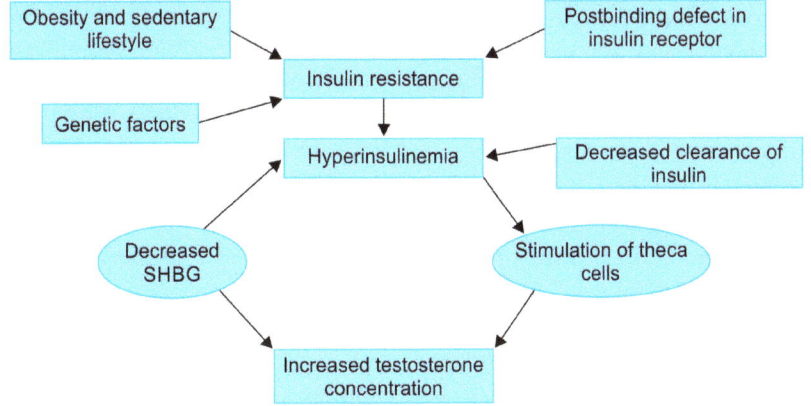

women with PCOS this response is exaggerated and prolonged.

The disposition index is used as a measure of beta-cell function and the ability of the body to dispose of a glucose level and is measured as the product of insulin sensitivity times the amount of insulin secreted in response to blood glucose levels. It is used to predict the risk of T2DM in women with PCOS in the future[5].

Hyperinsulinemia in PCOS may also result from decreased hepatic clearance along with the increased secretion of insulin (shown in **Flowchart 1**).

The hepatic insulin extraction (HIE) index is computed as a ratio of insulin to C-peptide plasma levels and used for measurement of impaired hepatic clearance of insulin.

MECHANISMS FOR THE ASSOCIATION OF INSULIN RESISTANCE IN POLYCYSTIC OVARY SYNDROME

Insulin as a Reproductive Hormone

Hyperinsulinemia causes hyperandrogenemia and anovulation in a woman with PCOS. Insulin receptors are present in both normal and polycystic human ovaries.[5] Observations from various studies revealed that selective IR is also present in the ovaries in PCOS. Insulin act as co-gonadotropin through its cognate receptor to modulate ovarian steroidogenesis and it regulates both pulsatile and surge secretion of gonadotropin-releasing hormone (GnRH)/LH. Prenatal programming of adult reproductive function may be mediated by insulin.

Insulin receptors are found in kisspeptin and pro-opiomelanocortin (POMC) neurons in the brain which is involved in puberty and fertility. It suggests the involvement of insulin in the central control of reproductive functions.

There is a need for well-defined experimental models, to determine the importance of insulin signaling in the central control of reproduction, and its mechanisms of action are independent of associated changes in metabolic signals.[5,6]

Metabolic Action of Androgens

The mechanisms of androgen actions in the ovary are complex and dynamic and start from fetal life till adulthood. This requires the cooperation of many cell-specific and follicle stage-specific factors. Therefore, both excess and deficiency of androgens can result in anovulation and infertility.

Androgens have a role in follicular development in the early stages, and insufficient or excessive androgen levels can cause defects in preantral follicles.

Excess of androgen results in follicle arrest and anovulation mainly through its actions on theca cells.[5]

Androgen receptors (ARs) act through both genomic and nongenomic pathways and enhance the growth and differentiation of granulosa cells as well as suppress apoptosis. In the dominant follicle, AR enhance steroid synthesis via extranuclear pathways.[5,6]

Genetic Susceptibility

Inheritance of hyperandrogenism, anovulation, and PCO suggests an underlying genetic predisposition for PCOS.

In some individuals, a heritable X-linked form of PCOS has been described which has different phenotypes. Studies on larger families suggested autosomal dominant inheritance, with premature balding as the male phenotype.

A high prevalence of hyperinsulinemia and hypertriglyceridemia was found in siblings and parents of women with PCOS.

Dyslipidemia was found in first-degree relatives of PCOS women.

Genome-wide association studies (GWAS) have started for the identification of several possible candidate genes, like *DENND1A* (differentially expressed in normal and neoplastic cell domain containing protein 1A) and *THADA* (thyroid adenoma-associated protein) genes.

An allele of a dinucleotide repeat D19S884 on chromosome 19p13.2, follistatin, and fibrillin-3 was linked and associated with the different PCOS reproductive phenotypes.

Polycystic ovary syndrome begins early in life and that metabolic changes precede reproductive abnormalities.[6] Currently, PCOS is identified as a polygenic disorder involving the interaction of numerous genomic variants and environmental factors.

CONCLUSION

Polycystic ovary syndrome is a major disorder affecting metabolic as well as reproductive function. IR of various degrees is common in cases of PCOS, especially in PCOS with obesity. IR is secondary to decreased insulin receptor signaling, caused by serine hyperphosphorylation of the receptor and insulin receptor substrate-1 (IRS1). The IR in PCOS is selective in skeletal muscles as well as in ovaries, affecting only metabolic actions but not the mitogenic functions. Insulin is an important reproductive hormone and insulin signaling in the central nervous system (CNS) is critical for proper ovulation. The proper balance of androgens is also important for follicular development. Abnormalities associated with PCOS start early in life and precede metabolic and reproductive abnormalities. PCOS is now recognized as a polygenic disorder caused by the interaction of numerous genomic variants and environmental factors.

REFERENCES

1. Achard C, Thiers J. Le virilisme pilaire et son association a l'insuffisance glycolytique (diabete des femmes a barb). Bull Acad Natl Med. 1921;86:51-64.
2. Kierland RR, Lakatos I, Szijarto L. Acanthosis nigricans: An analysis of data in twenty-two cases and a study of its frequency in necropsy material. J Invest Dermatol. 1947;9:299-305.
3. Kahn CR, Flier JS, Bar RS, Archer JA, Gorden P, Martin MM, et al. The syndromes of insulin resistance and acanthosis nigricans. N Engl J Med. 1976;294:739-45.
4. Burghen GA, Givens JR, Kitabchi AE. Correlation of hyperandrogenism with hyperinsulinism in polycystic ovarian disease. J Clin Endocrinol Metab. 1980;50: 113-6.
5. Diamanti-Kandarakis E, Dunaif A. Insulin resistance and the polycystic ovary syndrome revisited: an update on mechanisms and implications. Endocr Rev. 2012;33(6): 981-1030.
6. Taylor HS, Pal L, Seli E. Clinical Gynaecologic Endocrinology and Infertility, 9th edition. Philadelphia: Wolters Kluwer; 2020.

CHAPTER 9

Hirsutism and Hyperandrogenism in PCOS

K Geetha

■ INTRODUCTION

Females of all ages frequently present with hirsutism in the dermatology outpatient department (OPD), primarily for cosmetic reasons. About 5–10% of women are affected.[1] In contrast to being an isolated disorder known as idiopathic hirsutism (IH) or peripheral hirsutism, hirsutism may be a marker of other conditions, such as the polycystic ovary syndrome (PCOS), androgen-secreting tumors, nonclassical congenital adrenal hyperplasia (NCAH), or associated with syndromes of severe insulin resistance.[2]

■ DEFINITION

Hirsutism is defined as the development of androgen-dependent coarse pigmented terminal hair in women that follows a male-pattern distribution over the face, chest, abdomen, and back.

Hypertrichosis is the excessive hair growth limited to a normal pattern of distribution. It is frequently associated with the use of medications like antiepileptics, ciclosporin, etc.

■ PATHOPHYSIOLOGY

The interaction of the hair follicles with the transformation from vellus hair to terminal hair is associated with the circulating serum androgens and different growth factors that lead to hirsutism. Testosterone (ovarian origin), dehydroepiandrosterone sulfate (DHEAS) (adrenal origin), androstenedione (adrenal or ovarian origin), and dihydrotestosterone (DHT) (by conversion of testosterone intracellularly) are among the androgens that may be released in excess. The adrenal glands and peripheral tissues like hair follicles and external genitalia convert DHEAS, one of the aforementioned androgens, to androstenedione, testosterone, estrone, and estradiol **(Flowchart 1)**. Thus, hirsutism and virilization may result from adrenal hyperandrogenism.[3]

Due to the influence of androgens as well as an increase in the proportion of terminal hairs in the anagen or growth phase, the size and diameter of hair follicles increase. This extra testosterone in females increases hair growth in androgen-sensitive areas like upper lip, chin, mid sternum, upper abdomen, back, and buttocks.

Flowchart 1: Various types of androgens that cause transformation of vellus hair to terminal hair in hirsutism.

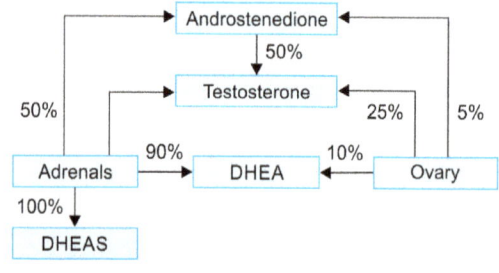

(DHEAS: dehydroepiandrosterone sulfate)

The fact that there is only a weak correlation between hair growth and serum testosterone levels, despite the fact that patients with hirsutism have an underlying androgen excess, suggests that other local factors and end organ sensitivity to androgens also play a part in the pathophysiology of hirsutism. It is primarily linked to an increase in free testosterone and a decrease in the levels of the sex hormone binding globulin (SHBG). Sometimes, increased testosterone to DHT conversion by the enzyme 5 alpha-reductase (5α-RA) in the hair follicles can also lead to hirsutism.[4]

CAUSES

The causes of hirsutism can be multiple as follows:
- Hyperproduction of androgens, of ovarian or adrenal origin, which includes PCOS, NCAH, or by hyperandrogenism of tumor-origin like androgen-secreting tumors
- Non-hyperandrogenic factors like medications, endocrinopathies, and other causes
- Idiopathic hirsutism

For approximately 75–85% of people with hirsutism, androgenic factors are the primary factor. About 75% of cases are caused by PCOS, which may afflict 5–10% of sexually active women and 20–25% of adolescent girls. It is a diverse condition marked by hyperplasia of the ovarian stroma and the termination of follicular maturation with an accumulation of tiny follicles under the cortex. In addition to menstrual cycle irregularities, weight gain, dyslipidemia, insulin resistance, acne, and acanthosis nigricans, hirsutism often develops throughout puberty.[1]

A partial 21-hydroxylase deficiency is the root cause of NCAH, which accounts for 2–8% of hirsutism cases. Hirsutism, oligomenorrhea, acne, infertility, alopecia, and primary amenorrhea are the main symptoms that appear after puberty. It is uncommon for ovarian or adrenal tumors to cause hyperandrogenism. Only 0.2% of all hirsutism cases are caused by it. Due to their independence, these androgen-secreting tumors are not reliant on the hypothalamic-pituitary axis. About 50% of them are malignant, and in these circumstances, plasma androgen levels are extremely high. They are also to account for hirsutism, a pelvic or abdominal mass, and the rapid beginning of virilization.[5]

Nonandrogenic causes of hirsutism are relatively uncommon and include medications such as androgens, glucocorticosteroids, progestins, estrogen antagonists (clomiphene, tamoxifen), minoxidil, cyclosporine, danazol, diazoxide, phenytoin, D-penicillamine, and interferon as well as endocrinopathies like Cushing syndrome, hyperthyroidism or hypothyroidism, hyperprolactinemia, and acromegaly.[6]

The hirsutism that is associated with regular menstruation, normal ovarian morphology, and normal plasmatic androgen levels is known as idiopathic hirsutism. After ruling out other causes, it is an exclusionary diagnosis. It accounts for roughly 10% of all hirsutism cases.[7]

APPROACH TO A PATIENT WITH HIRSUTISM

History and Physical Examination

An extensive history should be collected when a female patient has hirsutism, including the age of onset (adolescence, middle age, menopause), rate of onset (gradual or sudden), and any signs or symptoms of virilization (acne, deepening of voice, infrequent menstruation, loss of breast tissue or loss of normal female body contour, clitoromegaly, increased libido, increased muscle mass as in the shoulder gird). It is important to perform a detailed general physical and systemic examination, which includes palpating the abdomen for any ovarian masses. If a drug is the cause, a simple drug withdrawal should be beneficial. To determine the precise etiology in all other cases, laboratory analysis of the serum markers should be carried out.[8]

Scoring

In 1961, Ferriman and Gallwey developed a scoring system with 11 androgen-dependent locations. Later, the modified Ferryman–Gallwey (mFG) scoring system was adjusted to only include nine locations, and it is now regarded as the industry standard. A total hair growth score is calculated by adding the scores from each of the nine body areas, which range from 0 (no terminal hairs) to 4 (heavy terminal hair development). It is deemed abnormal if it is >7, with a maximum of 36 (**Fig. 1**). Although research done in various races has revealed that this cutoff value may not always be appropriate, traditionally, mFG score of 8 is considered hirsutism. The quantity and quality of hair on the sideburns, perineum, and perianal region are additional changes.[9]

■ MANAGEMENT

Women with moderate to severe hirsutism that has either recently manifested or is advancing rapidly require laboratory testing. Finding the underlying cause does not change management but identifies patients at risk for endometrial cancer, diabetes, infertility, and cardiovascular disease.

Some examples of blood indicators and diagnostic tests are as follows:[10]
- *Testosterone:* While it is normal for serum testosterone to rise in cases of benign pathology such as PCOS and CAH, it will be significantly higher (>200 ng/mL) in cases of adrenal or ovarian cancer.
- *DHEAS:* Elevated DHEAS (>700 µg/dL) always indicates a benign or malignant adrenal cause.
- *17-Hydroxyprogesterone:* It is found in CAH. The measurement should be taken between 0700 and 0900 hours during the menstrual cycle's early follicular phase. Levels of <200 ng/dL rule out the disease. Mildly elevated levels of 300–1,000 ng/dL necessitate an adrenocorticotropic hormone (ACTH) stimulation test. Cosyntropin (synthetic ACTH) 250 µg is given intravenously and levels of 17-hydroxyprogesterone are measured before and 1 hour after the injection. Poststimulation values (>1,000 ng/dL) constitute a positive test.
- 24-hour urine-free cortisol levels in women with Cushing's syndrome should be measured.
- A luteinizing hormone (LH)/follicle stimulating hormone (FSH) ratio >3 indicates PCOS.
- Prolactin levels would be elevated in hyperprolactinemia caused by hypothalamic disease or a pituitary tumor.
- *Serum thyroid stimulating hormone (TSH):* Hypophyseal hypothyroidism can be a cofactor in hirsutism, resulting in elevated TSH.
- Pelvic ultrasonography can be done to detect an ovarian neoplasm or a polycystic ovary, and magnetic resonance imaging (MRI) or computed tomography (CT) of the adrenal region is also useful for diagnosis.

The initial evaluation of a patient with hirsutism can be done as per **Flowchart 2**.[11]

Review Strategies and Expectations

Sometimes, hirsutism treatment is a matter of personal preference. Women have a wide

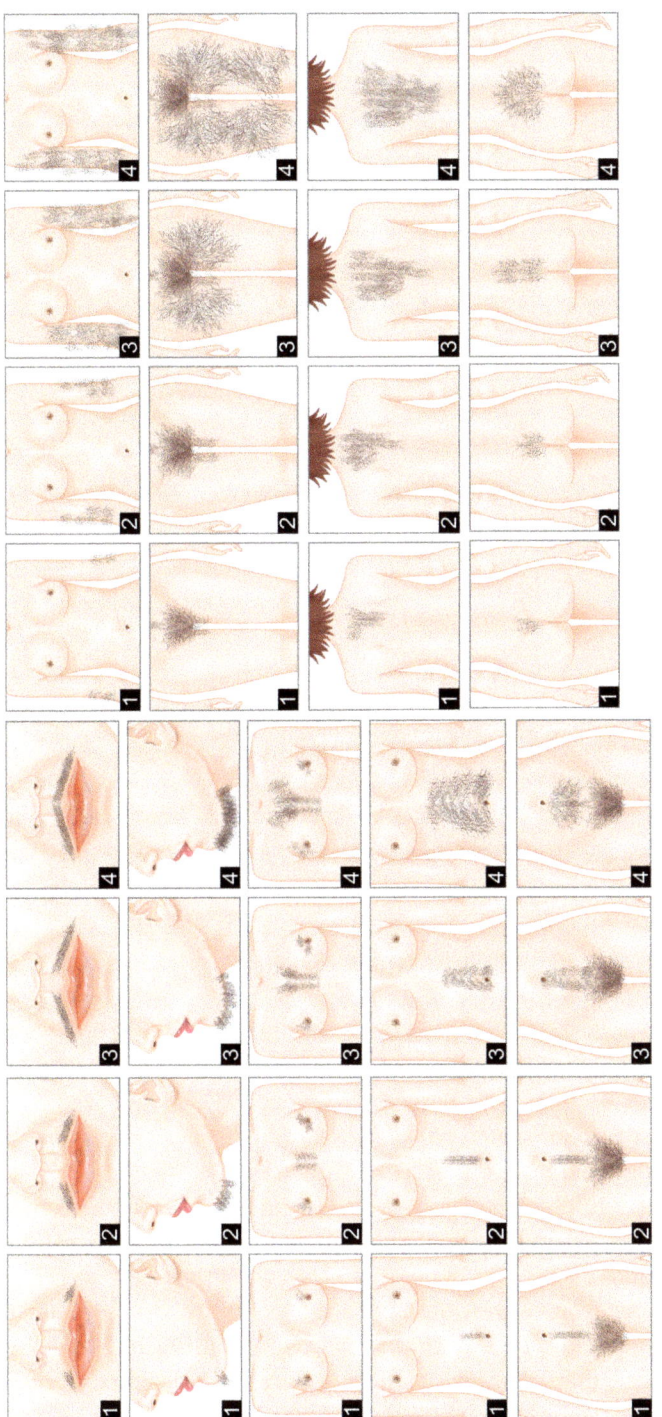

Fig. 1: Modified Ferryman–Gallwey (mFG) scoring system for hirsutism.

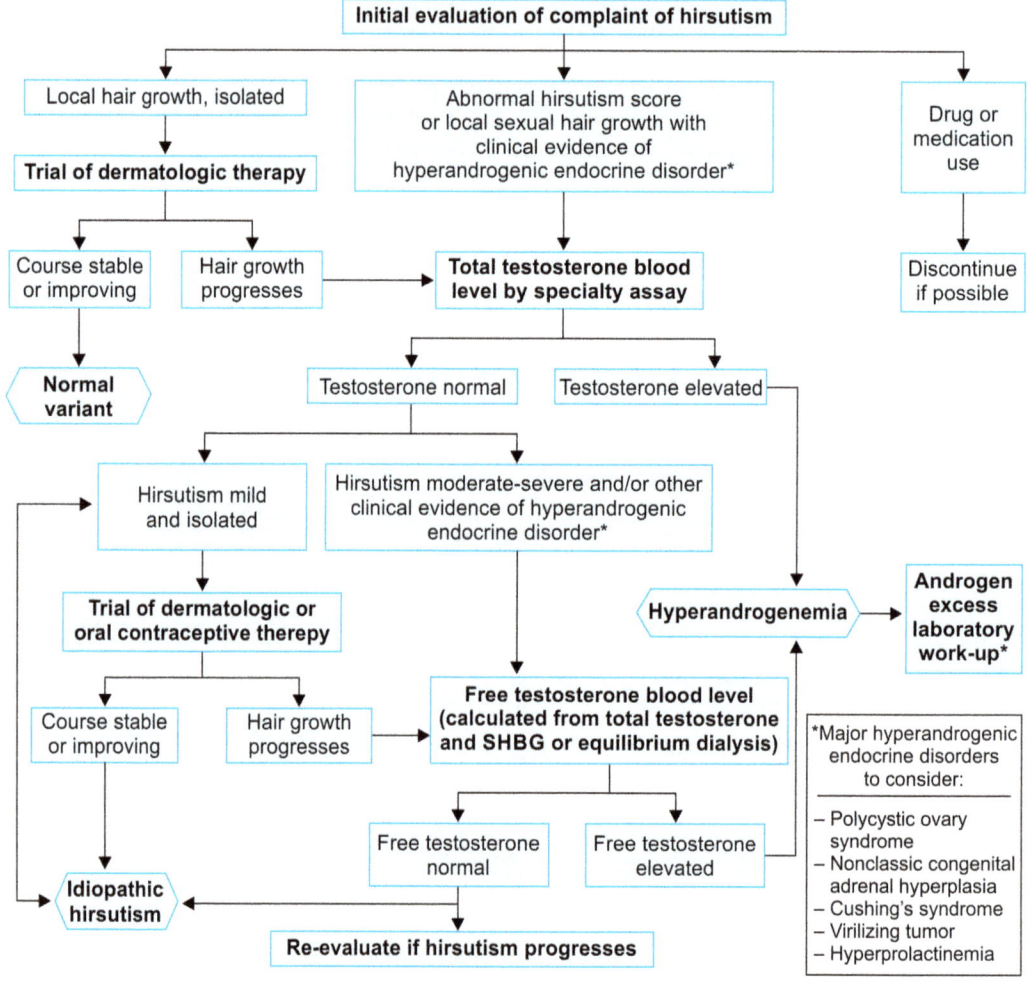

Flowchart 2: Initial evaluation of a patient with hirsutism.

variety of "normal" body hair densities. The development of body hair is greatly influenced by race and ethnicity. Women from Eastern Asia and Native America, for instance, typically have little body hair, whereas women from Southern Asia, the Middle East, and the Mediterranean region typically have moderate to abundant body hair.

Despite the fact that women typically have some facial and body hair, popular culture perpetuates the idea that women should have little to no body hair. Those who have hirsutism have significant rates of despair and anxiety that get better with treatment, regardless of weight or a PCOS diagnosis. Any woman who is bothered by her hair growth should discuss various treatments with her doctor.

Due to the average 6-month life span of hair follicles, hirsutism treatment calls for patience. Prior to observing a notable change, the majority of drugs require 6 months of use. The remaining hair can be mechanically removed or bleached in the meantime, and some women still combine these techniques with medicine.

In case there is a worry about an underlying condition, your provider will follow the course of your treatment and might repeat tests. A medication's dosage or kind may need to be changed if it is ineffective at first.

Duration of Treatment

Age-related declines in androgen hormone levels are observed in females. To control the hirsutism, women in their 20s may require multiyear treatment. Hormonal medication may no longer be necessary for some women in their 30s and 40s due to declining androgen levels, but this is not always the case. Hormonal therapies for hirsutism must be discontinued before becoming pregnant.

Weight loss, treatment for infertility, management of diabetes, and reduction of cardiovascular disease risk factors are all possible lifestyle modifications that may be part of PCOS treatment.

■ TREATMENTS

The treatment of hirsutism should be undertaken using combination therapy, including:
- Androgen suppression
- Peripheral androgen blockade
- Mechanical/cosmetic amelioration and destruction of the unwanted hairs.

The hirsute patient's treatment should also aim to reduce her risk of associated disorders such as endometrial hyperplasia or carcinoma, dysfunctional uterine bleeding, type 2 diabetes mellitus, and dyslipidemia, possibly through lifestyle changes, insulin sensitizers, and the use of lipid-lowering agents.

Androgen Receptor Blockers

As an androgen blocker, spironolactone (SPA) competes with DHT for binding to the androgen receptor. Additionally, ovarian androgen production is reduced by SPA, which also has varied progestational action. SPA inhibits the activity of 5α-RA and competes with androgens for SHBG. The recommended starting dose is 50 mg twice daily, while the maximum daily dose is 200 mg. At least 6 months must pass before any positive results are shown. With oral contraceptive pill (OCP) that offers effective contraception and also aids in reducing dysfunctional uterine hemorrhage, the use of SPA is advised. Polyuria and hypotension are unwanted side effects that might cause headaches, lethargy, or even fainting. Since individuals run the risk of developing life-threatening hyperkalemia when taking SPA with other potassium-sparing diuretics, thiazides, renal failure, or excessive potassium intake. Serum electrolytes and blood pressure should be checked 2–4 weeks after treatment begins. Dry skin and gastritis/dyspepsia are two minor adverse effects that are frequently linked to SPA use. Renal insufficiency, anuria, chronic renal impairment, hyperkalemia, pregnancy, and irregular uterine hemorrhage are all absolute contraindications to using SPA.[12]

Cyproterone acetate (CA) has strong progestogenic and antiandrogen properties. It has been used as a successful treatment for hirsutism because it causes a drop in the levels of circulating testosterone and androstenedione through a reduction in circulating LH. Ethinyl estradiol (EE) and CA can be found together in a tablet form (2 mg CA and 35 g EE).[13]

5-alpha Reductase Inhibitors

It has been discovered that the 5α-RA inhibitor finasteride is useful in treating IH. Type 2 5α-RA activity is significantly inhibited by finasteride. Finasteride will not be as effective as a 5α-RA inhibitor, particularly a "dual" type 1 and type 2 5α-RA inhibitor. 24 hours after oral treatment, this substance efficiently blocks the synthesis of DHT by 99%. A male fetus could potentially become feminized by any of these 5α-RA drugs. Therefore, patients taking these medications must use reliable contraception.[14]

Flutamide

The Food and Drug Administration has approved this androgen receptor blocker as an adjuvant therapy for prostate cancer. In doses of 500 mg/day, it is an efficient treatment for hirsutism. Up to 40% of the FG score is reduced. Along with liver enzyme abnormalities and, occasionally, fatal hepatotoxicity, side effects can include the appearance of greenish urine and severe dryness of the skin or scalp hair.[15]

Insulin Sensitizers

It has been shown that treating insulin resistance, primarily by losing weight or taking metformin or thiazolidinediones, improves hyperandrogenemia and ovulatory function in many PCOS-afflicted women. Its efficacy in treating hirsutism linked to PCOS, however, is less certain. Insulin-sensitizing medications may slightly alleviate PCOS-related hirsutism.[16]

Gonadotropin-releasing Hormone Agonists

For women with severe hirsutism, who do not respond to OC and antiandrogens, parenteral treatment is the only option. Long-acting gonadotropin-releasing hormone (GnRH) analogs lower testosterone production via lowering gonadotropin secretion, which in turn lowers ovarian stimulation. Additionally, less estrogen is produced. Consequently, treatment is typically combined with an oral contraceptive pill that contains estrogen and progestin.

Adrenal Suppression: Glucocorticoids

Corticosteroids have mostly been used to treat hirsutism brought on by CAH. They are utilized in a small dose of dexamethasone before bed.[17]

Biological Modifiers of Hair Follicular Growth

The topical cream (13.9%) eflornithine hydrochloride is a novel substance used to reduce or stop the growth of facial hair in females. A keratin synthesis enzyme is supposed to be inhibited, which prevents hair development. The formation of the polyamines that control cell migration, proliferation, and differentiation depends on the enzyme ornithine decarboxylase, which is a strong, irreversible inhibitor. The activation of ornithine decarboxylase production and the proliferation of hair matrix cells are linked to the binding of DHT to the androgen receptor. The cream is used twice daily to the face. Within 6-8 weeks, there is a noticeable improvement. For greater results, it can also be used in conjunction with laser therapy.[18]

MECHANICAL AND COSMETIC MEANS OF TREATING HIRSUTISM

Electroepilation and laser photothermolysis are two methods for permanently destroying the hair follicles that grow the undesirable hairs. Selective photothermolysis, a technique used in laser hair removal, involves targeting the hair follicle for thermal damage while sparing nearby tissues. Lasers for hair reduction include the following:[19]
- *Ruby laser (694 nm):* Synthetic ruby crystals are used to deliver red light, which is more effective for people with darker skin and darker hair.

- *Alexandrite laser (755 nm):* More penetration, beneficial for lighter hair
- *Diode laser (810 nm):* Deeper penetration, improved fluence, reduced epidermal damage, and safety for darker skin
- *Neodymium-doped yttrium aluminum garnet (Nd:YAG) laser (1,064 nm):* Improved penetration, reduced epidermal damage, and relatively less absorption of melanin
- *Intense pulse light (IPL) or broadband light (BBL) (500–1,200 nm):* A flash-lamp emits high-intensity pulses of polychromatic, noncoherent light. Different filters allow for the narrowing of the emitted wavelength band. It can be used on darker skin. Because of its larger spot size, it can cover larger areas; however, it is less expensive than a true laser but is less effective.

Multiple sessions will be required to treat all hair follicles at the time when they are most responsive to treatment because the hair matrix is only susceptible to laser treatment during the anagen phase of the hair development cycle. A minimum of four- to six treatments, spaced 4–6 weeks apart, are needed in the initial phase of hair removal therapy to produce satisfactory results. Patients may then require maintenance procedures once every 6–12 months as minor vellus hair regrowth is possible.

Many variables could influence the result, including the position of hair location (axillary and pubic hair respond better than hair on the extremities and chest), skin, and hair-tone (light skin of Fitzpatrick skin types I–IV with dark hair achieves the best results due to the lack of melanin in the skin and the abundance of melanin to absorb laser energy in the hair follicles), hair growth stage (anagen hair being most sensitive), type of laser used for therapy, hormonal status of the patient, and the treatment plan.[19]

TREATMENTS NOT ROUTINELY RECOMMENDED

Unwanted hairs may be temporarily reduced by shaving, bleaching, or chemical depilation. Shaving does not increase hirsutism, despite the possibility of a blunt hair end that may feel like stubble. Bleaching is advantageous, especially for sparse localized hair growth. Even though they are helpful, depilating treatments have the potential to cause persistent skin irritation and even aggravate hair growth if used excessively or carelessly. It is best to avoid using plucking and/or waxing on androgenized skin areas because these procedures not only do not kill the hair follicles, but can also cause folliculitis and damage to the hair shaft, leading to ingrown hairs and additional skin damage.

CONCLUSION

Hirsutism necessitates a thorough clinical evaluation and investigation in order to be treated. The majority of women are advised to use oral contraceptives for pharmacological therapy. If the response is inadequate after 6 months, an antiandrogen may be required. Unless adequate contraception is used, antiandrogen monotherapy is not recommended. Photoepilation with lasers is the preferred method of hair removal therapy for women.

REFERENCES

1. Mcknight E. The prevalence of "hirsutism" in young women. Lancet. 1964;1:410-3.
2. Agrawal NK. Management of hirsutism. Indian J Endocrinol Metab. 2013;17(Suppl 1): S77-82.
3. Deplewski D, Rosenfield RL. Role of hormones in pilosebaceous unit development. Endocr Rev. 2000;21(4):363-92.
4. Karrer-Voegeli S, Rey F, Reymond MJ, Meuwly JY, Gaillard RC, Gomez F. Androgen dependence of hirsutism, acne, and alopecia

in women: retrospective analysis of 228 patients investigated for hyperandrogenism. Medicine (Baltimore). 2009;88(1):32-45.
5. Hafsi W, Badri T. Hirsutism. [online] Available from: https://www.ncbi.nlm.nih.gov/books/NBK470417/ [Last accessed November 2022].
6. Saleh D, Yarrarapu SNS, Cook C. Hypertrichosis. [online] Available from: https://www.ncbi.nlm.nih.gov/books/NBK534854/ [Last accessed November 2022].
7. Lumezi BG, Berisha VL, Pupovci HL, Goçi A, Hajrushi AB. Grading of hirsutism based on the Ferriman-Gallwey scoring system in Kosovar women. Postepy Dermatol Alergol. 2018;35(6):631-5.
8. Sachdeva S. Hirsutism: Evaluation and treatment. Indian J Dermatol. 2010;55:3-7.
9. Aswini R, Jayapalan S. Modified Ferriman–Gallwey score in hirsutism and its association with metabolic syndrome. Int J Trichol. 2017;9:7-13.
10. Chang RJ, Katz SE. Diagnosis of polycystic ovary syndrome. Endocrinol Metab Clin North Am. 1999;28:397-408.
11. Kathryn A Martin, R Rox Anderson, R Jeffrey Chang, David A Ehrmann, Rogerio A Lobo, M Hassan Murad, et al. Evaluation and Treatment of Hirsutism in Premenopausal Women: An Endocrine Society Clinical Practice Guideline. J Clin Endocrinol Metab. 2018;103(4):1233-57.
12. Spritzer PM, Lisboa KO, Mattiello S, Lhullier F. Spironolactone as a single agent for long-term therapy of hirsute patients. Clin Endocrinol (Oxf). 2000;52:587-94.
13. Van der Spuy ZM, le Roux PA. Cyproterone acetate for hirsutism. Cochrane Database Syst Rev. 2003;2003(4):CD001125.
14. Faloia E, Filipponi S, Mancini V, Di Marco S, Mantero F. Effect of finasteride in idiopathic hirsutism. J Endocrinol Invest. 1998;21:694-8.
15. Cusan L, Dupont A, Gomez JL, Tremblay RR, Labrie F. Comparison of flutamide and spirolactone in the treatment of hirsutism: A randomized controlled trial. Fertil Steril. 1994;61:281-7.
16. Cosma M, Swiglo BA, Flynn DN, Kurtz DM, Labella ML, Mullan RJ, et al. Clinical review: Insulin sensitizers for the treatment of hirsutism: A systematic review and meta-analyses of randomized controlled trials. J Clin Endocrinol Metab. 2008;93:1135-42.
17. Rittmaster RS, Loriaux DL, Cutler GB Jr. Sensitivity of cortisol and adrenal androgens to dexamethasone suppression in hirsute women. J Clin Endocrinol Metab. 1985;61:462-6.
18. Malhotra B, Noveck R, Behr D, Palmisano M. Percutaneous absorption and pharmacokinetics of eflornithine HCl 13.9% cream in women with unwanted facial hair. J Clin Pharmacol. 2001;41:972-8.
19. Vaidya T, Hohman MH, Kumar D D. Laser Hair Removal. [online] Available from: https://www.ncbi.nlm.nih.gov/books/NBK507861/ [Last accessed November 2022].

CHAPTER 10

Psychological Aspects of PCOS

Deepa Chaudhary, Suman Chaudhary, Gaurav Rajender

■ INTRODUCTION

As the intricacies of the polycystic ovary syndrome (PCOS) are becoming comprehensible, we are able to appreciate the far-ranging, multisystem manifestations of this disorder. PCOS is not merely a gynecologic or dermatological disturbance or metabolic disorder. Reproductive (hyperandrogenism, anovulation, infertility, and pregnancy complications) and metabolic features (insulin resistance, impaired glucose tolerance, type 2 diabetes, and dyslipidemia) are well described.[1] Recent studies have thrown light on several psychological comorbidities of PCOS and its impact. The etiology of psychological features has not been well understood, but potential proposed mechanisms include obesity, insulin resistance, hyperandrogenemia, hypothalamic–pituitary–ovarian (HPO) axis abnormalities, and increased inflammatory markers. The high prevalence of PCOS (12–21%) poses health and economic burden[2] which requires greater cognizance and grasp of reproductive as well as psychological correlates of PCOS like emotional well-being, mood disorders, and health-related quality of life (HRQoL).[3-6] There is approximately threefold increased risk for depression, and risk for anxiety in women with PCOS may be even greater.[7] Recently (2018), routine screening for anxiety and depressive symptoms in all adolescents and women with PCOS at diagnosis was recommended by evidence-based guidelines on PCOS management.[8]

■ PSYCHOSOCIAL CONCERN RELATED TO POLYCYSTIC OVARY SYNDROME

Bodyweight and Body Image Disturbances

Body image is defined as an individual's psychological experience of the appearance and function of his/her body.[9] PCOS is linked with certain physical features such as acne, hirsutism, and obesity that might disturb body image.[10,11] Moreover high body mass index (BMI) is independently linked to greater body dissatisfaction in women with PCOS.[9,12,13] Taken together, these findings suggest that women with PCOS could be at a higher risk of body-image distress (BID). There are no clinical consensus recommendations of European Society of Human Reproduction and Embryology (ESHRE) about screening of BID but awareness in health professionals is required (Grade 3).

Recent cross-sectional study by Alur-Gupta et al. has proposed BID as an important component of PCOS to depression/anxiety pathway using a validated Multidimensional Body Self Relations–Appearance Subscale (MBSRQ-AS) and Stunkard Figure Rating

Scale (FRS).[14] This is a single study which identifies subjective experience such as body image as causal factor for mood disorders; more longitudinal studies are required to disentangle this vicious cycle. Routine psychological assessment of the body image in a patient with PCOS, alongside screening for depression and anxiety,[8,15] remains to be determined in future research. Lifestyle modification along with cognitive behavioral therapy (CBT) is the standard treatment.

Sexual and Relational Functioning

Data on sexual function and relational functioning women with PCOS are limited and often contradicting. Research in PCOS mainly focuses on infertility treatment rather than sexual well-being. Both sexual function and PCOS are complex biopsychosocial phenomena. Sexual function is affected by biological factors such as androgen levels, obesity, metabolic syndrome, and infertility as well as psychological factors such as depression, anxiety, body image, and self-esteem. Most of these factors are commonly present in women with PCOS and could be contributing to their sexual dysfunction. Psychosexual dysfunction refers to sexual problems or difficulties that have a psychological origin based in cognitions and/or emotions such as depression, low self-esteem, and negative body image. In considering screening tools, the female sexual function index (FSFI) and Arizona Sexual Experience Scale (ASEX) are commonly used to evaluate psychosexual dysfunction.

Pastoor et al.[16] in their largest meta-analysis on the effect of PCOS on sexual health assessed 1,925 articles and included only 18, which showed small impairment in sexual function, particularly arousal, lubrication, orgasm, and sexual satisfaction (sexual questionnaires), in PCOS. Sexuality was significantly impaired due to hirsutism ($p = 0.006$), body image ($p = 0.007$), and sexual attractiveness ($p < 0.001$). Satisfaction with sex life was impaired ($p < 0.001$), but sexual satisfaction was rated equally important in women with PCOS and controls. These findings imply that sexual function, sexual satisfaction, and psychosocial functioning need to be part of every clinical assessment of women with PCOS. ESHRE (2018) recommends:

- All health professionals should be aware of the increased prevalence of psychosexual dysfunction and should consider screening in adult women with PCOS (Grade 4).
- If psychosexual dysfunction is suspected, further assessment, referral, or treatment should follow as appropriate (Grade 4).

Health-related Quality of Life

Health-related quality of life is an important measure to assess the patient-related physical, social, and emotional effects of a chronic condition and its associated treatments. A meta-analysis of five studies using short form-36 (SF-36) and three studies using the WHO tool in adult women has shown that women with PCOS have lower quality of life (QoL) compared to women without PCOS. But tools like SF-36 or WHO tools are not ideal for PCOS as they do not consider the key dimensions of PCOS such as infertility and hirsutism.

Health-related quality of life in PCOS is measured using validated Polycystic Ovary Syndrome Questionnaire (PCOSQ), which is reliable and validated in several languages as an instrument for measuring HRQoL in women with PCOS. The PCOSQ has 26 items across emotions, body hair, weight, infertility, and menstrual abnormalities. Modified Polycystic Ovary Syndrome Health-Related

Quality of Life Questionnaire (MPCOSQ) has included acne dimension in it (PCOQ). MPCOSQ includes 30 items and seven-point Likert scale questions from six HRQoL areas or domains: emotional disturbances (eight items), hirsutism (five items), infertility (four items), weight (five items), menstrual (four items), and acne (four items) with higher values indicating higher QoL.[17,18] A recent meta-analysis has provided strong evidence that HRQoL is significantly impaired in hirsutism and mensuration domain of PCOS.[19] Hence, treatment of hyperandrogenism and menstrual irregularities will improve the psychological functioning as well as HRQoL in these patients.

Recent ESHRE recommendations: Health professionals should be aware of the impact of PCOS on QoL and should understand women's perception about the effect of symptoms on life to deliver meaningful outcomes when providing care (Grade-4 recommendation). If preferred, the MPCOSQ could be considered to assess the domains which have greatest impact on QoL and could guide treatment (not recommended in clinical practice but for research).

Stress and Coping Responses

Women with PCOS have high levels of stress, at least in part, due to clinical features of PCOS, including obesity, acne, hirsutism and also may be side effects of medication.[20,21] Various studies have suggested that high levels of stress are an underlying cause of the mood and anxiety disorders in these women.[22-26] Physiological reaction to stress was significantly high in women with PCOS in comparison to healthy women[23,27] and, moreover, they were hospitalized twice as often due to stress and self-harming behavior.[28]

Stress-coping mechanisms are an important mediator in the relationship between the experience of stress and any mental disorders resulting from it.[29] There are two basic strategies for coping with stress: active and passive coping **(Flowchart 1)**.

- Passive coping (concentrating on emotions) is the use of strategies for reducing

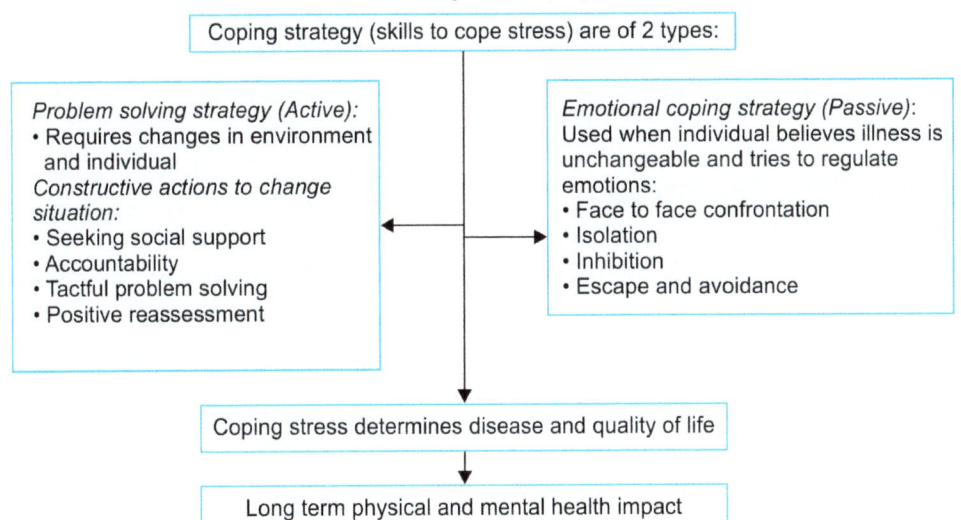

Flowchart 1: Strategies for coping with stress.

adverse emotions arising from a stressful situation; it may constitute a maladaptive strategy associated with anxiety and depression symptoms and leads to a worsening QoL.[30]
- Active coping (concentrating on the problem) is characterized by striving to resolve the problem and may protect psychosocial well-being.[31,32]

Until recently, coping strategies of women with PCOS were not commonly analyzed.[27,33-36] Benson et al. and Sigmon et al. showed that depression and anxiety are negative consequences of passive coping.[20,27]

Ego resiliency is a personality trait; it reduces the tendency of experiencing the anxiety and depression in stressful circumstances with flexible selection of coping strategies depending on requirement. It can be measured using ego-resiliency scale (14-item instrument). Women with PCOS usually have a low level of ego resiliency.

As the passive stress-coping strategies with a low level of ego resiliency are predictors of high levels of anxiety and depression in women with PCOS, an assessment of both in women with PCOS can help to identify people who are at risk of psychological well-being deterioration. It is also necessary to implement educational and therapeutic interventions to help women deal effectively with their illness.

PSYCHIATRIC DISORDERS

A recent meta-analysis of 57 studies of 172,040 females reported that those with PCOS were more likely to suffer from depression [odds ratio (OR): 2.79; 95% confidence interval (CI): 2.23-3.50], anxiety (OR: 2.75; 95% CI: 2.10-3.60), bipolar disorder (OR: 1.78; 95% CI: 1.43-2.23), and obsessive–compulsive disorder (OCD) (OR: 1.37; 95% CI: 1.22–1.55), but not social phobia or panic disorder.[37] Using various scales, the severity of symptoms of depression, anxiety, OCD, and somatization disorders was higher compared to women without PCOS.

Depression

Mood disorders include major depressive disorder (MDD), dysthymic disorder, and depression not otherwise specified based on Diagnostic and Statistical Manual of Mental Disorders, Fifth Edition, Text Revision (DSM-V TR). Daily fatigue, sleep disturbances, and diminished interest are the prominent symptoms in patients with PCOS. Various meta-analyses have found that prevalence of depression in women with PCOS is high, ranging from 28 to 64%.[3-5] Studies found that 14% of women suffering from PCOS reported suicidal ideation.

Cooney et al. in a meta-analysis of 23 studies with rigorous inclusion criteria including physician diagnosis of PCOS[7] showed increased moderate/severe depressive symptoms (OR: 4.18, 95% CI: 2.68-6.52) with a prevalence of depression of 36.6% in PCOS [interquartile range (IQR): 22.3, 50.0%] and 14.2% in controls (IQR: 10.7, 22.2%), independent of obesity and seen in both clinic and community recruits.

Anxiety

The prevalence of anxiety in women with PCOS ranges from 34 to 57%. Fears reported by hirsute women are mainly categorized as "social phobia" or anxiety-evoking situations, such as meeting strangers, attending parties, shopping, and mixing at work. A recent rigorous meta-analysis of 10 studies[6] showed increased moderate/severe anxiety symptoms in PCOS (OR: 5.38; 95% CI: 2.28–12.67), with a prevalence of 41.9% (IQR: 13.6, 52.0%) in PCOS and 8.5% (IQR: 3.3, 12.0%)

in controls. A large population-based study of 24,385 women with PCOS matched for sex, age, and country of birth to 10 controls showed increased anxiety disorder (OR: 1.37, CI: 1.32–1.43).[38]

The cause of depressive and anxiety symptoms in PCOS is not fully elucidated[39] as are the effects of PCOS treatments. While acne, hirsutism, infertility, and increased BMI have been linked to increased mood and distress, the evidence is inconsistent. Further potential contributors to depression and anxiety in PCOS include the chronic complex and frustrating nature of PCOS. Chronic conditions can cause related emotional distress, maladaptive coping skills, and low ego resiliency causing depression and anxiety.

Recent ESHRE guidelines have incorporated the following recommendations for the screening and treatment of depression and anxiety in PCOS:[40]

- Awareness in health professionals about high prevalence of moderate to severe anxiety and depressive symptoms in adults (more in adolescents)
- Routine screening of anxiety and depressive symptoms should be there in all adolescents and women with PCOS at diagnosis and if the screen is positive, health professionals should further assess and/or refer for assessment.
- If treatment is warranted, psychological therapy and/or pharmacological treatment should be offered to women with PCOS, informed by regional clinical practice guidelines.

EATING DISORDERS AND DISORDERED EATING

Eating disorders (ED), such as anorexia nervosa (AN), bulimia nervosa (BN), and binge eating disorder (BED), have high rates of medical complications. The prevalence for any ED diagnosis in women with PCOS ranges from 12 to 36%.[15] Although data of eating disorders in PCOS population is limited, apparently higher prevalence of eating disorders and disordered eating in women with PCOS, and the negative biopsychosocial consequences of it highlight the need to raise awareness of these conditions. EHSRE suggests:

- All health professionals and women should be aware of the increased prevalence of eating disorders and disordered eating associated with PCOS (Grade 2).
- If eating disorders and disordered eating are suspected, further assessment, referral, or treatment including psychological therapy could be offered, informed by regional clinical practice guidelines (Grade 2).

BIPOLAR AND OBSESSIVE–COMPULSIVE DISORDER

There is increased risk of clinical diagnosis of bipolar disorder and OCD in women with PCOS. But these findings are novel in comparison to the well-established increase in depression and anxiety, and very few studies, five on bipolar disorder and three on OCD were done. Further research is needed to bolster these findings and direct suggestions for clinicians are recommended.

CONCLUSION

Polycystic ovary syndrome can involve diverse clinical features that change across the life course. An interdisciplinary care model involves "the collaboration between a woman with PCOS and a care team who have shared goals for total well-being" and is founded on patient-centered care principles and is well suited to the PCOS context. For

models of care, women affected by PCOS may consult multiple health professionals such as:
- General practitioner/primary care physician
- Gynecologist
- Endocrinologist
- Infertility specialist
- Dietitian
- Dermatologist
- Psychologist
- Exercise physiologist.

Multidisciplinary care is increasingly required in chronic disease management, with improvements in health-related outcomes, yet presenting increased complexity, compartmentalization, and communication challenges.
- Provision of culturally appropriate, tailored, and high-quality information and education resources for women with PCOS with a respectful and empathetic approach and promote self-care and highlight peer support groups (Grade 4)
- Providing information and education resources to healthcare professionals about the recommended diagnostic criteria, appropriate screening for comorbidities, and effective lifestyle and pharmacological management (Grade 4)
- Information about polycystic ovarian disease (PCOD) should be comprehensive, evidence-based, and inclusive of the biopsychosocial dimensions of PCOS across the life span (Grade 4).
- Women's needs, communication preferences, beliefs, and culture should be considered and addressed through provision of culturally and linguistically appropriate resources and care according to women's needs, communication preferences, and beliefs (Grade 4).

▪ REFERENCES

1. Rotterdam ESHRE/ASRM-Sponsored PCOS consensus workshop group. Revised 2003 consensus on diagnostic criteria and longterm health risks related to polycystic ovary syndrome (PCOS). Hum Reprod. 2004; 19(1):41-7.
2. Lizneva D, Suturina L, Walker W, Brakta S, Gavrilova-Jordan L, Azziz R. Criteria, prevalence, and phenotypes of polycystic ovary syndrome. Fertil Steril. 2016;106(1):6-15.
3. Dokras A, Clifton S, Futterweit W, Wild R. Increased risk for abnormal depression scores in women with polycystic ovary syndrome: a systematic review and meta-analysis. Obstet Gynecol. 2011;117(1):145-52.
4. Barry JA, Kuczmierczyk AR, Hardiman PJ. Anxiety and depression in polycystic ovary syndrome: a systematic review and meta-analysis. Hum Reprod. 2011;26(9):2442-51.
5. Veltman-Verhulst SM, Boivin J, Eijkemans MJ, Fauser BJ. Emotional distress is a common risk in women with polycystic ovary syndrome: a systematic review and meta-analysis of 28 studies. Hum Reprod Update. 2012;18(6):638-51.
6. Dokras A, Clifton S, Futterweit W, Wild R. Increased prevalence of anxiety symptoms in women with polycystic ovary syndrome: systematic review and meta-analysis. Fertil Steril. 2012;97(1):225-30.e2.
7. Cooney LG, Lee I, Sammel MD, Dokras A. High prevalence of moderate and severe depressive and anxiety symptoms in polycystic ovary syndrome: a systematic review and meta-analysis. Hum Reprod. 2017;32(5):1075-91.
8. Teede HJ, Misso ML, Costello MF, Dokras A, Laven J, Moran L, et al. Recommendations from the international evidence-based guideline for the assessment and management of polycystic ovary syndrome. Hum Reprod. 2018; 33(9):1602-18.
9. Friedman KE, Reichmann SK, Costanzo PR, Musante GJ. Body image partially mediates the relationship between obesity and psychological distress. Obes Res. 2002;10(1):33-41.
10. Dumesic DA, Oberfield SE, Stener-Victorin E, Marshall JC, Laven JS, Legro RS. Scientific Statement on the Diagnostic Criteria,

Epidemiology, Pathophysiology, and Molecular Genetics of Polycystic Ovary Syndrome. Endocr Rev. 2015;36(5):487-525.
11. Dokras A. Cardiovascular disease risk in women with PCOS. Steroids. 2013;78(8): 773-6.
12. Son N. Assessment of body perception, psychological distress, and subjective quality of life among obese and nonobese subjects in Turkey. Niger J Clin Pract. 2017;20(10):1302-8.
13. Weinberger NA, Kersting A, Riedel-Heller SG, Luck-Sikorski C. Body Dissatisfaction in Individuals with Obesity Compared to Normal-Weight Individuals: A Systematic Review and Meta-Analysis. Obes Facts. 2016; 9(6):424-41.
14. Alur-Gupta S, Chemerinski A, Liu C, Lipson J, Allison K, Sammel MD, et al. Body image distress increased in women with polycystic ovary syndrome and mediates depression and anxiety. Fertil Steril. 2019;112(5):930-8. e1.
15. Dokras A, Stener-Victorin E, Yildiz BO, Li R, Ottey S, Shah D, et al. Androgen Excess-Polycystic Ovary Syndrome Society: position statement on depression, anxiety, quality of life, and eating disorders in polycystic ovary syndrome. Fertil Steril. 2018;109(5):888-99.
16. Pastoor H, Timman R, de Klerk C, M Bramer W, Laan ET, Laven JS. Sexual function in women with polycystic ovary syndrome: a systematic review and meta-analysis. Reprod Biomed Online. 2018; 37(6):750-60.
17. Cronin L, Guyatt G, Griffith L, Wong E, Azziz R, Futterweit W, et al. Development of a health-related quality-of-life questionnaire (PCOSQ) for women with polycystic ovary syndrome (PCOS). J Clin Endocrinol Metab. 1998;83(6):1976-87.
18. Barnard L, Ferriday D, Guenther N, Strauss B, Balen AH, Dye L. Quality of life and psychological well-being in polycystic ovary syndrome. Hum Reprod. 2007;22(8):2279-86.
19. Bazarganipour F, Taghavi SA, Montazeri A, Ahmadi F, Chaman R, Khosravi A. The impact of polycystic ovary syndrome on the health-related quality of life: A systematic review and meta-analysis. Iran J Reprod Med. 2015;13(2):61-70.
20. Benson S, Hahn S, Tan S, Mann K, Janssen OE, Schedlowski M, et al. Prevalence and implications of anxiety in polycystic ovary syndrome: Results of an internet-based survey in Germany. Hum Reprod. 2009; 24(6):1446-51.
21. Emeksiz HC, Bideci A, Nalbantoğlu, B.; Nalbantoğlu A, Çelik C, Yulaf Y, et al. Anxiety and depression states of adolescents with polycystic ovary syndrome. Turk J Med Sci. 2018;48(3):531-6.
22. Fatemeh B, Shahideh JS, Negin M. Health related quality of life and psychological parameters in different polycystic ovary syndrome phenotypes: a comparative cross-sectional study. J Ovarian Res. 2021;14(1):57.
23. Farrell K, Antoni MH. Insulin resistance, obesity, inflammation, and depression in polycystic ovary syndrome: biobehavioral mechanisms and interventions. Fertil Steril. 2010;94(5);1565-74.
24. Damone AL, Joham AE, Loxton D, Earnest A, Teede HJ, Moran LJ. Depression, anxiety and perceived stress in women with and without PCOS: a community-based study. Psychol Med. 2019;49(9):1510-20.
25. Light RS, Chilcot J, McBride E. Psychological Distress in Women Living with Polycystic Ovary Syndrome: The Role of Illness Perceptions. Womens Health Issues. 2021; 31(2):177-84.
26. Kumarapeli V, Seneviratne R, Wijeyaratne C. Health-related quality of life and psychological distress in polycystic ovary syndrome: a hidden facet in South Asian women. BJOG. 2011;118(3):319-28.
27. Benson S, Hahn S, Tan S, Janssen OE, Schedlowski M, Elsenbruch S. Maladaptive coping with illness in women with polycystic ovary syndrome. J Obstet Gynecol Neonatal Nurs. 2010;39(1):37-45.
28. Simon W. [Motivational factors and the psychotherapeutic change]. Psychiatr Pol. 2008;42:335-52.
29. Hahn S, Janssen OE, Tan S, Pleger K, Mann K, Schedlowski M, et al. Clinical and psychological correlates of quality-of-life in polycystic ovary syndrome. Eur J Endocrinol. 2005;153(6):853-60.

30. Ogińska-Bulik, N.; Zadworna-Cieślak, M. The role of mental toughness in coping with exam-related stress graduation. Education Research Review. 2015;2, 7.
31. Folkman S, Lazarus RS. The relationship between coping and emotion: implications for theory and research. Soc Sci Med.1988; 26(3);309-17.
32. Lechner L, Bolman C, van Dalen A. Definite involuntary childlessness: associations between coping, social support and psychological distress. Hum Reprod. 2007;22(1): 288-94.
33. Sigmon ST, Whitcomb-Smith SR, Rohan KJ, Kendrew JJ. The role of anxiety level, coping styles, and cycle phase in menstrual distress. J Anxiety Disord. 2004;18(2):177-91.
34. Carron R, Kooienga S, Boyle DK, Alvero R. Coping in Women With Polycystic Ovary Syndrome: Implications for Practitioners. J Nurse Pract. 2017;13:700-7.
35. Basirat Z, Faramarzi M, Chehrazi M, Amiri M, Ghofrani F, Tajalli Z. Differences between infertile women with and without PCOS in terms of anxiety, coping styles, personality traits, and social adjustment: a case–control study. Arch Gynecol Obstet. 2020;301(2): 619-26.
36. Kolahi L, Asemi N, Mirzaei M, Adibi N, Beiraghdar M, Mehr A. The relationship between quality of life and coping strategies in polycystic ovary syndrome patients. Adv Biomed Res. 2015;4:168
37. Brutocao C, Zaiem F, Alsawas M, Morrow AS, Murad MH, Javed A. Psychiatric disorders in women with polycystic ovary syndrome: a systematic review and meta-analysis. Endocrine. 2018;62(2):318-25.
38. Cesta CE, Månsson M, Palm C, Lichtenstein P, Iliadou AN, Landén M. Polycystic ovary syndrome and psychiatric disorders: Co-morbidity and heritability in a nationwide Swedish cohort. Psychoneuroendocrinology. 2016;73:196-203.
39. Hart R, Doherty DA. The potential implications of a PCOS diagnosis on a woman's long-term health using data linkage. J Clin Endocrinol Metab. 2015;100(3):911-9.
40. Monash University, Melbourne. (2018). International evidence-based guidelines for the assessment and management of polycystic ovary syndrome. [online] Available from: https://www.monash.edu/__data/assets/pdf_file/0004/1412644/PCOS_Evidence-Based-Guidelines_20181009.pdf [Last accessed November, 2022].

CHAPTER 11

Sleep Apnea and PCOS

Anand Srivastava, Parul Sinha

INTRODUCTION

Polycystic ovary syndrome (PCOS) is the most common endocrine disorder in premenopausal women and it affects approximately 5–8% of women.[1] Women with PCOS are at an increased risk for certain metabolic[2,3] and cardiovascular[4-6] disorders. Obstructive sleep apnea (OSA) is a newly identified and potentially very important disease that adds to this list of health risks. It is present at higher levels in PCOS women than in age- and weight-matched healthy women.[7] OSA was independently associated with adverse cardiovascular and metabolic outcomes in women without PCOS.[8,9]

Obstructive sleep apnea syndrome (OSAS) is characterized by recurrent complete (i.e., apnea) or partial (i.e., hypopnea) upper airway obstruction causing intermittent hypoxia, fragmented sleep, and poor sleep quality. Although snoring, witnessed apneas, daytime sleepiness, and cognitive impairment are common, women with OSA are more likely to present with insomnia, fatigue, or mood disturbances than snoring or daytime sleepiness.

PREVALENCE OF OBSTRUCTIVE SLEEP APNEA IN POLYCYSTIC OVARY SYNDROME

- The prevalence of OSA in the general adult population is approximately 17%.[10]
- The prevalence of OSA is low in premenopausal women and increases after menopause,[10-12] but is significantly more common than expected in women with PCOS.[13-15]
- OSA is estimated to be present, on an average, about 40%, in women with PCOS (reviewed in the study by Kahal et al.[16]).
- In a recent meta-analysis of 12 clinical studies that used polysomnography, it was seen that adult women with PCOS were found to be 9.7 times more likely to develop OSAS than women of similar age.[17]
- This association was not observed in adolescent girls, suggesting that increasing age may be an important determinant of OSA in PCOS.
- PCOS and OSAS[18] may be associated with other sleep disorders, such as difficulty initiating and maintaining sleep or insomnia.[19-21]
- A study was conducted on 40 women with PCOS to assess the frequency distribution of the risk for sleep apnea (derived from responses to the Berlin questionnaire) and sleep complaints derived from responses to the Pittsburgh Sleep Quality (PSQ) questionnaire and Epworth Sleepiness Scale (ESS). A single sleep complaint was defined as a PSQ index >5 or an ESS score of ≥10 **(Fig. 1)**.[22]

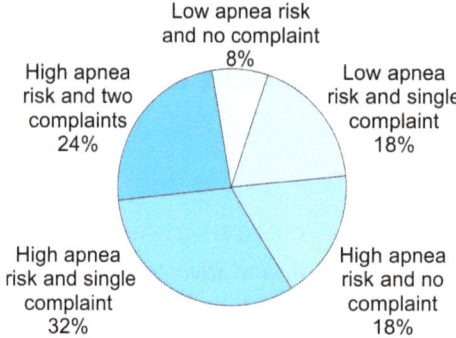

Fig. 1: Prevalence of obstructive sleep apnea in polycystic ovary syndrome.

OBSTRUCTIVE SLEEP APNEA PATHOPHYSIOLOGY IN POLYCYSTIC OVARY SYNDROME

Role of Sex Steroids in Causing OSA in PCOS

- Circulating sex steroids, i.e., estrogens, progestins, and androgens, may be responsible for the gender disparity in normal sleep architecture[23] as well as in the prevalence and severity of OSA.
- Androgens are thought to be "harmful" while estrogens and progestins are considered "protective" against the development of OSA.
- It has been shown by various studies that testosterone administration has an adverse effect on breathing during sleep and predisposes to OSA by influencing both the neural control of breathing[24] and upper airway mechanics.[25]
- A study by Zhou et al.[26] concluded that testosterone increases the apneic threshold in premenopausal women which facilitates central apnea leading to breathing instability during sleep.
- Therefore, androgen excess present in PCOS contributes to the higher prevalence of OSA in this disorder.

Role of Obesity in Causing OSA in PCOS

- High prevalence of OSA in PCOS is not only due to the elevated body mass index (BMI) but it also depends more on the degree of visceral adiposity as the visceral fat is metabolically more active.
- Women with PCOS have a high prevalence of visceral adiposity, as is evidenced by higher waist-to-hip circumferences than women without PCOS with matched BMI.
- The plausible reason for this is that high levels of androgen promote central obesity, which in turn leads to OSA.[16]

OSA in PCOS and its Effect on Insulin Resistance and Glucose Intolerance

- Recent studies have reported an association between the presence of OSA and fasting blood glucose[27] or insulin resistance in women with PCOS according to Homeostatic Model Assessment (HOMA) Index,[28] after statistical adjustments for BMI.
- Insulin resistance, as measured by HOMA index, was higher in adolescent PCOS girls with OSA than without OSA.[29]
- The risk and severity of OSA (respiratory events and hypoxia) is strongly correlated with insulin levels and measures of glucose tolerance.
- The presence and severity of OSA was found to predict insulin resistance and glucose intolerance in nondiabetic women with PCOS, after controlling for age, BMI, and ethnicity.[30]
- There may be potential mechanisms by which OSA may worsen metabolic outcomes, as explained in **Flowchart 1**, but further research is needed.
- Treatment of OSAS with continuous positive airway pressure (CPAP) in young and morbidly obese PCOS women

Flowchart 1: Potential mechanisms linking obstructive sleep apnea (OSA) to adverse metabolic consequences.

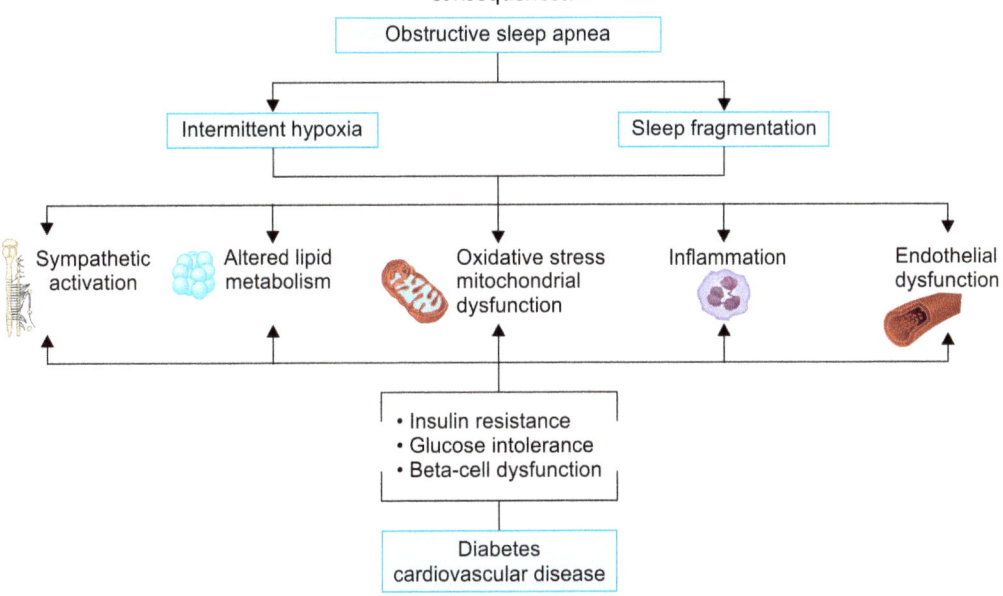

improves their metabolic and cardiovascular outcomes.[31]
- The beneficial effects were greater with longer hours of CPAP use and were less in those with higher levels of obesity.

DIAGNOSIS AND MANAGEMENT OF OBSTRUCTIVE SLEEP APNEA

Diagnostic Assessment

- Obstructive sleep apnea is not a clinical diagnosis and requires objective tests to make a diagnosis.
- Diagnostic testing of OSA should be performed on patients with excessive daytime sleepiness (EDS) on most of the days and those who have at least two of the following clinical features of OSA: habitual loud snoring, witnessed apnea, gasping or choking during sleep, and diagnosed systemic hypertension.[32]
- Most sleep specialists do not routinely use assessment tools because the history and physical examination are considered to be superior.
- But the most commonly used tools are the STOP-Bang questionnaire or its variants and the ESS **(Tables 1 and 2; Box 1)**.
- The STOP-Bang questionnaire is commonly used by physicians during

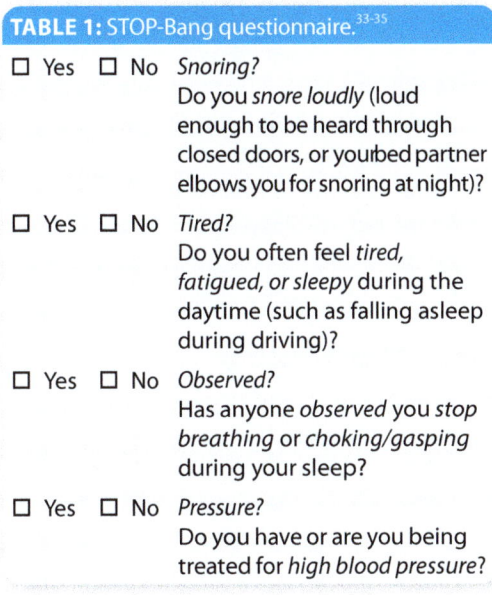

TABLE 1: STOP-Bang questionnaire.[33-35]

☐ Yes ☐ No	*Snoring?* Do you *snore loudly* (loud enough to be heard through closed doors, or your bed partner elbows you for snoring at night)?
☐ Yes ☐ No	*Tired?* Do you often feel *tired, fatigued, or sleepy* during the daytime (such as falling asleep during driving)?
☐ Yes ☐ No	*Observed?* Has anyone *observed* you *stop breathing* or *choking/gasping* during your sleep?
☐ Yes ☐ No	*Pressure?* Do you have or are you being treated for *high blood pressure*?

Contd...

Contd...

☐ Yes ☐ No Body mass index more than 35 kg/m²?
☐ Yes ☐ No Age older than 50 years old?
☐ Yes ☐ No • Neck size large (measured around Adam's apple)?
              • Is your shirt collar 16 inches or larger?
☐ Yes ☐ No Gender (biologic sex) = Male?

Scoring criteria:
- Low risk of OSA: Yes to 0–2 questions
- Intermediate risk of OSA: Yes to 3–4 questions
- High risk of OSA: Yes to 5–8 questions

(OSA: obstructive sleep apnea)

TABLE 2: Enhanced STOP-Bang interpretation.

Risk category	Risk factors
Low risk	Yes to 0–2 of the questions
Intermediate risk	Yes to 3–4 of the questions
High risk	Yes to 5–8 of the questions
High risk	Yes to 2 or more of 4 STOP questions and body mass index (BMI) >35 kg/m²
High risk	Yes to 2 or more of 4 STOP questions and neck circumference ≥16 inches (≥40 cm)
High risk	Yes to 2 or more of 4 STOP questions and male gender (biologic sex)

preoperative evaluation to assess the risk of undiagnosed OSA.
- Other evaluation tools include the Berlin Score and the Sleep Apnea Clinical Score, but none of these diagnostic tools should be used to replace a sleep apnea testing.

Sleep Apnea Testing

- In-laboratory polysomnography [PSG; either full-night (i.e., diagnostic only) or split-night (i.e., diagnostic and therapeutic with positive airway pressure)] is the gold standard diagnostic test.
- In patients in whom uncomplicated OSA is suspected and the pretest probability

BOX 1: Epworth sleepiness scale (ESS): Key questions in evaluating the tired patient.

Key questions in the evaluation of a patient who complains of sleepiness, tiredness, fatigue, or low energy

Questions about sleepiness:
- Do you feel sleepy during the day?
- Is daytime sleepiness a problem for you?
- Is it difficult to keep your eyes open at times during the day?
- Do you struggle to stay awake during the day?
- Do you take naps?
- How often and how long do you nap during the day?
- Do you fall asleep at times you do not want to (i.e., watching a movie, reading a book, or on long drives)?

Questions about tiredness, fatigue, and low energy:
- Do you lack the energy to go about your daily activities?
- Do you tire easily, or sooner than others, when you are active?
- Do you feel physically or mentally exhausted?

Questions to differentiate sleepiness from related complaints:
- Does your problem bother you more if you sit to read for an hour, or if you go out shopping for an hour?
- Which of the following is the single most important problem for you: Sleepiness, tiredness, fatigue, or lack of energy?
- Which of the following most interferes with your ability to accomplish what you would like to: sleepiness, tiredness, fatigue, or lack of energy?
- Which of the following is the one problem you would most like to address effectively: sleepiness, tiredness, fatigue, or lack of energy?

Sources: Adapted from Bodkin CL, Manchanda S. Office evaluation of the "tired" or "sleepy" patient. Semin Neurol. 2011;31:42; Chervin RD. Sleepiness, fatigue, tiredness, and lack of energy in obstructive sleep apnea. Chest. 2000;118:372.

is estimated as moderate or severe, unattended home sleep apnea testing (HSAT) with a type 3 device is a reasonable alternative to in-laboratory PSG.
- Several factors influence the choice between home and in-laboratory testing as depicted in **Flowchart 2**.

Flowchart 2: Algorithm for sleep apnea testing.

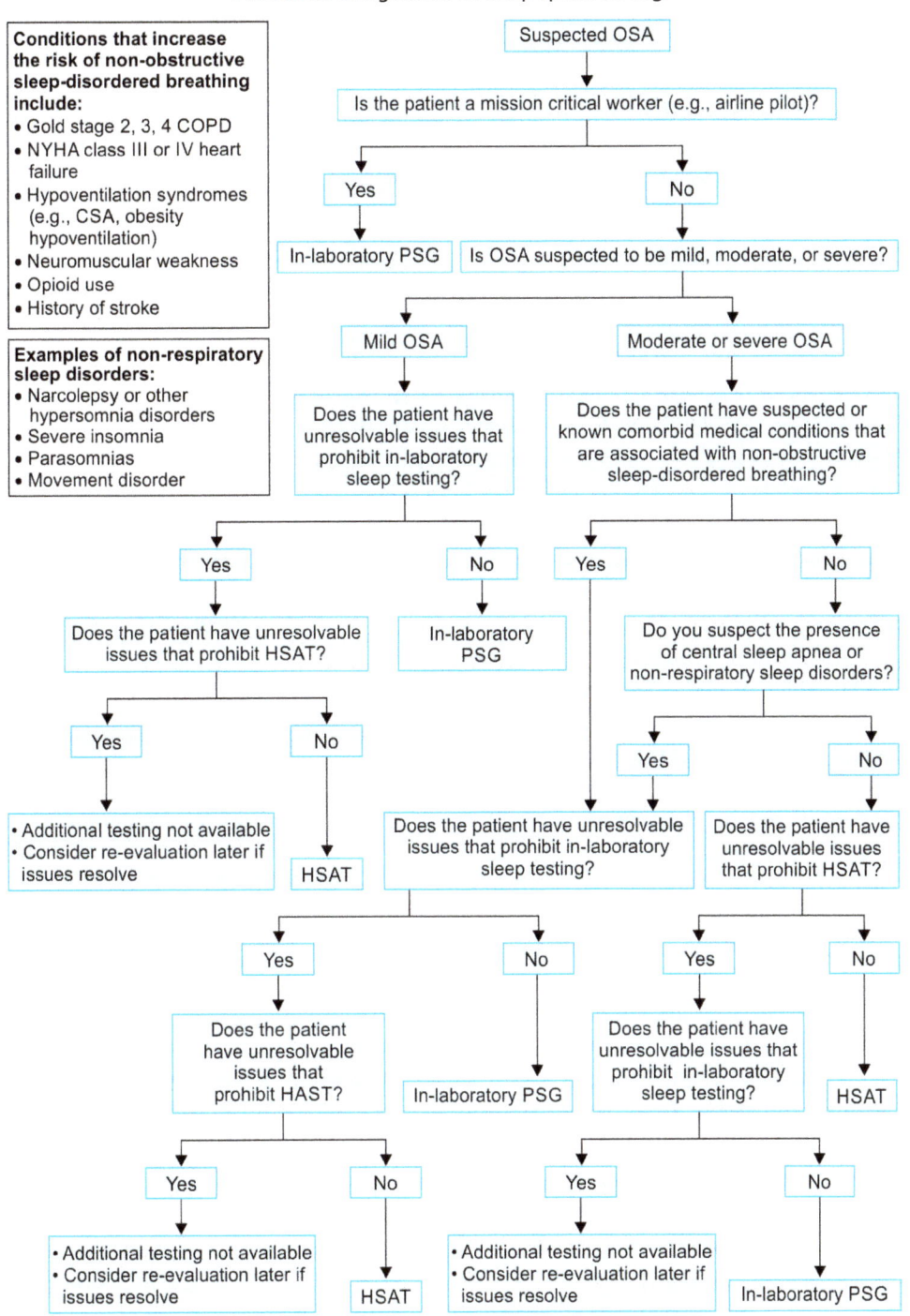

(COPD: chronic obstructive pulmonary disease; NYHA: New York Heart Association; OSA: obstructive sleep apnea; HSAT: home sleep apnea testing; PSG: polysomnography)

BOX 2: Clinical guidelines/recommendations for obstructive sleep apnea (OSA) screening for women with polycystic ovary syndrome (PCOS) (Endocrine Society, 2013).

- Screening overweight/obese adolescents and women with PCOS for symptoms suggestive of OSA and, when identified, obtaining a definitive diagnosis using polysomnography. If OSA is diagnosed, patients should be referred for institution of appropriate treatment
- It seems wise at this moment to screen sleep disorders by clinical questionnaires in obese women with PCOS. In the case of clinical suspicion resulting from these questionnaires, patients should be referred to a center of sleep disorders for polysomnography and further evaluation

BOX 3: International evidence-based guideline for the assessment and management of polycystic ovary syndrome (PCOS) 2018.

- Screening should only be considered for obstructive sleep apnea (OSA) in PCOS to identify and alleviate related symptoms, such as snoring, waking unrefreshed from sleep, daytime sleepiness, and the potential for fatigue to contribute to mood disorders. Screening should not be considered with the intention of improving cardiometabolic risk, with inadequate evidence for metabolic benefits of OSA treatment in PCOS and in general populations
- A simple screening questionnaire, preferably the Berlin tool, could be applied and if positive, referral to a specialist is considered
- A positive screen raises the likelihood of OSA; however, it does not quantify symptom burden and alone does not justify treatment. If women with PCOS have OSA symptoms and a positive screen, consideration can be given to be referral to a specialist center for further evaluation

CONCLUSION

- Polycystic ovary syndrome is one of the most common endocrine disorders affecting women.
- Recent evidence suggests that sleep disturbances appear to be an important feature in PCOS and that OSAS is significantly more common than anticipated in women with PCOS.
- However, the high prevalence of OSA is not well documented by clinicians managing PCOS patients.
- The androgen excess, subnormal estrogen levels, and visceral fat appear to be associated with an increased risk of OSA in PCOS, and there may be a strong association between OSA severity, glucose intolerance, and insulin resistance.
- Various questionnaires are available to screen for this entity, but the final diagnosis is made by sleep apnea testing.

REFERENCES

1. Knochenhauer ES, Key TJ, Kahsar-Miller M, Wagonner W, Boots LR, Azziz R. Prevalence of polycystic ovary syndrome in unselected black and white women of the southeastern United States: a prospective study. J Clin Endocrinol Metab. 1998;83(9):3078-82.
2. Ehrmann DA, Barnes RB, Rosenfield RL. Polycystic ovary syndrome as a form of functional ovarian hyperandrogenism due to dysregulation of androgen secretion. Endocr Rev. 1995;16(3):322-53.
3. Dunaif A, Segal KR, Futterweit W, Dobrjansky A. Profound peripheral insulin resistance, independent of obesity, in polycystic ovary syndrome. Diabetes. 1989;38(9):1165-74.
4. Talbott E, Guzick D, Clerici A, Berga S, Detre K, Weimer K, et al. Coronary heart disease risk factors in women with polycystic ovary syndrome. Arterioscler Thromb Vasc Biol. 1995;15(7):821-6.
5. Talbott E, Clerici A, Berga SL, Kuller L, Guzick D, Detre K, et al. Adverse lipid and coronary heart disease risk profiles in young women with polycystic ovary syndrome: results of a case-control study. J Clin Epidemiol. 1998; 51(5):415-22.
6. Talbott EO, Guzick DS, Sutton-Tyrrell K, McHugh-Pemu KP, Zborowski JV, Remsberg

KE, et al. Evidence for association between polycystic ovary syndrome and premature carotid atherosclerosis in middle-aged women. Arterioscler Thromb Vasc Biol. 2000; 20(11):2414-21.
7. Fogel RB, Malhotra A, Pillar G, Pittman SD, Dunaif A, White DP. Increased prevalence of obstructive sleep apnea syndrome in obese women with polycystic ovary syndrome. J Clin Endocrinol Metab. 2001;86(3):1175-80.
8. Punjabi NM, Polotsky VY. Disorders of glucose metabolism in sleep apnea. J Appl Physiol (1985). 2005;99(5):1998-2007.
9. Wolk R, Somers VK. Sleep and the metabolic syndrome. Exp Physiol. 2007;92(1):67-78.
10. Bixler EO, Vgontzas AN, Lin HM, Ten Have T, Rein J, Vela-Bueno A, et al. Prevalence of sleep-disordered breathing in women: effects of gender. Am J Respir Crit Care Med. 2001;163(3 Pt 1):608-13.
11. Shahar E, Redline S, Young T, Boland LL, Baldwin CM, Nieto FJ, et al. Hormone replacement therapy and sleep-disordered breathing. Am J Respir Crit Care Med. 2003; 167(9):1186-92.
12. Young T, Finn L, Austin D, Peterson A. Menopausal status and sleep-disordered breathing in the Wisconsin Sleep Cohort Study. Am J Respir Crit Care Med. 2003; 167(9):1181-5.
13. Ehrmann DA. Polycystic ovary syndrome. N Engl J Med. 2005;352(12):1223-36.
14. Vgontzas AN, Legro RS, Bixler EO, Grayev A, Kales A, Chrousos GP. Polycystic ovary syndrome is associated with obstructive sleep apnea and daytime sleepiness: role of insulin resistance. J Clin Endocrinol Metab. 2001;86(2):517-20.
15. Gopal M, Duntley S, Uhles M, Attarian H. The role of obesity in the increased prevalence of obstructive sleep apnea syndrome in patients with polycystic ovarian syndrome. Sleep Med. 2002;3(5):401-4.
16. Kahal H, Kyrou I, Tahrani AA, Randeva HS. Obstructive sleep apnoea and polycystic ovary syndrome: A comprehensive review of clinical interactions and underlying pathophysiology. Clin Endocrinol (Oxf). 2017;87(4):313-19.
17. Helvaci N, Karabulut E, Demir AU, Yildiz BO: Polycystic ovary syndrome and the risk of obstructive sleep apnea: a meta-analysis and review of the literature. Endocr Connect. 2017;6(7):437-45.
18. Kumarendran B, Sumilo D, O'Reilly MW, Toulis KA, Gokhale KM, Wijeyaratne CN, et al. Increased risk of obstructive sleep apnoea in women with polycystic ovary syndrome: a population-based cohort study. Eur J Endocrinol. 2019;180(4):265-72.
19. Hung JH, Hu LY, Tsai SJ, Yang AC, Huang MW, Chen PM, et al. Risk of psychiatric disorders following polycystic ovary syndrome: a nationwide population-based cohort study. PLoS One. 2014;9(5):e97041.
20. Moran LJ, March WA, Whitrow MJ, Giles LC, Davies MJ, Moore VM. Sleep disturbances in a community-based sample of women with polycystic ovary syndrome. Hum Reprod. 2015;30(2):466-72.
21. Mo L, Mansfield DR, Joham A, Cain SW, Bennett C, Blumfield M, et al. Sleep disturbances in women with and without polycystic ovary syndrome in an Australian National Cohort. Clin Endocrinol (Oxf). 2019;90(4):570-8.
22. Tasali E, Van Cauter E, Ehrmann DA. Relationships between sleep disordered breathing and glucose metabolism in the polycystic ovary syndrome. J Clin Endocrinol Metab. 2006;91(1):36-42
23. Driver HS, Dijk DJ, Werth E, Biedermann K, Borbély AA. Sleep and the sleep electroencephalogram across the menstrual cycle in young healthy women. J Clin Endocrinol Metab. 1996;81(2):728-35.
24. White DP, Schneider BK, Santen RJ, McDermott M, Pickett CK, Zwillich CW, et al. Influence of testosterone on ventilation and chemosensitivity in male subjects. J Appl Physiol (1985). 1985;59(5):1452-7.
25. Cistulli PA, Grunstein RR, Sullivan CE. Effect of testosterone administration on upper airway collapsibility during sleep. Am J Respir Crit Care Med. 1994;149(2 Pt 1):530-2.
26. Zhou XS, Rowley JA, Demirovic F, Diamond MP, Badr MS. Effect of testosterone on the

apneic threshold in women during NREM sleep. J Appl Physiol (1985). 2003;94(1):101-7.
27. Chatterjee B, Suri J, Suri JC, Mittal P, Adhikari T. Impact of sleep-disordered breathing on metabolic dysfunctions in patients with polycystic ovary syndrome. Sleep Med. 2014;15(12):1547-53.
28. Tock L, Carneiro G, Togeiro SM, Hachul H, Pereira AZ, Tufik S, et al. Obstructive sleep apnea predisposes to nonalcoholic Fatty liver disease in patients with polycystic ovary syndrome. Endocr Pract. 2014;20(3):244-51.
29. Nandalike K, Agarwal C, Strauss T, Coupey SM, Isasi CR, Sin S, et al. Sleep and cardiometabolic function in obese adolescent girls with polycystic ovary syndrome. Sleep Med. 2012;13(10):1307-12.
30. Tasali E, Van Cauter E, Hoffman L, Ehrmann DA: Impact of obstructive sleep apnea on insulin resistance and glucose tolerance in women with polycystic ovary syndrome. J Clin Endocrinol Metab. 2008;93(10):3878-84.
31. Tasali E, Chapotot F, Leproult R, Whitmore H, Ehrmann DA: Treatment of obstructive sleep apnea improves cardiometabolic function in young obese women with polycystic ovary syndrome. J Clin Endocrinol Metab. 2011; 96(2):365-74.
32. Kapur VK, Auckley DH, Chowdhuri S, Kuhlmann DC, Mehra R, Ramar K, et al. Clinical Practice Guideline for Diagnostic Testing for Adult Obstructive Sleep Apnea: An American Academy of Sleep Medicine Clinical Practice Guideline. J Clin Sleep Med. 2017;13(3):479-504.
33. Chung F, Yegneswaran B, Liao P, Chung SA, Vairavanathan S, Islam S, et al. STOP questionnaire: a tool to screen patients for obstructive sleep apnea. Anesthesiology. 2008;108(5): 812-21.
34. Chung F, Subramanyam R, Liao P, Sasaki E, Shapiro C, Sun Y. High STOP-Bang score indicates a high probability of obstructive sleep apnoea. Br J Anaesth. 2012;108(5): 768-75.
35. Chung F, Yang Y, Brown R, Liao P. Alternative scoring models of STOP-bang questionnaire improve specificity to detect undiagnosed obstructive sleep apnea. J Clin Sleep Med. 2014;10(9):951-8.

CHAPTER 12

Role of Micronutrients in PCOS

Priti Kumar, Sangeeta Rai

■ INTRODUCTION

Polycystic ovary syndrome (PCOS) is one of the most common endocrine and metabolic disorders in the females of reproductive age.[1] Its prevalence is approximately in the range of 4–21% throughout the world.[2] PCOS increases the risk factor for the development of metabolic syndrome affecting a woman all throughout her life.[1] These women present with irregular menses, chronic oligo-/anovulation, and hyperandrogenism, along with other metabolic features of obesity, insulin resistance, hyperinsulinemia, dyslipidemia, type 2 diabetes, inflammation, and oxidative stress. It also increases the long-term risk for the development of endometrial cancer and cardiovascular diseases.[1] Till date the exact cause of PCOS is unknown, but many studies have shown the association of genetic factor and unhealthy lifestyle and environment in the pathogenesis of PCOS.[3]

There is an essential role of minerals in female reproductive function. Minerals can be associated with ovulation, metabolism, and hormone management. There are over 60 minerals in varying amounts in the human cells. Each of them plays an important role in various processes in the human body.[4] Minerals are components of enzymes or coenzymes that control a wide range of energetic and metabolic reactions and act as compounds or coordinators of specific cellular functions in major body tissues.[5] So far, most studies on minerals and reproductive function, especially reproductive hormones, have been based on concentrations of minerals in human serum[6-8] or in animal models.[6,9]

There are only individual studies devoted to studying the composition of macro- and microelements in women with PCOS. Many authors observe higher levels of Cu, Zn,[10] Ca, and Mn[5] in women with PCOS.

■ MICRONUTRIENTS

Selenium

Selenium (Se) is one of the indispensable minerals bestowed by antioxidant properties, which acts against the free oxygen radicals in reactive oxygen species (ROS).[11] It is a trace element, which is functional as an integral part of *selenoproteins*, ultimately helping in redox processes as an efficient antioxidant.[12] Not only this, Se has also got *insulin-like properties* (it acts as an insulin-like agent), antihyperlipidemic effect [i.e., Se helps out in lowering bad cholesterol (low-density lipoprotein, LDL) and very-low-density lipoprotein (VLDL)] and has got protective role against insulin resistance.[12]

There is a possibility that via Se supplementation, diabetes can be prevented, since it has been found that Se increases the gene expression in beta cells of the pancreas while downregulating cyclooxygenase-2 (COX-2) and P-selectin expression.[13] Studies have also shown that high consumption of Se leads to decreased risk of oxidative stress and inflammation-induced diseases by alterations in the lipid metabolism.[11]

In PCOS patients, the serum level of Se is found to be lower than the normal patients.[11] There are certain studies which point toward the improvement in the insulin metabolism, triglycerides, and VLDL in patients of PCOS taking Se.[11] Se may have stimulatory effect on the insulin signaling pathway leading to diminished insulin resistance.[13] PCOS patients are most prone to developing lipid abnormality (dyslipidemia) because of insulin resistance and hyperandrogenism.[13] Beneficial effects of Se have been reported on dyslipidemia, but still a lot needs to be done to search the protective effects of Se on lipid profile.[13]

Polycystic ovary syndrome patients show features of insulin resistance, which in turn results into hyperinsulinemia, ultimately leading to higher androgen production and hence increased luteinizing hormone/follicle stimulating hormone (LH/FSH) ratio.[13,14] These conditions have certain phenotypic manifestations in PCOS patients like acne, hirsutism, etc.[11] It has been reported that Se supplementation leads to decreased acne and hirsutism in such patients; not only this, it also leads to higher pregnancy rates in them.[13]

There are promising results of Se supplementation on body mass index (BMI). It is believed to decrease the BMI and weight of the patients with PCOS and this occurs by affecting the concentration of insulin, which in turn results in the reduction of insulin-like growth factors (IGFs) and their binding proteins.[13] This is of significance since, obesity is considered as a great risk factor for PCOS. Also, obesity is believed to aggravate the severity of PCOS.[13]

Proinflammatory cytokines and markers of oxidative stress are found to be elevated in PCOS patients.[13,14] Also, these patients possess lower *total antioxidant capacity* (TAC) as compared to the normal individuals.[13,15] Se supplementation in PCOS patients has been found to have a significant role in the improvement in plasma malondialdehyde There is a thin line of difference between Se deficiency and toxicity; therefore, it is recommended to have an optimal dose of Se (to mitigate the complications induced in PCOS).[13]

Overall, it can be said that Se is nutritionally essential for humans because it has got vital roles in multiple dimensions such as reproduction, protection from oxidative damage and infection, and DNA synthesis.[16] Besides, Se has been reported to reduce thyroid antibody levels.[16]

Carotenoids

Carotenoids have got a significant role in the improvement of oxidative stress.[2] Besides, studies have shown the improving effects of carotenoids on insulin resistance.[2]

Chromium

Chromium (Cr) is an essential trace element in glucose and insulin homeostasis.[17] It intensifies the insulin effect. Hence, it has got a crucial role in glucose and lipid metabolism.[3] It also improves insulin sensitivity.[7] In PCOS patients, Cr supplementation has been reported to have beneficial impacts on glycemic control, in improvement of cardiovascular diseases and oxidative stress state.[18] Because of its ability to improve insulin sensitivity, Cr can be of great usage for the improvement of PCOS symptoms in adult patients.[19]

Chromium [especially chromium picolinate (CrPic)] is a safe and highly tolerable trace element provided by dietary intake and supplementation.[14,16] CrPic has been reported to be the widely prescribed supplement for proper insulin activity and function.[18] Also, CrPic consists of a trivalent Cr, a trace element combined with picolinic acid to improve its gut absorption.[13] In PCOS patients, it has been found that Cr has potential effects on the body composition, involving reduction in the fat mass and also causing increment in the lean body mass.[16] Hence, beneficial effect of Cr supplementation on BMI (kg/m^2) has been reported in PCOS women.[15]

In a meta-analysis, it has been found that Cr supplementation is associated with decrement in the serum insulin and free testosterone levels, along with improvement in the body weight of PCOS patients.[16]

There is a variegated influence of Cr supplementation. Cr supplementation resulted in the reduction of serum high sensitivity-C-reactive proteins [(hs-CRP); the reduction in the level of hs-CRP signifies lowered inflammation]. It also resulted in the upregulation in the gene expression of peroxisome proliferator-activated receptor gamma (PPAR-γ), glucose transporter 1 (GLUT-1), LDL receptor (LDL-R) and down-regulated the gene expression of interleukin-1 (IL-1). PPAR-γ is the central regulator of insulin, glucose and lipid metabolism, which is widely expressed in the adipose tissue.

When it comes to PCOS in adolescents, Cr supplementation has been observed to show promising results.[13] No side effects were found following Cr consumption in PCOS women.[15] Because of these facts, this mode of treatment sounds very promising in near future.

It reduces triglyceride levels in humans and in rats, it leads to an increment in high-density lipoprotein (HDL) and reduction in the level of LDL, along with improved platelet hyperaggregability.[16]

After the course of Cr treatment/supplementation, there are certain positive effects reported in PCOS patients:
- Decrease in the ovarian volume
- Significant reduction in the number of follicles between 2 and 9 mm
- Decrement in the level of free testosterone.[18]

Certain reviews and research papers suggest that an optimum dose of CrPic, i.e., a daily dose of 1,000 µg of CrPic in adolescent girls with PCOS for a tenure of 6 months, has shown a significant improvement in the regular menstrual cyclicity, along with the decrease in number of ovarian follicles between 2 and 9 mm as well as decrease in the level of free testosterone.[19]

Zinc

Zinc (Zn) is one of the basic components of superoxide dismutase enzyme and a cofactor for antioxidative enzymes.[9] It plays an important role in glucose and hormone metabolism. It has a significant role in reducing insulin resistance and inflammatory markers.[9] It has been reported that the concentration of Zn in insulin-resistant PCOS women was found to be lower than the healthier ones.[10] Zn has a role in the development of PCOS and its long-term metabolic complications through its involvement in glucose metabolism, synthesis, secretion, and signaling of insulin.[17] Zn is a stabilizer of the insulin complex in beta-cell secretory granules.[18] Many studies have shown that women with PCOS have low levels of Zn compared to healthy people. It is unclear whether this is caused by improper intake or absorption, increased excretion, or the need for Zn.[19,20] It is also observed that in the case of Zn deficiency, insulin is less stable and degrades faster.[18] The reference range of Zn in red blood cells is 8–14.5 (μg/g). Several human studies have shown that Zn supplementation lowers total cholesterol, LDL, and triglycerides and increases HDL levels.[21-23] A randomized controlled trial (RCT) in 2015 found that zinc sulfate supplementation of 220 mg daily over 8-week period improved both insulin and glucose markers in women with PCOS. Rich sources are pumpkin seeds, tofu, lentils, chickpeas, spinach, and yoghurt.

Vitamin D

Vitamin D is a secosteroid hormone with similar activity to that of progesterone.[11] It is not active until it is converted into 1,25-dihydroxy (OH) vitamin D in the proximal convoluted tubule (PCT) region of the nephrons. It is a two-step process: firstly it is converted to 25-OH vitamin D in the liver with the help of 25-hydroxylase and then to 1,25-OH vitamin D in the PCT, in the presence of alpha-1-hydroxylase.

Metformin is an oral hypoglycemic drug with its established role in the regulation of menstrual cycle irregularity in PCOS patients deficient/insufficient in vitamin D. It has been found that supplementation with calcium and vitamin D has got a supporting effect along with metformin in PCOS.[9,10] Besides, vitamin D supplementation has been reported to reduce insulin resistance and hyperandrogenism in PCOS patients.[6] Hence, vitamin D-level supplementation helps in control of symptoms in PCOS patients.

Vitamin D indeed has myriad of roles to play, one of which is attenuation of the harmful effects of advanced glycation end products (AGEs) in PCOS women and it does so by enhancing androgen synthesis and via improvisation in the abnormal folliculogenesis.[19]

A number of studies have shown that vitamin D metabolism not only affects glucose and insulin metabolism, but also plays a pivotal role in the improvement of type 2 diabetes mellitus.[2]

The exact cause of PCOS is still unknown, but micro- and macroelements have been shown to be important in the pathogenesis and metabolism of PCOS. Abnormal mineral content may serve as an indicator of illness.[6,7]

Vitamin D and calcium deficiency are found to potentiate development of obesity. Moreover, in women with PCOS, it has been demonstrated that an increased body weight has got a negative impact on 25-OH vitamin D and 1,25-OH vitamin D concentrations. Calcium and vitamin D consumption results in a decrease in the BMI.[11,17]

Vitamin D supplementation has been proven to play a vital role in the treatment of PCOS patients, apart from its role in the improvement of insulin resistance and infertility.[20]

REFERENCES

1. Pittas AG, Lau J, Hu FB, Dawson-Hughes B. The role of vitamin D and calcium in type 2 diabetes. A systematic review and meta-analysis. J Clin Endocrinol Metab. 2007; 92(6):2017-29.
2. Muscogiuri G, Sorice GP, Prioletta A, Policola C, Della Casa S, Pontecorvi A, et al. 25-Hydroxyvitamin D concentration correlates with insulin-sensitivity and BMI in obesity. Obesity (Silver Spring). 2010; 18(10):1906-10.
3. Zemel MB. Role of calcium and dairy products in energy partitioning and weight management. Am J Clin Nutr. 2004;79(5): 907S-12S.
4. Namvar K. Effect of laparoscopic ovarian cauterization on Zn, Fe and Mg serum level in PCOS patient. Women's Health Gynecol. 2017;3(4):72.

5. Günalan E, Yaba A, Yılmaz B. The effect of nutrient supplementation in the management of polycystic ovary syndrome-associated metabolic dysfunctions: A critical review. J Turk Ger Gynecol Assoc.2018;19(4):220-32.
6. Tatarchuk TF, Kosei NV, Vetokh HV, Gunkov SV. Serum micro- and macroelements levels in women with polycystic ovary syndrome associated with pelvic inflammatory disease. Reprod Endocrinol. 2016;27:26-9.
7. Muneyyirci-Delale O, Nacharaju VL, Altura BM, Altura BT. Sex steroid hormones modulate serum ionized magnesium and calcium levels throughout the menstrual cycle in women. Fertil Steril 1998;69(5): 958-62.
8. Pine M, Lee B, Dearth R, Hiney JK, Dees WL. Manganese acts centrally to stimulate luteinizing hormone secretion: a potential influence on female pubertal development. Toxicol Sci. 2005;85:880-85.
9. Coskun A, Arikan T, Kilinc, M, Arikan DC, Ekerbiçer HÇ. Plasma selenium levels in Turkish women with polycystic ovary syndrome. Eur J Obstet Gynecol Reprod Biol. 2013;168(2):183-6.
10. Basini G, Tamanini C. Selenium stimulates estradiol production in bovine granulosa cells: Possible involvement of nitric oxide. Domest Anim Endocrinol. 2000;18(1):1-17.
11. Young KA, Engelman CD, Langefeld CD, Hairston KG, Haffner SM, Bryer-Ash M, et al. Association of plasma vitamin D levels with adiposity in Hispanic and African Americans. J Clin Endocrinol Metab. 2009;94(9):3306-13.
12. Panidis D, Balaris C, Farmakiotis D, Rousso D, Kourtis A, Balaris V, et al. Serum parathyroid hormone concentrations are increased in women with polycystic ovary syndrome. Clin Chem. 2005;51(9):1691-7.
13. Rotterdam ESHRE/ASRM-Sponsored PCOS Consensus Workshop Group. Revised 2003 consensus on diagnostic criteria and long-term health risks related to polycystic ovary syndrome. Fertil Steril. 2004;81(1):19-25.
14. Mahmoudi T, Gourabi H, Ashrafi M, Yazdi RS, Ezabadi Z. Calciotropic hormones, insulin resistance, and the polycystic ovary syndrome. Fertil Steril. 2010;93(4);1208-14.
15. Firouzabadi Rd, Aflatoonian A, Modarresi S, Sekhavat L, MohammadTaheri S. Therapeutic effects of calcium & vitamin D supplementation in women with PCOS. Complementary Ther Clin Pract. 2012;18(2): 85-8.
16. Eshre R. ASRM-Sponsored PCOS Consensus Workshop Group Revised 2003 consensus on diagnostic criteria and long-term health risks related to polycystic ovary syndrome. Fertil Steril. 2004;81(1):19-25.
17. Al-Jeborry MM. Some Altered Trace Elements in Patients with Polycystic Ovary Syndrome. J Adv Med Med Res. 2017;20(3):1-10.
18. Donner T; Sarkar S. In: Feingold KR, Anawalt B, Boyce A (Eds). Insulin—Pharmacology, Therapeutic Regimens and Principles of Intensive Insulin Therapy. South Dartmouth, MA, USA: MDText.com, Inc.; 2000.
19. Benaglia L, Paffoni A, Mangiarini A, Restelli L, Bettinardi N, Somigliana E, et al. Intrafollicular iron and ferritin in women with ovarian endometriomas. Acta Obstet Gynecol Scand. 2015;94(6):646-53.
20. Zheng, G, Wang L, Guo Z, Sun L, Wang L, Wang C, et al. Association of Serum Heavy Metals and Trace Element Concentrations with Reproductive Hormone Levels and Polycystic Ovary Syndrome in a Chinese Population. Biol Trace Elem Res. 2015;167:1-10.
21. Pisoschi AM, Pop A. The role of antioxidants in the chemistry of oxidative stress: A review. Eur J Med Chem. 2015;97:55-74.
22. Khalaf BH, Ouda MH, Alghurabi HS, Shubbar AS. Zinc and copper levels and their correlation with polycystic ovary syndrome biochemical changes. Int J Pharm Sci Res. 2018;9(7):3036-41.
23. Afkhami-Ardekani M, Karimi M, Mohammadi SM, Nourani F. Effect of zinc sulfate supplementation on lipid and glucose in type 2 diabetic patients. Pak J Nutr. 2008;7(4): 550-3.

CHAPTER 13

Gut Microbiome and PCOS

Ruchika Garg, Soniya Dhiman, Akanksha Gupta

■ INTRODUCTION

Polycystic ovary syndrome (PCOS) is thought to have a multifactorial origin including genetic factors, neuroendocrine, lifestyle, immune, and recently studied metabolic dysfunctions in the gut.

Gut microbes can impart their effect by various ways. Some of them are explained in the following text.

GUT MICROBES AND METABOLIC DYSFUNCTION

Gut microbiota encompasses about 10^{14} microorganisms and commensals residing within the human intestinal tract. Studies have closely linked the gut microbiome with the level of human metabolism. Continuously changing dynamics of intestinal flora might lead to a variety of endocrine and metabolic diseases. Bäckhed et al. found that implanting normal microbiota, harvested from the distal intestine of adult germ-free (GF) C57BL/6 mice, produces a 60% increase in body fat content and insulin resistance (IR) within 14 days despite reduced food intake.[1] Vrieze et al. demonstrated that the reverse is also true by transferring gut microbiota from lean donors to males with metabolic syndrome which leads to a decrease in IR in 6 weeks.[2]

These studies highlighted the role of gut microbiota in IR which may subsequently lead to PCOS in women.

Tremellen and Pearce proposed a hypothesis called DOGMA (dysbiosis of gut microbiota), which explains a possible sequence of events in the pathogenesis of PCOS as explained in **Flowchart 1**.[3]

The tiny microbes residing in the gut, most notably *Lactobacillus*, Firmicutes, and *Bacteroides*, followed by Actinomycete, Proteobacteria, and *Clostridium*, are responsible for normal physiology, immunity, metabolism, and nutrition. Any alteration in the number or diversity of these microbes causes multifactorial alterations in human metabolism. Using a letrozole-induced PCOS mouse model, Kelley et al. demonstrated significant diet-independent changes in the gut microbial community, suggesting that gut microbiome dysbiosis may also occur in PCOS women.[4]

A landmark study done by Qi et al. established a major understanding about the role of gut microbes in PCOS.[5] They compared PCOS cohort with non-PCOS controls in terms of diversity of gut microbiota and found that *Bacteroides vulgatus* colonization was significantly increased in PCOS cohort as compared to controls. It was also observed that conjugated bile salts [tauroursodeoxycholic acid (TUDCA) and glycodeoxycholic acid (GDCA)] were also reduced in PCOS women as compared to controls. The likely cause is that *B. vulgatus*

Flowchart 1: Pathogenesis of polycystic ovary syndrome (PCOS) by dysbiosis of gut microbiota.

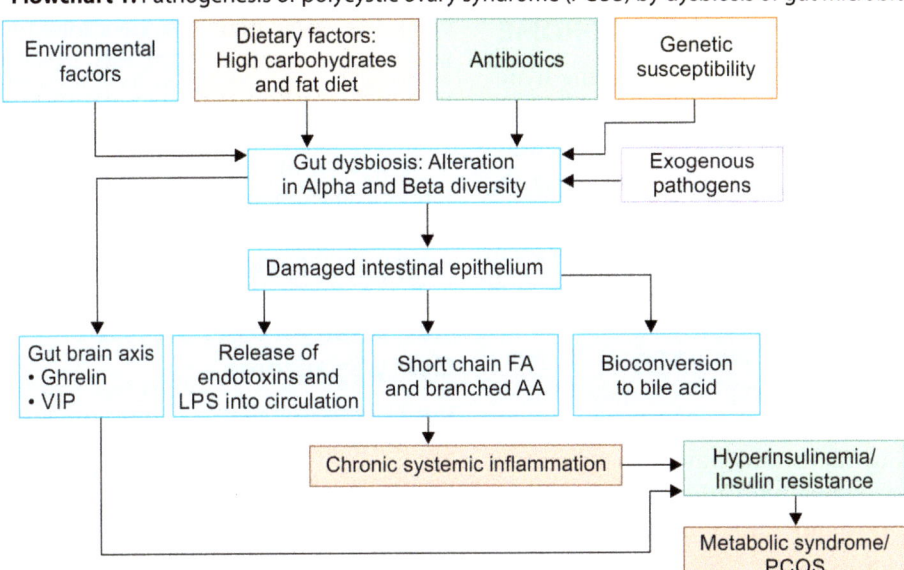

(AA: amino acids; FA: fatty acids; LPS: lipopolysaccharide; VIP: vasoactive intestinal peptide)

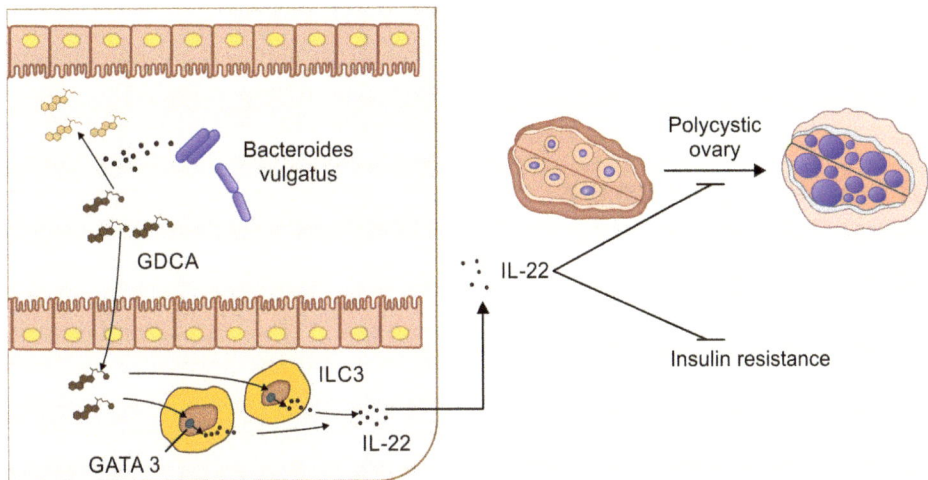

Fig. 1: Role of *Bacteroides* in pathogenesis of insulin resistance and polycystic ovary syndrome (PCOS). (GDCA: glycodeoxycholic acid; ILC3: innate lymphoid cells; IL: interleukin)

produces intestinal bile salt hydrolases. Another major finding of the study was the decreased levels of interleukin-22 (IL-22), in intestinal cells in mice with induced PCOS morphology, which has a role in increasing ovarian functioning and decreasing IR. It was also noted that supplementing the bile acids and IL-22 reversed the colonization of *B. vulgatus* and its effects mediated by them in PCOS mice, as shown in **Figure 1**.

Hence, we can say that the gut microbiota definitely has a role in the pathogenesis of PCOS and can be a potential therapeutic target.

CHRONIC INFLAMMATION AND POLYCYSTIC OVARY SYNDROME

Tremellen and Pearce[3] proposed the hypothesis of the "gut barrier endotoxemia-inflammation mechanism" for explaining the pathogenesis of PCOS. Notable is the role of lipopolysaccharide (LPS) produced by intestinal flora which has an endotoxin effect and leads to the early development of inflammatory and metabolic diseases.

Actually, LPS binding protein (LBP) binds to CD14 toll-like receptor complex (TRL-4) on the surface of innate immune cells, activating them and hence the resulting immune system activation interferes with insulin receptor function, causing serum insulin levels to rise.[6] Also gut synthesis of serum tumor necrosis factor-alpha (TNF-α) and IL-6, which is mediated by endotoxin-induced activation of macrophages in gut, leads to chronic low-grade systemic inflammation leading to IR and hence PCOS.[7]

GUT BIODIVERSITY AND ITS ALTERATION IN POLYCYSTIC OVARY SYNDROME

There are two kinds of gut microbe diversity: alpha (α) and beta (β). The α and β diversity define the microbiome changes: α diversity is considered as an index of the health of an ecosystem and indicates the number of species present in a community that occupy a given environment in a specific community, whereas β diversity represents how similar one community is to another.[8]

Zeng et al.[9] demonstrated in their study that *Bacteroidaceae* was prolific in the IR and PCOS with no-insulin resistance (NIR)-PCOS group, while the *Prevotellaceae* dramatically decreased in PCOS patients. It was also seen that clinical parameter levels, including IR, sex hormones, and inflammation, were positively associated with the abundance of *Bacteroidaceae*, but negatively associated with that of *Prevotellaceae*.[9] Qi et al. also proved the increase in *B. vulgatus* as a pathognomonic of PCOS. *Lactobacillus* and *Bifidobacterium* are known as good bacteria having gut-protective effects which are decreased in PCOS.[5]

Gut–brain Axis in Polycystic Ovary Syndrome

It was seen by Liu et al.[10] that the levels of gut hormones like ghrelin and peptide YY are decreased in PCOS women likely due to *Bacteroides*. These gut hormones have a negative correlation with IR and BMI.

Sex Hormones and Polycystic Ovary Syndrome

The contrast between gut microbiomes of women and men was highlighted in many studies (described below). It is seen that women have more α diversity than men and fewer *Bacteroides* as compared to men whereas men have more *Prevotella* and *Bacteroides* as compared to women likely under the influence of respective sex hormones.[11,12] The correlation between gut microbes and sex hormones was studied by Torres et al., where it was seen that hyperandrogenism, total testosterone, and hirsutism were negatively correlated with α diversity. Moreover, the α diversity in polycystic ovarian morphology (PCOM) was intermediate between healthy and PCOS women.[13]

The study by Insenser et al. has shown a positive correlation between α diversity and testosterone levels and a negative correlation with estradiol concentrations, suggesting that sex hormones might be involved in the modification of gut microbiome.[14]

Short-chain Free Fatty Acids and Polycystic Ovary Syndrome

Butyrate acts as an important short-chain free fatty acid (SCFA) in protecting the intestinal barrier by acting as a source of energy for intestinal cells and having an anti-inflammatory function. SCFAs protect intestinal barrier integrity by acting on β cells of the pancreas to promote insulin secretion, thus improving the metabolism of PCOS. Zhang et al. proposed that *Bifidobacterium* and *Faecalibacterium* from probiotics increase SCFA which binds to enteroendocrine cells and releases ghrelin and peptide YY which further acts on hypothalamus and ameliorates the PCOS symptoms.[15]

■ TREATMENT

Now in the light of gut microflora and their underlying role in chronic inflammation in the gut leading to PCOS, newer treatment options have been provided such as probiotics, prebiotics, and synbiotics in the management of PCOS. Utilizing the knowledge of genetics and species of the gut flora and their subsequent roles in the pathogenesis of metabolic syndrome, IR, PCOS, and infertility has provided a new horizon in the management of PCOS.

Diet

The age-old management of PCOS consists of lifestyle modification including not only exercise but also a high fiber and low carbohydrate diet. These factors are mediated by acting on the tiny inhabitants of individuals. It is seen that high fat and carbohydrate diets increase the colonization of *Bacteroides*, *Clostridium*, and *Enterobacter* species which further increases the inflammatory state in the body, thus leading to IR and hyperandrogenism.

In their review, Singh et al.[16] described the microbiome and its modification through diet, with the influence on inflammatory bowel disease (IBD), obesity, type 2 diabetes, cardiovascular disease, cancer, and its response to immunotherapy. They reported that animal-based proteins increase *Bacteroides*, *Alistipes*, and *Bilophila* and reduce counts of *Bifidobacterium* leading to an increased risk of cardiovascular disease. On the opposite, plant proteins increase *Bifidobacterium* and *Lactobacillus*, and decrease *Bacteroides fragilis* and *Clostridium perfringens*, with the positive health outcome of increasing SCFA's levels consequently decreasing inflammation. The authors also reported that a high-fat diet increases counts of *Bacteroides* and *Clostridium*, *Bacteroides*, and *Enterobacteria* associated with inflammation. Regarding carbohydrates, it has been suggested that high levels of glucose, fructose, and sucrose increase *Bifidobacterium* and reduce *Bacteroides*. Nondigestible carbohydrates, such as whole grain and wheat bran, seem linked to an increase in *Bifidobacterium* and *Lactobacilli*.[16]

Probiotics, Prebiotics, and Synbiotics

Probiotics are tiny microbes which are beneficial to the gut and they perform antioxygenic, antimicrobial, and anti-inflammatory effects, improving metabolic parameters, modulating intestinal microbiota, and regulating the immune system metabolism, also known as the good bacteria. In many clinical trials and randomized controlled trials (RCTs), it has been seen that by supplementing probiotics like *Bifidobacterium*, *Lactobacillus*, etc., for a period of 8-12 weeks in PCOS women, a statistically significant improvement in triglyceride levels, HOMA-IR, BMI, etc., was seen.[17-19]

Prebiotics are selectively fermented ingredients that allow specific changes in the gut microflora which confer benefits upon the host's well-being and health, whereas synergist combinations of probiotics and prebiotics are called synbiotics.

Fecal Microbiota Transplantation

Transplantation of *B. vulgatus*-infected fecal microbes in mice resulted in ovarian dysfunction, IR, changes in bile acid metabolism, decreased secretion of IL-22, and infertility.[20]

Newer innovative treatment options for the treatment of PCOS after the significant role of gut microbiota on the table is FMT. However no clinical reports are available for the same; only few trials on mice have been done till now.[21]

Hence, the newer options of fecal microbiota transplantation (FMT) are still in research settings and need definite results to be recommended clinically.

Interleukin-22 Transplantation

As shown by Qi et al. in their study, IL-22 increases the brown fat and thereby increases insulin sensitivity. IL-22 was substituted in the PCOS mice model and beneficial results were seen.[5] This treatment model is still in research setting.

■ FUTURE RESEARCH

Since less is known about the clinical implications of the studies as of now, and many of the hypotheses for causation of PCOS are yet to be proven by studies, it provides a research opportunity in the direction of working on the clinical utility of gut microflora replenishment for treating or managing PCOS.

Wang et al. in his study[22] found that unlike healthy women, vaginal microflora in women with PCOS does not show cyclical changes in the menstrual cycle inciting a new research direction in PCOS.

■ REFERENCES

1. Bäckhed F, Ding H, Wang T, Hooper LV, Koh GY, Nagy A, et al. The gut microbiota as an environmental factor that regulates fat storage. Proc Natl Acad Sci USA. 2004; 101(44):15718-23.
2. Vrieze A, Van Nood E, Holleman F, Salojärvi J, Kootte RS, Bartelsman JFWM, et al. Transfer of Intestinal microbiota from lean donors increases insulin sensitivity in individuals with metabolic syndrome. Gastroenterology. 2012;143(4):913-6.e7.
3. Tremellen K, Pearce K. Dysbiosis of Gut Microbiota (DOGMA)—a novel theory for the development of Polycystic Ovarian Syndrome. Med Hypotheses. 2012;79(1): 104-12.
4. Kelley ST, Skarra DV, Rivera AJ, Thackray VG. The Gut Microbiome Is Altered in a Letrozole-Induced Mouse Model of Polycystic Ovary Syndrome. PLoS One. 2016;11(1):e0146509.
5. Qi X, Yun C, Sun L, Xia J, Wu Q, Wang Y, et al. Gut microbiota–bile acid–interleukin-22 axis orchestrates polycystic ovary syndrome. Nat Med. 2019;25(8):1225-33.
6. Hersoug LG, Møller P, Loft S. Gut microbiota-derived lipopolysaccharide uptake and trafficking to adipose tissue: implications for inflammation and obesity. Obes Rev. 2016; 17(4):297–312.
7. Wellen KE, Hotamisligil GS. Inflammation, stress, and diabetes. J Clin Invest. 2005;115(5): 1111-9.
8. Thackray VG. Sex, Microbes, and Polycystic Ovary Syndrome. Trends Endocrinol Metab. 2019;30(1):54-65.
9. Zeng B, Lai Z, Sun L, Zhang Z, Yang J, Li Z, et al. Structural and functional profiles of the gut microbial community in polycystic ovary syndrome with insulin resistance (IR-PCOS): a pilot study. Res Microbiol. 2019; 170(1):43-52.

10. Liu R, Zhang C, Shi Y, Zhang F, Li L, Wang X, et al. Dysbiosis of Gut Microbiota Associated with Clinical Parameters in Polycystic Ovary Syndrome. Front Microbiol. 2017;8:324.
11. Haro C, Rangel-Zúñiga OA, Alcalá-Díaz JF, Gómez-Delgado F, Pérez-Martínez P, Delgado-Lista J, et al. Intestinal Microbiota Is Influenced by Gender and Body Mass Index. PLoS One. 2016;11(5):e0154090.
12. Chen T, Long W, Zhang C, Liu S, Zhao L, Hamaker BR. Fiber-utilizing capacity varies in Prevotella-versus Bacteroides-dominated gut microbiota. Sci Rep. 2017;7(1):2594.
13. Torres PJ, Siakowska M, Banaszewska B, Pawelczyk L, Duleba AJ, Kelley ST, et al. Gut Microbial Diversity in Women With Polycystic Ovary Syndrome Correlates With Hyperandrogenism. J Clin Endocrinol Metab. 2018;103(4):1502-11.
14. Thursby E, Juge N. Introduction to the human gut microbiota. Biochem J. 2017; 474(11):1823-36.
15. Zhang J, Sun Z, Jiang S, Bai X, Ma C, Peng Q, et al. Probiotic Bifidobacterium lactis V9 Regulates the Secretion of Sex Hormones in Polycystic Ovary Syndrome Patients through the Gut-Brain Axis. mSystems. 2019;4(2):e00017-19.
16. Singh RK, Chang HW, Yan D, Lee KM, Ucmak D, Wong K, et al. Influence of diet on the gut microbiome and implications for human health. J Transl Med. 2017;15(1):73.
17. Ahmadi S, Jamilian M, Karamali M, Tajabadi-Ebrahimi M, Jafari P, Taghizadeh M, et al. Probiotic supplementation and the effects on weight loss, glycaemia and lipid profiles in women with polycystic ovary syndrome: a randomized, double-blind, placebo-controlled trial. Hum Fertil (Camb). 2017; 20(4):254-61.
18. Shoaei T, Heidari-Beni M, Tehrani H, Feizi A, Esmaillzadeh A, Askari G. Effects of Probiotic Supplementation on Pancreatic β-cell Function and C-reactive Protein in Women with Polycystic Ovary Syndrome: A Randomized Double-blind Placebo-controlled Clinical Trial. Int J Prev Med. 2015;6:27.
19. Ghanei N, Rezaei N, Amiri GA, Zayeri F, Makki G, Nasseri E. The probiotic supplementation reduced inflammation in polycystic ovary syndrome: A randomized, double-blind, placebo-controlled trial. J Funct Foods. 2018;42:306-11.
20. Torres PJ, Ho BS, Arroyo P, Sau L, Chen A, Kelley ST, et al. Exposure to a Healthy Gut Microbiome Protects Against Reproductive and Metabolic Dysregulation in a PCOS Mouse Model. Endocrinology. 2019; 160(5):1193-204.
21. Guo Y, Qi Y, Yang X, Zhao L, Wen S, Liu Y, et al. Association between Polycystic Ovary Syndrome and Gut Microbiota. PLoS One. 2016;11(4):e0153196.
22. Wang L, Zhou J, Gober HJ, Leung WT, Huang Z, Pan X, et al. Alterations in the intestinal microbiome associated with PCOS affect the clinical phenotype. Biomed Pharmacother. 2021;133:110958.

CHAPTER 14

Endocrine Disruptors in PCOS

Neha Kapoor, Ruchika Garg, Poonam Goyal

What are Endocrine Disrupting Chemicals?

Endocrine disrupting chemicals (EDCs) are chemicals that may interfere with the body's endocrine system inducing adverse developmental, reproductive, neurologic, and immune effects in both humans and animals.

Endocrine disrupting chemicals consist of a plethora of consumer products—natural and man-made, found in daily products such as plastic food bottles, cans, detergents, toys, cosmetics, and pesticides.

These can mimic, block, or interfere with the way the body's hormones work.

Endocrine disrupting chemicals' exposure can happen anywhere and come from the air we breathe, the food we eat, and the water we drink. EDCs can also enter the body through the skin and transfer from mother to fetus (transplacental) or mother to infant (via breastfeeding).

Examples include bisphenol A (BPA), phthalates, pesticides, and polychlorinated biphenyls (PCPs).

■ BISPHENOL A

Bisphenol A is a high-volume production, plastic monomer used widely for manufacturing polycarbonated plastics, polyvinyl chlorides, dental sealants, and epoxy linings for canned food goods.

Molecular structure consists of a phenol group and may possess halogen group substitution by chlorine and bromine; therefore, they can mimic steroid hormones and interfere with the synthesis, secretion, transport, metabolism, binding action, or elimination of natural hormones that are present in the body.[1]

The ester bond linking BPA monomers to the polymers used for packaging is susceptible to hydrolysis, promoting migration into foods and beverages and allowing gastrointestinal exposure. Dermal exposures result from contact with thermal receipts, paper money, and paper products.

Mechanism of Action (Flowchart 1)

Bisphenol A is an estrogenic endocrine disruptor in vitro and in vivo.
- It is a weak ligand for the classic estrogen receptors alpha (ERα) and beta (ERβ) with binding affinities that are 1,000–10,000 times lower than endogenous estradiol (E2).[2]
- Potent ligand for the orphan estrogen-related receptor gamma (ERRγ) and for nonclassic membrane-bound G-coupled protein receptor.
- It acts as antiandrogen.[3]
- It is human pregnancy X receptor (HPXR) agonist.

Polycystic ovary syndrome (PCOS)-like symptoms were first documented in the historical literature in the 1700s, long before

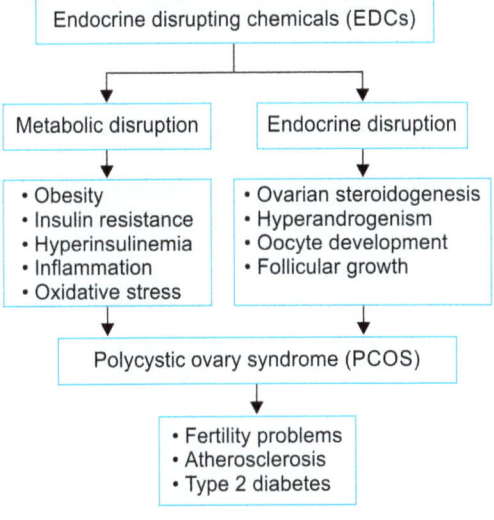

Flowchart 1: Mechanism of action of endocrine disrupting chemicals.

Reproductive Disruption

The mechanism by which BPA affects ovarian function appears to be bidirectional.

- In vitro studies have provided evidence that exposure of rat ovarian theca interstitial cells to BPA results in elevated testosterone synthesis, by upregulation of enzyme 17-β-hydroxylase enzyme.
- Androgens interfere with BPA clearance in the liver leading to increased serum levels of BPA.
- BPA acts as a potent sex hormone binding globulin (SHBG) binder and displaces androgens resulting in increased levels of free androgens.
- BPA inhibits testosterone catabolism, thereby leading to elevated androgen levels.

the surge of modern chemistry; thus, EDCs are certainly not the primary causal agent in PCOS.

In humans, cross-sectional data suggests that BPA concentrations are higher in women with PCOS than in reproductively healthy women, but the direction of causality has not been established.

Evidence from rat models has demonstrated that exposure to high doses of BPA during the neonatal period resulted in a PCOS-like phenotype in adulthood, including increased serum testosterone and estrogen levels and reduced progesterone and ovarian cysts. Also, BPA exposure leads to altered gonadotropin-releasing hormone (GnRH) pulsatility and pituitary GnRH signaling which may be crucial in PCOS development.[4]

Therefore, EDCs impact on female ovulation, directly at the level of gonads and indirectly via alterations of the hypothalamic–pituitary–ovarian (HPO) axis.

Metabolic Disruption

Bisphenol A acts on hormone systems involved in obesity, metabolism, and insulin regulation.

- BPA affects adipocyte differentiation, inhibits adiponectin release, and increases expression of genes involved in adipocyte differentiation.[5]
- It activates glucocorticoid receptor which in turn leads to upregulation of 11-β-HSD (hydroxysteroid dehydrogenase)-1 enzymes which catalyze conversion of cortisone to cortisol, ultimately promoting adipogenesis
- BPA disturbs pancreatic physiology by stimulating pancreatic β cells, increasing insulin production resulting in hyperinsulinemia.[6]

■ REFERENCES

1. Rutkowska AZ, Diamanti-Kandarakis E. Polycystic ovary syndrome and environmental toxins. Fertil Steril. 2016;106(4): 948-58.

2. Barrett ES, Sobolewski M. Polycystic ovary syndrome: do endocrine-disrupting chemicals play a role? Semin Reprod Med. 2014;32(3):166-76.
3. Bloom MS, Mok-Lin E, Fujimoto VY. Bisphenol A and ovarian steroidogenesis. Fertil Steril. 2016;106(4):857-63.
4. Sartain CV, Hunt PA. An old culprit but a new story: bisphenol A and "NextGen" bisphenols. Fertil Steril. 2016;106(4):820-6.
5. Brieño-Enríquez MA, Larriba E, Del Mazo J. Endocrine disrupters, microRNAs, and primordial germ cells: a dangerous cocktail. Fertil Steril. 2016;106(4):871-9.
6. Kandaraki E, Chatzigeorgiou A, Livadas S, Palioura E, Economou F, Koutsilieris M, et al. Endocrine disruptors and polycystic ovary syndrome (PCOS): elevated serum levels of bisphenol A in women with PCOS. J Clin Endocrinol Metab. 2011;96(3):E480-4.

CHAPTER 15

Protisol/Nutraceuticals in PCOS

Neharika Malhotra, Narendra Malhotra, Ramesh Patodia

INTRODUCTION

Nutraceuticals: These are substances which have established nutritional function, e.g., vitamins, minerals, amino acid, fatty acid.

Herbals/photochemicals: Herbs or botanical products.

Dietary supplements: Probiotics, prebiotics, antioxidants, enzymes, etc.

Polycystic ovarian syndrome (PCOS) is one of the most common hormonal disorders among women of reproductive age. Globally, its prevalence rate is 10–80%. In an adolescent woman, the prevalence is as high as 36%. Its manifestations are different in different age groups. The clinical features may however change throughout the life span, starting from adolescence to postmenopausal age **(Fig. 1)**. Therefore, PCOS is considered a lifespan disorder today.

Major concerns for which a patient needs a doctor's help are (1) hirsutism and its clinical signs—androgen excess, (2) amenorrhea and menstrual irregularities, (3) unexplained infertility, and (4) obesity and related features **(Flowchart 1)**.

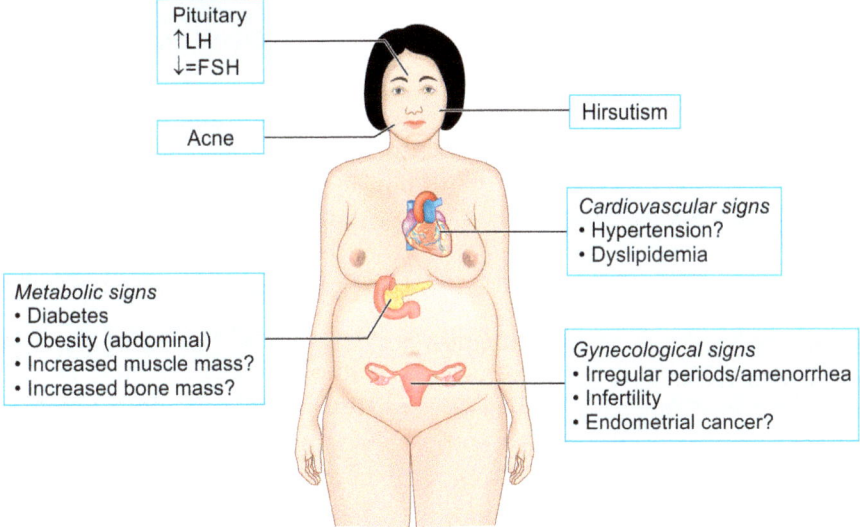

Fig. 1: PCOS woman.
(FSH: follicle-stimulating hormone; LH: luteinizing hormone)

Flowchart 1: Pathophysiology.

```
Excess excretion of
inositols in PCOS
        │
        ▼
Inositols ↓ Glucose ↑ Insulin ↑ ──────▶ LH ↑ FSH ↓
(Glucose/insulin > 4.5)                 (LH/FSH>2.5)
        ↑
        ▼
     Obesity    • Androgen
                • Testosterone ↑ SHBG ↓ Progesterone ↓
                • Estrogen
                        │
                        ▼
            Hirsutism | Acne | Low ovulation

    Also deficient in folate, vitamin D, magnesium, zinc...
```

(FSH: follicle-stimulating hormone; LH: luteinizing hormone; PCOS: polycystic ovarian syndrome; SHBG: sex hormone binding globulin)

■ HOW PROTISOL WORKS

A woman suffering from PCOS is deficient in m-inositol (due to excess excretion), protein, folic acid, vitamin D, zinc, magnesium, and other micronutrients. Protisol reverses the metabolic imbalance by supplementing the following nutrients.

- M-inositol—4 g/day, the quantity body produces per day
- Pea protein
- Folic acid
- Vitamin D
- Zinc
- Magnesium
- 25 vitamins

■ AIM AND OBJECTIVES

There is an ongoing study of 132 patients who were diagnosed to have PCO features in the last 2½ months. They were given plant protein-based powder Protisol in dose of four scoops with water twice daily (before breakfast and dinner) for the first month until improvement in symptoms appeared, followed by four scoops with water once daily (before breakfast). Our aim was to study improvement in features such as weight, acne, hirsutism, menstrual irregularities, and blood sugar levels.

At the start of the study, we did basic physical examination to record their BP, weight, body mass index (BMI), and features of androgen excess and conducted investigations to check blood sugar (fasting), follicle-stimulating hormone (FSH), luteinizing hormone (LH), anti-mullerian hormone (AMH), and testosterone levels. Patients were counseled regarding lifestyle modification and diet management. All patients were followed up at 1- and 2-month interval, and outcomes were studied.

■ RESULTS

- Out of a total of 132 patients, 123 patients came for follow-up **(Table 1)**.
- Out of 123 patients, 101 patients had weight loss in the first 2 months, ranging from 1 to 2.5 kg **(Fig. 2)**.
- 52 patients who were previously having prolonged cycles or bleeding on withdrawal started having period without withdrawal after 2 months of Protisol.

TABLE 1: Case study.

Total number of patients registered till date	Number of patients who came for follow-up	Follow-up parameters studied				
		Weight loss	Improvement in menstrual pattern	Acne improvement	Hirsutism improvement	Blood sugar control
132	123	101	52	18	10	36

Number of patients	Weight loss 1–1.5 kg	Weight loss 2 kg	No weight loss
123	80	21	22

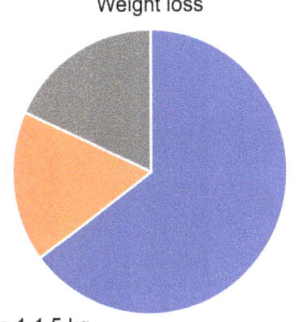

Fig. 2: Weight loss in study cases.

- Out of 89 patients who had acne, 18 patients showed improvement in acne after the first month **(Fig. 3)**.
- Hirsutism improved in 10 patients out of a total of 78 patients presenting with hirsutism.
- 90 patients had slightly raised fasting blood sugar levels. With Protisol, 36 reported normal fasting sugar levels.
- 14 patients were taken up for in vitro fertilization (IVF) **(Fig. 4)**.
- 33 patients were taken up intrauterine insemination (IUI) **(Fig. 4)**.
- Only two patients reported an increase in weight after treatment
- Significant reduction in testosterone levels was seen in long-term management **(Figs. 5A and B)**.

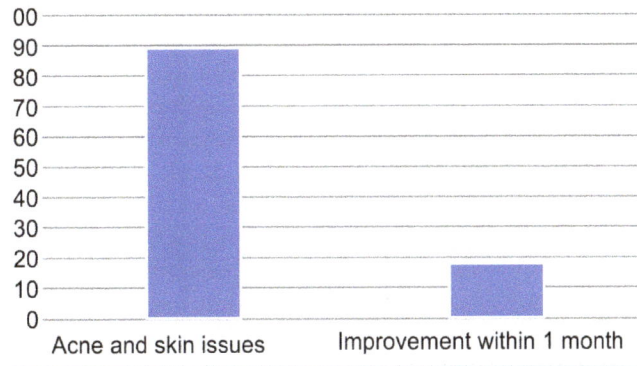

Fig. 3: Skin issues with polycystic ovarian syndrome.

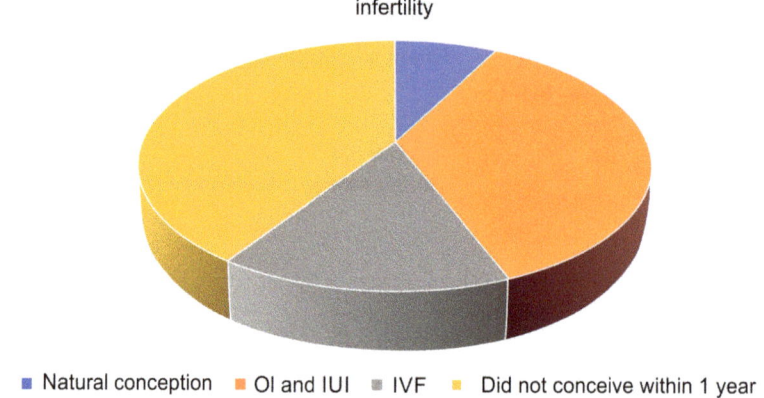

Fig. 4: Infertility in polycystic ovarian syndrome case study.
(IUI: intrauterine insemination; OI: ovulation induction; IVF: in vitro fertilization)

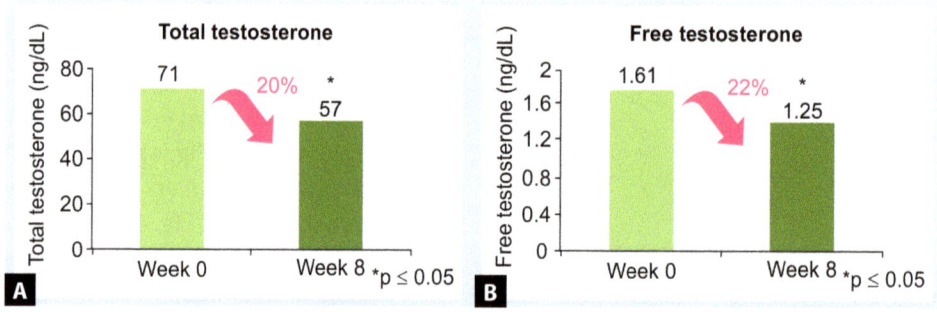

Figs. 5A and B: (A) Total testosterone; (B) Free testosterone.

DISCUSSION

Polycystic ovarian syndrome compromises other pathological conditions that strongly modify the phenotype and play a dominant role in the pathophysiology of the disorders, including insulin resistance (IR) and hyperinsulinemia, obesity, and metabolic disorders, all favoring together with androgen excess, an increased susceptibility to develop type 2 diabetes mellitus (T2DM) and possibly cardiovascular diseases (CVD). PCOS by itself may also have a genetic component.

Polycystic ovarian syndrome patients are also at an increased risk for premature arteriosclerosis, obesity, IR, T2DM, and endometrial cancer. Therefore, PCOS has significant implication for health and quality of life of such patients

- Inositol and its metabolites belong to B complex vitamins. Inositol-derived metabolites have essential roles in insulin sensitivity as second messengers, lipid synthesis, signal transduction, oocyte maturation, oogenesis, cell morphogenesis, and cytoskeleton organization.
- Randomized controlled studies involving inositol supplementation in women with PCOS show that inositol provides improvement in almost all pathologic conditions in PCOS such as recovery of reproductive abnormalities, decreased androgen levels, and improved insulin levels.

- Combined treatment of inositol isomers such as myoinositol (MI) and D-chiroinositol (DCI) should be applied at a certain ratio which is known as a physiologic ratio (MI:DCI— 4:1).
- 4 g of myoinositol is the recommended daily dosage.
- Addition of folic acid, vitamin D, Mg, and Zn has shown improvement in PCOS.
- Protein is also crucial when managing PCOS through diet. Aside from supporting muscle growth, metabolism, and providing sustained energy, protein also helps in regulating blood sugar, insulin production, and control weight.

Whole plant-based proteins have advantages over animal protein. They are free of cholesterol and saturated fats, high in fiber, vitamins and minerals, phytochemicals, and essential amino acids. They are also free from residual hormones which may be present in animal proteins.

CONCLUSION

- With two doses of 2 g each, a patient gets 4 g of MI/day, which is the minimum recommended dosage for treatment of PCOS.
- Protein deficiency is one of the causes of PCOS. Pea-based protein is one of the best plant proteins. Moreover, synergistic action of inositols with protein, folic acid, and 25+ vitamins improves its efficacy in management of PCOS.
- Protisol promotes normal hormone and lipid levels for regular menstrual cycles, improves egg quality, increases sex hormone binding globulin (SHBG) levels and thereby decreased testosterone levels, improves insulin sensitivity, decreases LH levels, induces weight loss, effectively manages hirsutism, induces ovulation, and prevents gestational diabetes.

REFERENCES

1. Günalan E, Yaba A, Yılmaz B. The effect of nutrient supplementation in the management of polycystic ovary syndrome-associated metabolic dysfunctions: A critical review. J Turk Ger Gynecol Assoc. 2018;19(4): 220-32.
2. Arentz S, Smith CA, Abbott J, Bensoussan A. Nutritional supplements and herbal medicines for women with polycystic ovary syndrome; a systematic review and meta-analysis. BMC Complement Altern Med. 2017;17:500.
3. Espinola MSB, Bartelli M, Bizzarri M, Unfer V, Lagana AS, Visconti B, et al. Nutritional supplements and herbal medicines for women with polycystic ovary syndrome; a systematic review and meta-analysis. J Reprod Immunol. 2021;144:103271.

CHAPTER 16

Clinical Spectrum of PCOS

Vidya Thobbi, Parul Sinha

INTRODUCTION

- Polycystic ovary syndrome (PCOS) is a widespread medical condition that affects multiple aspects of a woman's overall health, with long-term consequences.
- Considerable variability in clinical manifestations coupled with lack of generally accepted diagnostic criteria makes it difficult to identify a definitive etiology for this disease.
- With multifactorial etiology combining genetic and environmental factors, PCOS patients are at increased risk of developing type 2 diabetes, dyslipidemia, endometrial cancer, and cardiovascular disease.
- The clinical picture of PCOS consists of hyperandrogenism, oligomenorrhea, and typical ovarian ultrasound morphology.
- Identifying the different symptoms of PCOS at different stages of life will of course help orchestrate individual treatment strategies and prevent long-term metabolic effects.
- Treatment options depend on the type and extent of the disorder and whether the patient is trying to conceive.[1]

Polycystic ovary syndrome can cause:
- Short-term cosmetic and menstrual problems in adolescents.
- Infertility and pregnancy complications in the reproductive age group.
- Long-term sequelae due to metabolic and cardiovascular effects and endometrial cancer in postmenopausal group.

CRITERIA FOR DIAGNOSIS

The criteria for diagnosis in adolescents are same as that of adult criteria, but these overlap with the physiological changes during adolescence **(Table 1)**.

National Institutes of Health (NIH) Criteria (1990)

- Clinical/biochemical hyperandrogenism
- Oligo-/amenorrhea anovulation

TABLE 1: PCOS phenotypes included in specific diagnostic criteria.

Diagnostic criteria	PCOS phenotype			
	AE+ OD	AE + PCOM	PCOM+ OD	AE +PCOM+ OD
NIH 1990	+			
Rotterdam 2003/2006	+	+	+	+
AE-PCOS society 2006	+	+		+
NIH 2012	+	+	+	+

All criteria recommend exclusion of other causes. (AE: androgen excess; OD: ovulatory dysfunction; PCOM: polycystic ovary morphology; PCOS: polycystic ovary syndrome; NIH: National Institutes of Health).

Rotterdam Criteria (2003)

Any two of the following three:
1. Clinical/biochemical hyperandrogenism.
2. Oligo-/amenorrhea anovulation.
3. Polycystic ovarian morphology on ultrasonography (USG).

Androgen Excess Society (AES) Criteria (2006)

- Clinical/biochemical hyperandrogenism.
- Oligomenorrhea/polycystic ovary morphology (PCOM) on USG.

Pediatric Endocrine Society (PES) Criteria

- Clinical/biochemical hyperandrogenism.
- Oligo-/anovulation.

In December 2012, the NIH's Evidence-based Methodology Workshop on Polycystic Ovary Syndrome recommended upholding the broad, inclusionary Rotterdam criteria while specifically identifying the distinct PCOS phenotype.

- A biochemical and clinical hyperandrogenism of ovarian origin and to a lesser extent adrenal is evident in about 60–80% of PCOS patients.
- Ovarian hyperandrogenism is primarily due to an intrinsic steroidogenic defect in ovarian thecal cells.
- Extraovarian factors such as high luteinizing hormone (LH) and insulin levels and low follicle-stimulating hormone (FSH) levels, as well as intraovarian factors such as anti-Müllerian hormone (AMH) and inhibin can exacerbate the hyperandrogenic state.
- High androgen levels are also considered as one of the possible causes of insulin resistance in PCOS.
- Intrauterine and postpartum androgen excess may increase visceral obesity and insulin resistance.
- Drugs with antiandrogenic activity can improve insulin resistance.
- Insulin resistance and compensatory hyperinsulinemia contribute to all three major clinical features of this syndrome: hyperandrogenemia, ovarian dysfunction, and metabolic alterations.
- Increased pulsatility of LH increases circulating levels of LH and stimulates ovarian cortical synthesis of androgens.
- Elevated LH levels are partly due to negative feedback changes acting on the hypothalamic–pituitary axis by androgens.
- Insulin potentiates the stimulation of androgen production by ovarian theca cells and, to a lesser extent, the adrenal cortex, in synergy with LH.
- Insulin is also implicated in the ovarian dysfunction by increasing the expression of LH receptors on the granulosa cells.
- PCOS patients have altered inositol metabolism and there is an association between insulin resistance and inositol deficiency.
- In females with PCOS, conversion of myo-inositol to D-chiro-inositol is reduced at the muscle tissue level due to reduced epimerase activity. This hypothesis draws attention to the importance of myo-inositol and D-chiro-inositol supplementation to restore normal ovarian function.

CLINICAL FEATURES[2]

Menstrual irregularities: Usually associated with anovulation which causes oligomenorrhea (less than nine menstrual cycles per year; cycles of average duration exceeding 36–40 days). Anovulation is accompanied by secondary amenorrhea (absence of menses for 3 or more consecutive months) in 30% of cases.

- *Hyperandrogenism:* The most characteristic clinical manifestations are hirsutism and acne.

- Total testosterone best reflects the androgen levels and can be measured on any day of the menstrual cycle.
- Other laboratory tests are:
  - Free androgen index (FAI) is the ratio of total testosterone to sex hormone-binding globulin (SHBG).
  - Androstenedione is the immediate precursor of testosterone, produced by the ovaries, adrenal glands, and peripheral tissues. Women with PCOS may have elevated levels of androstenedione even when the total testosterone is normal.
  - Dehydroepiandrosterone-sulfate (DHEA-S) is mostly derived from the adrenal glands and is elevated in approximately 20–30% of PCOS patients.

A recent study has shown that androstenedione and total testosterone level helps to better assess the risk of developing metabolic syndrome in women with PCOS.

Polycystic Ovary Morphology

According to the Rotterdam criteria:
- The Ovaries are defined as "Polycystic" when at least one ovary has 12 or more follicles with an average diameter 2–9 mm, regardless of their disposition, and/or a total ovarian volume >10 mL^3.
- Should be examined with a transvaginal probe and must be evaluated in both longitudinal and transverse scanning plane.
- A single ovary with these characteristics is sufficient, when evaluated in the follicular phase and in the absence of any hormonal treatment.
- Peripheral distribution of the follicles and hypertrophy of the ovarian stroma may be present but are not required for diagnosis.

Other clinical spectra associated with PCOS include:[3]
- *Endometrial cancer:*
  - PCOS is associated with an incremental risk of endometrial cancer with aggravating effect from inter-related comorbidities including obesity, and potential influence from PCOS treatments.
  - Pathophysiology is associated with uninhibited estrogen in the context of anovulation and is preventable.
  - The risk of endometrial cancer is 2–6 times higher in women with PCOS, predominantly adenocarcinomas (>95%) including type I and type II cancers, with type I higher in PCOS.
  - Routine screening for endometrial hyperplasia or cancer in PCOS is advisable but endometrial surveillance by transvaginal sonography (TVS) or endometrial biopsy is recommended for PCOS women with thickened endometrium, prolonged amenorrhea, unopposed estrogen exposure, or abnormal vaginal bleeding, on the basis of clinical suspicion.

Mental health issues:
  - Health-related quality of life (HRQoL) is a well-recognized and important health problem, especially in chronic diseases and is associated with physical, social, and emotional effects of a condition and its associated treatments.
  - Assessment is self-reported and can be measured with a variety of tools.
- *Obesity and weight gain:*
  - Insulin resistance affects 75% of lean women and 95% of overweight women.
  - It is exacerbated by excess weight increasing prevalence and severity of metabolic, reproductive, and psychological features of PCOS.

- Women with PCOS have universally reported that excess weight causes significant distress and anxiety.
- Weight was also a highly ranked, prioritized outcome by both health professionals and women during the guideline development process.
- Overall, lifestyle interventions that reduce even as little as 5% of total body weight have been shown to provide health, metabolic, reproductive, and psychological benefits in overweight women with PCOS.
- Psychological comorbidities of PCOS with overweight/obesity include anxiety, depression, decreased HRQoL, sexual dissatisfaction, low self-esteem, and psychological distress.
- Mental health should also be considered when assessing and managing obesity, especially in PCOS.
- Weight assessments should take into account associated prejudices, negative body image, and/or low self-esteem, and assessments should be conducted respectfully.

CONCLUSION

Polycystic ovary syndrome encompasses a wide range of symptoms and signs which have short-term and long-term effects and may affect each and every phase of life. Thus, its identification and its prompt treatment can help evade short-term miseries and long-term effects.

REFERENCES

1. ESHRE. (2018). International evidence-based guideline for the assessment and management of polycystic ovary syndrome (PCOS). [online] Available from: https://www.eshre.eu/Guidelines-and-Legal/Guidelines/Polycystic-Ovary-Syndrome [Last accessed November, 2022].
2. Alsadi B. (2019). Clinical Features of PCOS. [online] Available from: https://www.intechopen.com/chapters/70216 [Last accessed November, 2022].
3. Taylor HS, Pal L, Seli E (Eds). Speroff's Clinical Gynecologic Endocrinology and Infertility, 9th edition. Wolters Kluwer; 2019.

CHAPTER 17

PCOS in Peri and Post Menopause

Dolly Mehra

■ INTRODUCTION

Polycystic ovary syndrome (PCOS) is the most common endocrinopathies diagnosed in the reproductive age women, but it can continue to have impact on the postmenopausal health of women. PCOS has been redefined as a reproductive and metabolic disorder after the recognition of the important role of insulin resistance in the pathophysiology of the syndrome.[1] PCOS has been associated with significant adverse sequelae that affect overall long-term health and well-being.[2] With increasing age, it is presumed that PCOS evolves from a reproductive disease to a metabolic disorder like obesity, dyslipidemia, diabetes mellitus, metabolic syndrome, hypertension (HT), cardiovascular disease (CVD), and neoplasm.[3]

■ HORMONAL CHANGES IN THIS AGE GROUP

Menopause is cessation of menstruation due to loss of ovarian follicular activity. Number of ovarian primordial follicles decrease with increasing age up to about age 38, followed by a steeper decline. During this period, several hormonal and metabolic changes take place. Early in the menopause transition, when the cycles are irregular, the initial hormonal change is decrease in inhibin B level in early follicular phase. In late perimenopause estradiol and inhibin A level falls, inhibin B remains low, and serum-follicle-stimulating hormone (S-FSH) levels are markedly increased.[4] Serum androgen levels appear to fall with age rather than any relationship with menopause. Ovarian androgen secretion decline with age in both healthy and in women with PCOS, but levels remain high until the late reproductive years in PCOS.[5,6] Hyperandrogenism seen in PCOS women persists after the menopausal transition. Insulin acts synergistically with the luteinizing hormone to increase androgen production in the theca cell of the ovary.[7] The adrenal androgen secretion also remain high up to menopause in women with PCOS, indicating that hyperandrogenism persists for a long time in women with PCOS.[8] This long lasting hyperandrogenism magnify the unfavorable hormonal and metabolic changes related to menopause and expose these women with PCOS to increased health risk.

Hyperandrogenism plays an important role in pathophysiology of PCOS and is associated with altered body fat distribution, dyslipidemia, hyperinsulinemia because of insulin resistance, along with anovulation and infertility.[9]

The various metabolic disturbances in PCOS may be related to a higher risk of developing CVD.[10] In addition to impaired carbohydrate and lipid metabolism, chronic inflammatory markers, reflected by elevated levels may cause additional risk of CVD.[11] Insulin resistance and hyperandrogenism may also be associated with predisposition to arterial HT in women with PCOS.[12]

AGE OF MENOPAUSE IN POLYCYSTIC OVARY SYNDROME

Age of menopause varies between women and this difference may be due to difference in original number of follicles or difference in depletion of follicles with aging.

Women with PCOS have higher anti-Mullerian hormone (AMH) levels.[13] Attempts have been made to calculate menopausal age of women with or without PCOS based on AMH levels earlier in life and postulated menopausal age of women with PCOS, was approximately 2 years later than in non-PCOS.[14] Forslund et al. demonstrated that women with PCOS reached menopause 4 years later than their age matched controls.[15] S-FSH levels and proportion of women with S-FSH levels <50 IU\L were lower in women with PCOS.

DIAGNOSING POLYCYSTIC OVARY SYNDROME IN THIS AGE GROUP

It is difficult to diagnose PCOS when a woman has already reached menopause. Few modalities are useful.
- On ultrasound (USG) polycystic ovaries (PCO) morphology persists into menopause, the hypoechoic structures on USG in postmenopause PCOS corresponds to inclusion cysts and vascular structures rather than follicles.
- Testosterone levels may not be higher, but other measures of androgen excess like free androgen index (FAI) and human chorionic gonadotropin-stimulated androstenedione and 17-hydroxyprogesterone levels remain high.[16-18]
- Lipid profile worsens as PCOS women age. Low-density lipoprotein (LDL) and cholesterol levels are similar in middle-aged women with or without PCOS, but high-density lipoprotein (HDL) levels are lower and triglycerides levels are higher in women with PCOS.[19]
- Waist circumference, body mass index (BMI), homeostasis model assessment (HOMA), and triglycerides levels increase in PCOS women as they reach 40–50 years of age.[16,20,21]

SPECIFIC CLINICAL FEATURES

Specific clinical features of polycystic ovary syndrome are:
- *Endometrial cancer:* Women with PCOS are at increased risk of developing endometrial cancer particularly endometrioid carcinoma.[22] Endometrial hyperplasia, the precancerous stage of endometrial cancer, is associated with PCOS. Increased risk of malignancy is due to prolonged exposure of endometrium to unopposed estrogen because of anovulation **(Fig. 1)**.
- *Ovarian malignancy:* NorthEast Cerebrovascular Consortium (NECC) study reported an association between PCOS and borderline serous ovarian cancers **(Table 1)**, the association was strongest in

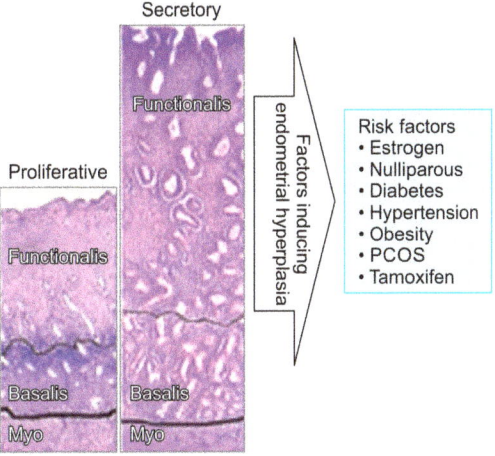

Fig. 1: PCOS and endometrial cancer.

TABLE 1: PCOS and ovarian cancer.	
Prevalence	• 2.7% increased risk in women with PCOS • 9% lifetime risk of developing an endometrial cancer in women with PCOS
Pathogenesis	• Anovulation leads to prolonged exposure to unopposed estrogen • Ovulation induction drugs and synthetic progestins act on secretory endometrium
Surveillance	• TVS for examining endometrial thickness • Endometrial biopsy

(PCOS: polycystic ovary syndrome; TVS: transvaginal sonography)

women with BMI >25,[23] hypothesized due to increased androgen exposure.[22]

- *Other malignancy:* Some studies have shown higher prevalence of kidney, colon, and brain cancers among women with PCOS.[22]
- *Metabolic syndrome*: A combination of disorders like abdominal obesity, insulin resistance, impaired glucose tolerance (IGT), HT, and dyslipidemia which increases risk of type 2 diabetes mellitus (T2DM), CVD, and endometrial cancer. Higher prevalence of metabolic syndrome is seen in women with PCOS than in the general women of similar age **(Flowchart 1).**[24]

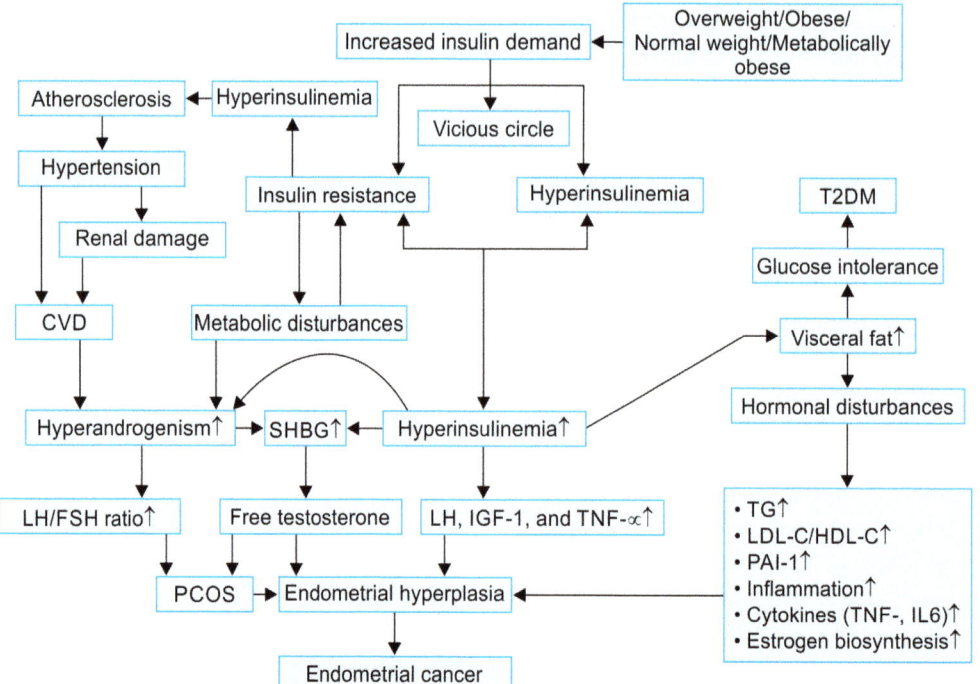

Flowchart 1: Association of polycystic ovary syndrome with metabolic syndrome and other long-term consequences.

(CVD: cardiovascular disease; FSH: follicle-stimulating hormone; HDL-C: high-density lipoprotein cholesterol; IL: interleukin; IGF-I: insulin like growth factor-I; LH: luteinizing hormone; LDL-C: low-density lipoprotein cholesterol; PAI-1: plasminogen activator inhibitor-1; PCOS: polycystic ovary syndrome; SHBG: sex hormone-binding globulin; T2DM: type 2 diabetes mellitus; TNF: tumor necrosis factor)

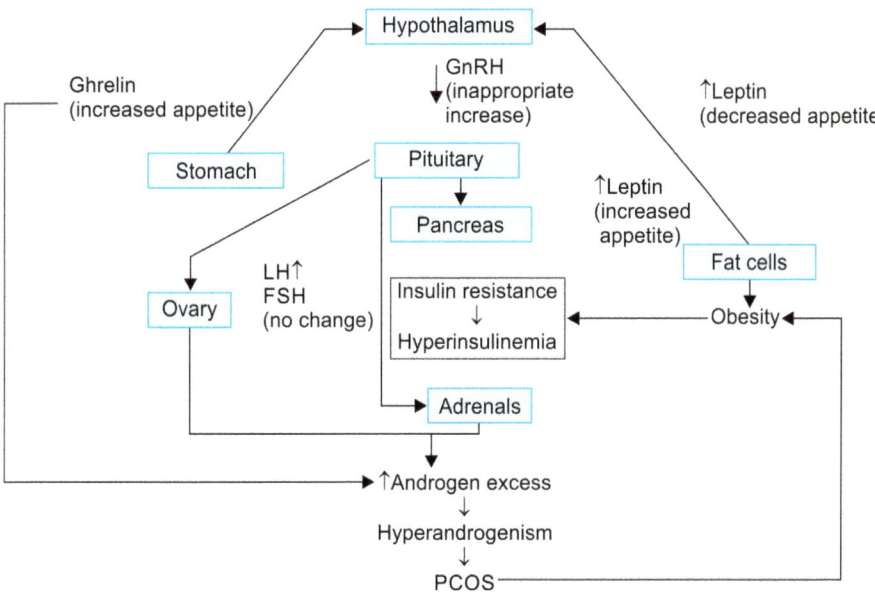

Flowchart 2: Obesity and polycystic ovary syndrome.

(FSH: follicle-stimulating hormone; GnRH: gonadotropin-releasing hormone; LH: luteinizing hormone; PCOS: polycystic ovary syndrome)

- *Obesity:* PCOS and obesity has a bidirectional relationship as women with PCOS are more inclined to weight gain and excess weight gain increases PCOS prevalence.[25] Obesity and metabolic syndrome are also correlated **(Flowchart 2)**.
- *Dyslipidemia:* Represented by hypertriglyceridemia and low HDL cholesterol levels and small dense LDL cholesterol particles are typically seen in women with PCOS postulated to be due to insulin resistance **(Fig. 2)**.
- *T2DM:* PCOS is an independent risk factor for development of glucose intolerance followed by T2DM,[26] according to level A evidence attributed by the European Society for Human Reproduction and Embryology (ESHRE)/American Society for Reproductive Medicine (ASRM) statement of the third PCOS consensus workshop group.

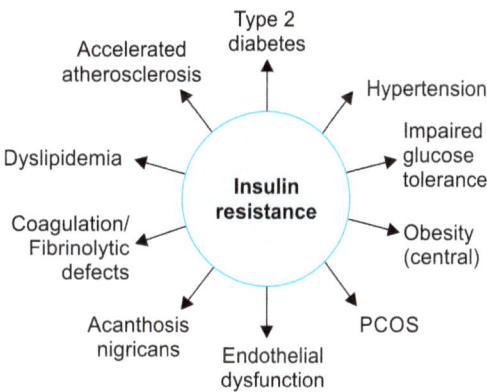

Fig. 2: Insulin resistance.
(PCOS: polycystic ovary syndrome)

The likelihood of developing T2DM increased as BMI, fasting blood sugar levels increased and decreased as sex hormone-binding globulin (SHBG) levels increased.[27]

- *Nonalcoholic fatty liver disease (NAFLD):* NAFLD prevalence is increased in women with PCOS.[28] NAFLD is a chronic liver disease extending from fatty infiltration to end stage liver disease. Women with premenopausal NAFLD are diagnosed with PCOS. Androgen excess and insulin resistance found in PCOS may be the contributing factor.

- *CVD:* Women with PCOS are at increased risk for CVD, classic risk factors for CVD like HT, dyslipidemia, diabetes, and obesity along with nonclassic risk factors like C-reactive protein (CRP), homocysteine, and tumor necrosis factor alpha are seen in women with PCOS.[29]

Women with hyperandrogenic PCOS have a bad cardiometabolic profile with high prevalence for CVD risk factors as compared to women with nonhyperandrogenic PCOS.[30,31]

- *Mental health:* Women with PCOS carry higher risk of developing depression, anxiety, low self-esteem, negative body image, and psychosexual dysfunction.[32] Long-term health-related concerns compromise the quality of life (QoL) and adversely affect mood and psychological wellbeing.[33] High prevalence of eating disorders is also seen in women with PCOS.
- *Disturbed sleep patterns:* PCOS women are more likely to suffer from sleep disordered breathing like obstructive sleep apnea and excessive daytime sleepiness **(Flowchart 3)**.

MANAGEMENT

Polycystic ovary syndrome is associated with long-term health consequences **(Fig. 3)**. Peri- and postmenopausal screening of these women helps to identify risk factors early and hence treated promptly.

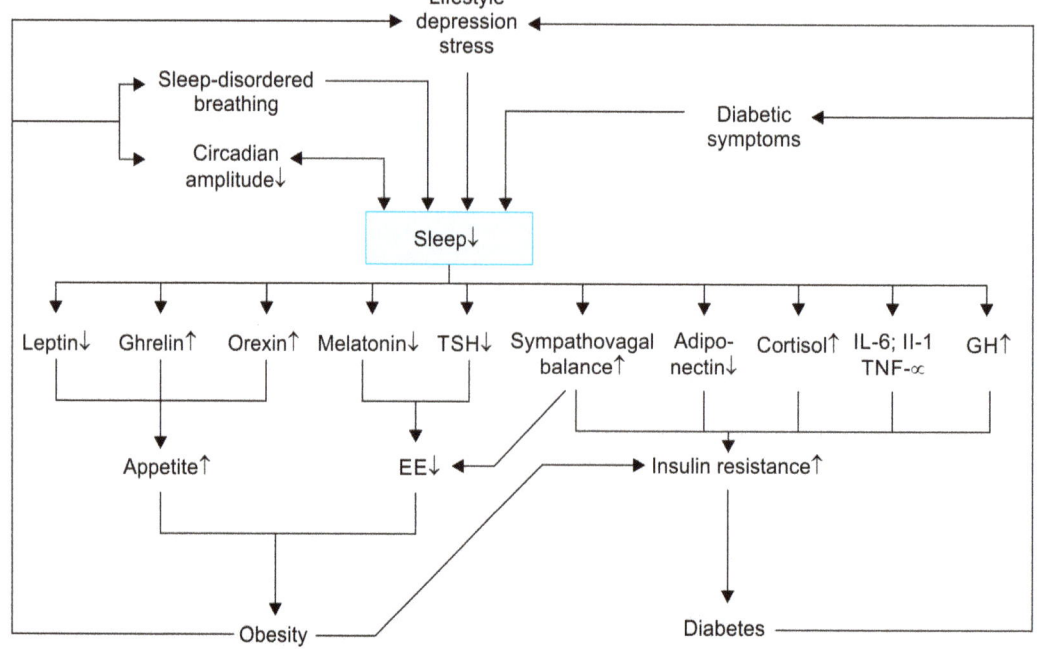

Flowchart 3: Disturbed sleep patterns: A cause of metabolic disorder in women with polycystic ovary syndrome.

(EE: ethinylestradiol; GH: growth hormone; IL: interleukin; OSA: obstructive sleep apnea; TSH: thyroid-stimulating hormone; TNF: tumor necrosis factor)

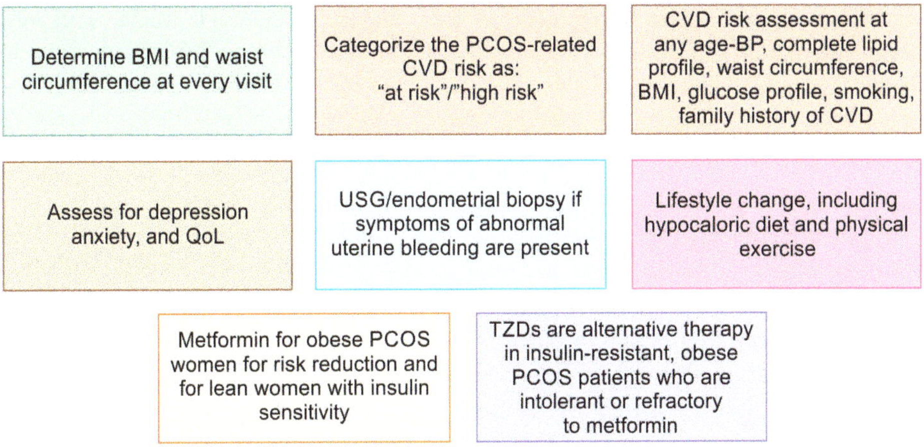

Fig. 3: Management of long-term health consequences of PCOS.
(BMI: body mass index; BP: blood pressure; CVD: cardiovascular disease; PCOS: polycystic ovary syndrome; QoL: quality of life; TZDs: thiazolidinedione; USG: ultrasound)

Few recommendations to be followed are:
- BMI and waist circumference should be measured at every visit and lifestyle modifications discussed.
- Periodic CVD risk assessment and reassessment as age advances. CVD risk assessment by blood pressure (BP), complete lipid profile, waist circumference, BMI, glucose profile, history of cigarette smoking, and family history of early CVD.
- "At risk" for PCOS women with risk factors like obesity, cigarette smoking, HT, dyslipidemia, subclinical vascular disease, IGT, metabolic syndrome and\ or T2DM, overt vascular and renal disease should be identified.
- Invasive and noninvasive tests may be used to assess endothelial function like carotid intima media thickness (CIMT) and coronary artery calcification (CAC) scores for CVD surveillance.
- PCOS women particularly in peri- and postmenopausal phase should be assessed for mental health like depression, anxiety, and QoL. Holistic management is required, experts from the field should be involved in management.
- Psychological treatment is recommended for eating disorders and continuous positive airway pressure (CPAP) for obstructive sleep apnea particularly in obese women.
- Transvaginal sonography (TVS) or endometrial biopsy should be done for screening of endometrial cancer. Borderline ovarian tumors can be detected on USG.
- Lifestyle changes in form of hypocaloric diet and physical exercise to be considered for management of peri- and postmenopausal PCOS women particularly with obesity. Same advice is offered for women with NAFLD.
- Insulin sensitizing agents may be considered, if need arises but lifestyle modification is the first-line therapy in PCOS women with metabolic risks.[34] Metformin is considered for prevention of diabetes in women with PCOS and IGT when lifestyle modification is not successful and/or as an adjuvant to general lifestyle modification. Thiazolidinediones can be considered as an alternative therapy in insulin resistant, obese PCOS

women who are intolerant or refractory to metformin or in PCOS women with severe insulin resistance due to genetic disorder.

■ CONCLUSION

Polycystic ovary syndrome is associated with long-term health consequences. Obesity and insulin resistance are the major pathologic factors. Screening peri- and postmenopausal women with PCOS for identifying risk factors and promptly treating these health issues is important. Lifestyle modification is the cornerstone. Awareness programs for the same should be conducted. Multidisciplinary approach is recommended for these women.

■ REFERENCES

1. Vassilatou E. Nonalcoholic fatty liver disease and polycystic ovary syndrome. World J Gastroenterol. 2014;20(26):8351-63.
2. Wild RA. Long-term health consequences of PCOS. Hum Reprod Update. 2002;8(3): 231-41.
3. Azziz R, Carmina E, Chen Z, Dunaif A, Laven JS, Legro RS, et al. Polycystic ovary syndrome. Nat Rev Dis Primers. 2016;11:16057.
4. Burger HG, Hale GE, Dennerstein L, Robertson DM. Cycle and hormone changes during perimenopause: The key role of ovarian function. Menopause. 2008;15(4 Pt 1):603-12.
5. Piltonen T, Koivunen R, Ruokonen A, Tapanainen JS. Ovarian age-related responsiveness to human chorionic gonadotropin. J Clin Endocrinol Metab. 2003;88:3327-32.
6. Piltonen T, Koivunen R, Perheentupa A, Morin-Papunen L, Ruokonen A, Tapanainen JS. Ovarian age-related responsiveness to human chorionic gonadotropin in women with polycystic ovary syndrome. J Clin Endocrinol Metab. 2004;89:3769-75.
7. Erhmann DA. Polycystic ovary syndrome. N Engl J Med. 2005;352:1223-36.
8. Puurunen J, Piltonen T, Jaakkola P, Ruokonen A, Morin-Papunen L, Tapanainen JS. Adrenal androgen production capacity remains high up to menopause in women with polycystic ovary syndrome. J Clin Endocrinol Metab. 2009;94:1973-8.
9. Legro RS, Kunselman AR, Dunaif A. Prevalence and predictors of dyslipidemia in women with polycystic ovary syndrome. Am J Med. 2001;111:607-13.
10. Chen MJ, Yang WS, Yang JH, Chen CL, Ho HN, Yang YS. Relationship between androgen levels and blood pressure in young women with polycystic ovary syndrome. Hypertension. 2007;49:1442-7.
11. Orio F Jr, Palomba S, Cascella T, Di Biase S, Manguso F, Tauchmanovà L, et al. The increase of leukocytes as a new putative marker of low-grade chronic inflammation and early cardiovascular risk in polycystic ovary syndrome. J Clin Endocrinol Metab. 2005;90:2-5.
12. Palomba S, Santagni S, Falbo A, et al. Complications and challenges associated with polycystic ovary syndrome: current perspectives. Int J Womens Health. 2015;7: 745-763.
13. Tehrani FR, Solaymani-Dodaran M, Hedayati M, Azizi F. Is polycystic ovary syndrome an exception for reproductive aging? Hum Reprod. 2010;25:1775-81.
14. Minooee S, Ramezani Tehrani F, Rahmati M, Mansournia MA, Azizi F. Prediction of age at menopause in women with polycystic ovary syndrome. Climacteric. 2018;21:29-34.
15. Forslund M, Landin-Wilhelmsen K, Schmidt J, Brännström M, Trimpou P, Dahlgren E. Higher menopausal age but no differences in parity in women with polycystic ovary syndrome compared with controls. Acta Obstet Gynecol Scand. 2019;98:320-6.
16. Puurunen J, Piltonen T, Morin-Papunen L, Perheentupa A, Järvelä I, Ruokonen A, et al. Unfavorable hormonal, metabolic, and inflammatory alterations persist after menopause in women with PCOS. J Clin Endocrinol Metab. 2011;96:1827-34.
17. Alsamarai S, Adams JM, Murphy MK, Post MD, Hayden DL, Hall JE, et al. Criteria for polycystic ovarian morphology in polycystic ovary syndrome as a function of age. J Clin Endocrinol Metab. 2009;94:4961-70.

18. Schmidt J, Brännström M, Landin Wilhelmsen K, Dahlgren E. Reproductive hormone levels and anthropometry in postmenopausal women with polycystic ovary syndrome (PCOS): A 21-year follow-up study of women diagnosed with PCOS around 50 years ago and their age-matched controls. J Clin Endocrinol Metab. 2011;96:2178-85.
19. Krentz AJ, von Mühlen D, Barrett-Connor E. Searching for polycystic ovary syndrome in postmenopausal women: Evidence of a dose-effect association with prevalent cardiovascular disease. Menopause. 2007;14:284-92.
20. Carmina E, Campagna AM, Lobo RA. A 20-year follow-up of young women with polycystic ovary syndrome. Obstet Gynecol. 2012;119:263-9.
21. Pasquali R, Gambineri A, Anconetani B, Vicennati V, Colitta D, Caramelli E, et al. The natural history of the metabolic syndrome in young women with the polycystic ovary syndrome and the effect of long-term oestrogen-progestogen treatment. Clin Endocrinol (Oxf) 1999;50:517-27.
22. Harris HR and Terry KL. Polycystic ovary syndrome and risk of endometrial, ovarian, and breast cancer: a systematic review. Fertil Res Pract. 2016; 2:14.
23. Harris H, Titus L and Cramer D. Long and irregular menstrual cycles, polycystic ovary syndrome, and ovarian cancer risk in a population-based case–control study. Int J Cancer. 2017;140(2):285-91.
24. Carmina E, Napoli N, Longo RA, et al. Metabolic syndrome in polycystic ovary syndrome (PCOS): lower prevalence in southern Italy than in the USA and the influence of criteria for the diagnosis of PCOS. Eur J Endocrinol. 2006;154:141-5.
25. Teede HJ, Joham AE, Paul E, et al. Longitudinal weight gain in women identified with polycystic ovary syndrome: results of an observational study in young women. Obesity. 2013;21(8):1526–32.
26. Fauser BC, Tarlatzis BC, Rebar RW, et al. Consensus on women's health aspects of polycystic ovary syndrome (PCOS): the Amsterdam ESHRE/ASRM-Sponsored 3rd PCOS Consensus Workshop Group. Fertil Steril. 2012;97(1):28-38.
27. Gambineri A, Patton L, Altieri P, et al. Polycystic ovary syndrome is a risk factor for type 2 diabetes: results from a long-term prospective study. Diabetes. 2012;61(9): 2369-2374.
28. Bedogni G, Miglioli L, Masutti F, et al. Prevalence of and risk factors for nonalcoholic fatty liver disease: the dionysos nutrition and liver study. Hepatology. 2005;42:44-52.
29. Toulis KA, Goulis DG, Mintziori G, et al. Meta-analysis of cardiovascular disease risk markers in women with polycystic ovary syndrome. Hum Reprod Update. 2011; 17(6):741-60.
30. Fauser BC, Tarlatzis BC, Rebar RW, et al. Consensus on women's health aspects of polycystic ovary syndrome (PCOS): the Amsterdam ESHRE/ASRM-Sponsored 3 PCOS Consensus Workshop Group. Fertil Steril. 2012;97(1):28-38.
31. Daan NM, Louwers YV, Koster MP, et al. Cardiovascular and metabolic profiles amongst different polycystic ovary syndrome phenotypes: who is really at risk? Fertil Steril. 2014;102(5):1444-1451.
32. Deeks A, Gibson-Helm M, Teede H. Anxiety and depression in polycystic ovary syndrome (PCOS): a comprehensive investigation. Fertil Steril. 2010;93:2421-23.
33. Teede H, Deeks A, and Moran L. Polycystic ovary syndrome: a complex condition with psychological, reproductive and metabolic manifestations that impacts on health across the lifespan. BMC Med. 2010;8:41.
34. Knowler WC, Barrett-Connor E, Fowler SE, et al. Diabetes Prevention Program Research Group Reduction in the incidence of type 2 diabetes with lifestyle intervention or metformin. N Engl J Med. 2002;346(6):393-403.

CHAPTER 18

Cancer in PCOS

Sarita Kumari, Neerja Bhatla

■ INTRODUCTION

Polycystic ovary syndrome (PCOS) is a complex reproductive, endocrine, and metabolic disorder that affects 5-15% of women worldwide.[1] Its pathological profile includes, variably, hyperandrogenism, ovulatory dysfunction, polycystic ovarian morphology, and is often accompanied by insulin resistance and obesity. Speert in 1984 noted a recurrent presence of cystic ovaries in young women (<40 years old) with endometrial cancer (EC).[2] Given the widespread distribution of this disorder and the modifiable metabolic profile, determination of the gynecological oncological risk in this population is important for early detection and establishing preventive measures.

■ BREAST CANCER

In 2009, Chittenden et al. published the first systematic review of available literature to determine the risk of developing gynecological cancers in women with PCOS. The aggregated data of three studies with 23,842 women failed to determine an elevated risk of breast cancer (BC) in women with PCOS.[3] Three further meta-analysis also failed to demonstrate an association.[4-6]

The Danish National Patient Register was used to identify 12,070 women in whom PCOS was diagnosed when they of age 9-49 years during 1977-2012. These women were followed till 2012, but did not have a higher incidence of BC than the general Danish population.[7] Similarly, a cohort of 14,764 women aged 15-50 years between 1985 and 2009 determined from a Swedish register found the adjusted hazard ratio (aHR) between PCOS and BC as 0.85 [95% confidence interval (CI) 0.64-1.13], suggesting no association.[8] Another large cohort study of 8,155 women with PCOS from Taiwan also failed to demonstrate any association.[9] A possible cofounding factor is the widespread use of oral contraceptive pills for women with PCOS to control menstrual irregularities. Oral contraceptives, although protective for endometrial and ovarian cancer (OC), may result in a small short-term increase in BC risk in current or recent users of approximately one extra BC for every 7,690 women using hormonal contraception for 1 year.[10] However, 10 years after cessation of use the risk of BC returns to the same risk as those who had never used oral contraceptives.[11]

■ ENDOMETRIAL CANCER

Hyperandrogenism, insulin resistance, and the inflammatory state characteristic of PCOS contribute to endometrial hyperplasia and dysplasia. Hyperandrogenism leads to generation of reactive oxygen species, dysregulates cell death, and leads to endometrial hyperplasia. Insulin resistance also contributes to endometrial inflammation and progesterone resistance. Anovulation results in long periods of unexposed estrogen exposure.[12]

Way back in 2010, Fearnley et al. found a fourfold increased risk of EC in women aged under 50 with PCOS, in a case control study (156 cases, 398 controls) in Australia [odds ratio (OR) 4.0, 95% CI 1.7-9.3].[13] This risk was diminished when adjusted for body mass index (OR 2.2, 95% CI 0.9-5.7) and was slightly greater when restricted to type I cancers.

In view of a lack of clarity in the published literature at that point of time, Haoula et al. performed a systematic review to determine the exact strength of association between PCOS and EC. 14 comparative and noncomparative data suggested that women with PCOS were more likely to develop EC. Five comparative studies suggested an OR of 2.89 (95% CI 1.52-5.48).[14] In the Danish cohort of 12,070 women, there was a fourfold increased risk for EC [N = 16, standardized incidence ratio (SIR) = 3.9; 95% CI = 2.2-6.3], and the large majority of cases being type 1 (N = 14, SIR = 4.7; 95% CI = 2.6-7.9).[7] Subsequently, an increased risk of EC was also described in the Swedish cohort study (HR 2.62; 95% CI 1.58-4.35).[8] A similar cohort study in women from Taiwan detected EC in 11 patients (11/8,155) of the PCOS cohort compared to three patients (3/32,620) in the comparison group (aHR = 17.7, 95% CI = 4.9-64.2). Patients with PCOS had a significantly higher risk of EC in the first 5 years of follow-up (aHR = 6.29, 95% CI = 1.02-8.7). The incidence was 49.2/100,000 person-years between 5 and 10 years of follow-up and after >10 years, no statistically significant difference in the incidence of EC was observed between the groups.[9] This is depicted in **Figure 1**.

Several studies report an association with PCOS and EC, however, overlapping risk factors such as obesity, diabetes, and nulliparity must be taken into account.

OVARIAN CANCER

The link between PCOS and OC has not been consistent. The Danish registry study has reported a nonsignificant increase in OC (SIR = 1.8; 95% CI = 0.8-3.2), but this finding is limited by small numbers (only 10 cases of OC). The Swedish cohort reported an increased probability (HR = 2.16; 95% CI = 1.30-3.59).[8] The Taiwan cohort study did not demonstrate an increased risk.[9] In the New England Case-Control (NECC) study of OC, 2,041 women with epithelial OC and 2,100 controls were retrospectively reviewed for history of irregular menstrual cycles, cycle length >35 days or self-reported PCOS. Logistic regression analysis revealed no difference in the OC risk in women who reported irregular or prolonged cycles or a diagnosis of PCOS.[15]

OTHERS

In the Swedish cohort, PCOS was positively associated with an increased overall cancer risk (fully aHR 1.15; 95% CI 1.00-1.33). Excess cancer risks other than endometrium and ovary were as follows: endocrine gland (HR 1.92; 95% CI 1.21-3.06), pancreas (HR 3.40; 95% CI 1.41-8.20), kidney (HR 3.07; 95% CI 1.27-7.39), and skeletal and hematopoietic system (HR 1.69; 95% CI 1.05-2.72).[8] The Danish registry also reported a higher risk of kidney, colon, and brain cancer but without adjusting for confounding factors.[7]

CONCLUSION

The link between PCOS and gynecological cancer is debatable because of the heterogenicity of studies published till date, the varying definitions used to diagnose this syndrome and the clinical overlap with other risk factors such as hyperandrogenism, obesity, and diabetes. There is little to no data

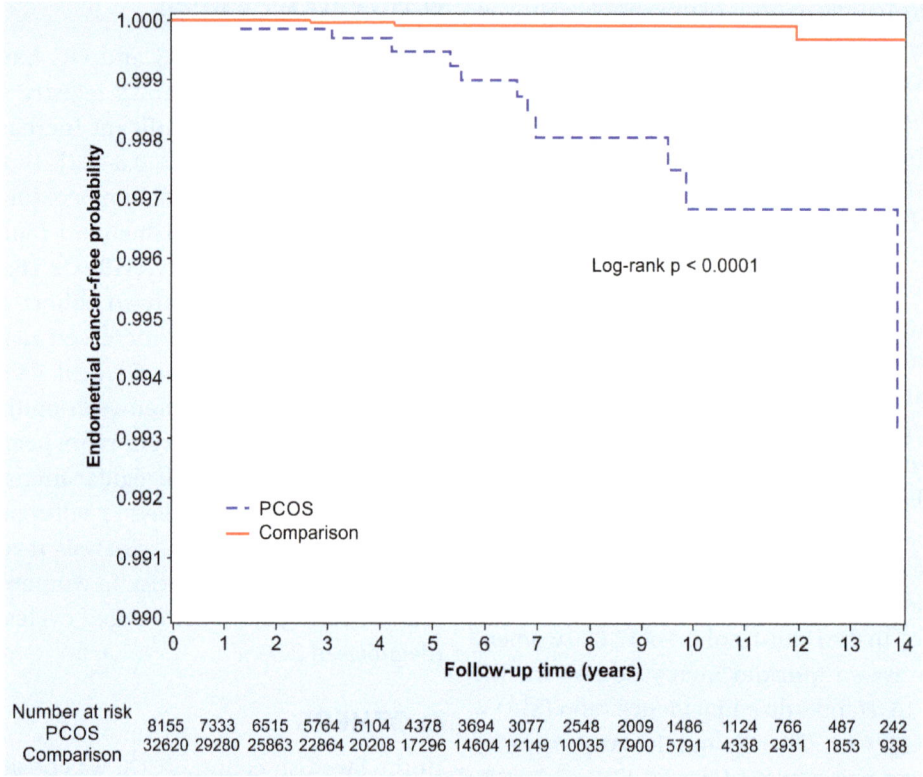

Fig. 1: Comparison of Kaplan–Meier survival estimates for endometrial cancer in women with and without polycystic ovary syndrome (PCOS).
Source: Ding DC, Chen W, Wang JH, Lin SZ. Association between polycystic ovarian syndrome and endometrial, ovarian, and breast cancer: A population-based cohort study in Taiwan. Medicine. 2018;97(39):e12608.

TABLE 1: Summary of studies on the risk of gynecologic cancers in women with polycystic ovary syndrome.

Author, year of publication	Type of study	Sample size	Findings	Additional comments
Fearnley et al., 2010	Case control	156 cases, 398 controls	Increased risk of EC	Risk reduced after BMI adjustment
Haula et al., 2012	Meta-analysis	5 comparative studies	Increased risk of EC	
Gottschau et al., 2015	Population-based cohort	12,070 Danish women	• Increased risk of EC • No association with BC and OC	Majority cases type 1
Yin et al., 2019	Population-based cohort	14,764 Swedish women	• Increased risk of EC • No association with BC • Increased risk of OC	
Ding et al., 2018	Population-based cohort	8,155	• Increased risk of EC • No association with BC and OC	Highest in first 5 years of follow-up

(BMI: body mass index; BC: breast cancer; EC: endometrial cancer; OC: ovarian cancer)

linking PCOS to cervical or vulvar cancers, till date. However, an increased risk of EC in women with PCOS appears established and as women are often diagnosed at a young age, they constitute an opportunity to implement preventive lifestyle modifications. **Table 1** summarizes the key messages from the published data on the risk of gynecologic cancers in women with PCOS.

■ REFERENCES

1. Azziz R. Introduction: Determinants of polycystic ovary syndrome. Fertil Steril. 2016; 106(1):4-5.
2. Speert H. Carcinoma of the endometrium in young women. Surg Gynecol Obstet. 1949;88(3):332-6.
3. Chittenden B, Fullerton G, Maheshwari A, Bhattacharya S. Polycystic ovary syndrome and the risk of gynaecological cancer: A systematic review. Reprod Biomed Online. 2009;19(3):398-405.
4. Shobeiri F, Jenabi E. The association between polycystic ovary syndrome and breast cancer: A meta-analysis. Obstet Gynecol Sci. 2016;59(5):367.
5. Harris HR, Terry KL. Polycystic ovary syndrome and risk of endometrial, ovarian, and breast cancer: A systematic review. Fertil Res and Pract. 2016;2(1):14.
6. Barry JA, Azizia MM, Hardiman PJ. Risk of endometrial, ovarian and breast cancer in women with polycystic ovary syndrome: A systematic review and meta-analysis. Hum Reprod Update. 2014;20(5):748-58.
7. Gottschau M, Kjaer SK, Jensen A, Munk C, Mellemkjaer L. Risk of cancer among women with polycystic ovary syndrome: A Danish cohort study. Gynecol Oncol. 2015; 136(1):99-103.
8. Yin W, Falconer H, Yin L, Xu L, Ye W. Association between polycystic ovary syndrome and cancer risk. JAMA Oncol. 2019; 5(1):106.
9. Ding DC, Chen W, Wang JH, Lin SZ. Association between polycystic ovarian syndrome and endometrial, ovarian, and breast cancer: A population-based cohort study in Taiwan. Medicine. 2018;97(39): e12608.
10. Mørch LS, Skovlund CW, Hannaford PC, Iversen L, Fielding S, Lidegaard Ø. Contemporary hormonal contraception and the risk of breast cancer. N Engl J Med. 2017;377(23): 2228-39.
11. IARC Working Group on the Evaluation of Carcinogenic Risks to Humans. Combined estrogen-progestogen contraceptives and combined estrogen-progestogen menopausal therapy. IARC Monogr Eval Carcinog Risks Hum. 2007;91:1-528.
12. Xue Z, Li J, Feng J, Han H, Zhao J, Zhang J, et al. Research progress on the mechanism between polycystic ovary syndrome and abnormal endometrium. Front Physiol. 2021; 12:788772.
13. Fearnley EJ, Marquart L, Spurdle AB, Weinstein P, Webb PM; Australian Ovarian Cancer Study Group and Australian National Endometrial Cancer Study Group. Polycystic ovary syndrome increases the risk of endometrial cancer in women aged less than 50 years: An Australian case-control study. Cancer Causes Control. 2010;21(12):2303-8.
14. Haoula Z, Salman M, Atiomo W. Evaluating the association between endometrial cancer and polycystic ovary syndrome. Hum Reprod. 2012;27(5):1327-31.
15. Harris HR, Titus LJ, Cramer DW, Terry KL. Long and irregular menstrual cycles, polycystic ovary syndrome, and ovarian cancer risk in a population-based case-control study: Menstrual cycle, PCOS, and ovarian cancer. Int J Cancer. 2017;140(2): 285-91.

CHAPTER 19

Lifestyle Interventions in PCOS

Prerna Keshan

INTRODUCTION

In the modern era, the most common metabolic and reproductive endemic comes by the name polycystic ovary syndrome (PCOS). The endocrinal complexity of this syndrome makes it very widely researched. Not being a disease to be cured but being a disorder to be rectified, a lot needs to be said and emphasized about lifestyle management in this otherwise distressing syndrome proper. The hypothalamic-pituitary-ovarian (HPO) axis of the reproductive cycle is disrupted leading to anovulation, infertility, and more so obesity. Here comes the role of exercise, diet, and lifestyle[1] modification (LSM) to combat the adverse effects on reproductive functions and to aid medical therapy for PCOS.

WHAT DIET?

A lot has been discussed over years for a stipulated diet[2] for PCOS. The PCOS manifestations can up to a wide extent be taken care of with a sustainable form of dietary changes that targets the impaired insulin sensitivity of PCOS. Definitely diet only cannot fix all the symptoms of PCOS, but it provides relief to a great extent in improving menstrual cycle length and ovulation frequency. No specific dietary routine can be considered the best in PCOS, but exclusion of processed refined food and inclusion of natural alternatives should be sought for.

A proper diet is one that has a favorable effect on the lipids and insulin intake of these women and improves the insulin sensitivity which is the crux of the entire pathophysiology of PCOS. Proper diet implies balanced and nutritious diet comprising of complex carbohydrates, proteins, and limited intake of fat. The mantra towards rescue from PCOS is not fad dieting or starving on calories but maintenance of nourishment and enjoyable diet pattern which is not distressing and can be gradually incorporated into lifestyle.

Diet should include a combination of the following:

- *Dietary fiber:* Increase in dietary fiber improves insulin sensitivity and hence helps fight PCOS naturally. 21–25 g of fiber should be included in daily diet for better clinical outcomes. High fiber containing foods are:
  - Beans
  - Lentils
  - Berries
  - Broccoli
  - Green peas
  - Chia seeds
  - Nuts like almonds and pistachios
- *Food stuff that reduces inflammation:* An ongoing silent inflammation takes place in PCOS patients which aggravates the production of androgenic hormones and further escalates the PCOS pathophysiology. Hence anti-inflammatory food items

help combat this excess androgenic effects and improves reproductive outcomes. Some food items of this category are:
- Tomatoes
- Green leafy vegetables like kale and spinach
- Fish with high fatty acid content like salmon, sardines, and mackerel
- Nuts like almonds and walnuts
- Olive oil

- *Whole grains:* Recommendation of balanced diet including whole grains as carbohydrates has a lot of added advantages over refined carbohydrates like maintenance of the glycemic index. This category may include whole grain cereal, bread oatmeal, brown rice, and wheat pasta.
- *Fatty acids:* 30% of calories should be consumed as fats. Saturated fats should be abstained from as they may end up in nutrient malabsorption. Oil and food enriched with vitamin E are a good dietary source toward maintaining insulin sensitivity. Low-fat milk and yoghurt should be preferred over whole milk.
- *Lean protein:* About 30% of the calories should come from lean protein.

PROPORTION OF CARBOHYDRATES IN POLYCYSTIC OVARY SYNDROME

- Simple or refined carbohydrates as in junk food and sugary beverages, fried snacks, or bakery stuff should be avoided, as these food stuff impair the glycemic index and adversely affects insulin sensitivity.
- *Complex carbohydrates:* 30–40% of calories should come from complex carbohydrates like whole grains, fruits like apple, peach, orange, sweet lime, pomegranate, and vegetables like carrot, lettuce, celery, cucumber, and legume that are fiber rich and also have a very low-glycemic index.

The carbohydrate intake should be spread through the day aiming to three meals with 45 g carbohydrates and two to three nutritious snacks including 15–20 g carbohydrates in each.

DIET CHART—LOW FAT, ADEQUATE PROTEIN, HIGH FIBER DIET

Recommended meal plan: 1,500 kcal diet

Time	Menu
Early morning (7 am)	Green tea 1 cup without sugar + soaked almonds four to five in number
Breakfast (8 am)	• *Besan Chilla*—2 (made without oil) with roasted *Bengal gram dhal* or onion *chutney* or tomato or ginger *chutney* 2 tablespoon OR • Vegetable *poha*—1 *katori* with *pudina chutney* + boiled/poached egg white—2 OR • Oats/oat bran/muesli any other whole cereal—10 g (made with 150 mL toned milk, with a pinch of cinnamon and assorted cut fruits (100 g), no sugar + boiled/poached egg whites—2
Midmorning (11 am)	Fruits: guava—1 OR peeled apple—1 OR pomegranate seeds/papaya/kiwi—1 *katori* (100 g) and nuts (almonds—10 + walnut—1 + tablespoon of flax seeds)
Lunch (1 pm)	Boiled vegetable salad cucumber, carrot, lettuce, tomato, etc. 1 *katori* AND rice/brown rice/quinoa—1 *katoris* AND *dal* with vegetables or greens—1 *katori* (made with 30 g) OR steamed fish/fish curry—75 g AND vegetable curry—1 *katori* (gravy and not fried and no roots and tubers like potatoes can be mixed vegetable curry (100 g) AND toned milk curd/yoghurt—1 cup (100 mL milk)

Contd...

Contd...

Time	Menu
Evening (4 pm)	Green tea—1 cup without sugar
Evening (5 pm)	Fruit—1 any from above OR plain flaked rice—1 small cup OR plain puffed rice—1 small cup with roasted Bengal gram OR *bhelpuri/muri* with sprouts—1 *katori*
Dinner (8 pm)	Boiled vegetable salad cucumber, carrot, tomatoes, etc. 1 *katori* AND boiled broken wheat/millet (*dalia*)/rice—1 *katori* AND vegetable curry—1 *katori* (gravy and not fried) AND skimmed/toned milk curd/yoghurt—1 cup (100 mL)
Bed time (10 pm)	Thin buttermilk—1 cup

Note:
- Low-fat *paneer*/chicken/fish/tofu can be included in the diet at least three to four times in a week, if preferable prepared with less oil, not fried and eat only pieces.
- 1 *phulka* and 1 cup of rice are prepared from 30 g of whole wheat flour or raw rice.
- Dal (30 g) can be made with red gram or green gram/*kabuli channa, lobia*, kidney beans.

MEASUREMENT

1 teaspoon (level)	4 g/5 mL
1 tablespoon (level)	14 g/15 mL
Glass	250 mL
Cup (medium size)	180–200 mL
Bowl/*katori* (medium size)	150–160 mL/200 g (cooked)

EXERCISES TARGETED TOWARD POLYCYSTIC OVARY SYNDROME

It is of paramount importance that diet has to stipulated as per the physical activity of the person. Exercise improves the glycemic index by improving insulin sensitivity and can help in managing weight of the individual. Now, it is very important to understand that we need not revert to army style exercise maneuvers to build an impact on our physique, rather we need to have a gradual and sustainable form of exercise that is equally goal attainable and enjoyable at the same time.

The crux of the entire exercise pattern should be a sense of wellbeing and not amounting to physical and mental strain under any circumstances. The various modes of exercise can be:

- *Mind:* Body exercises[3] like yoga, tai chi, qi gong, and pilates for peace of mind and soul as well as wellness of the body, it improves ovulation, imparts positive mental health, allays anxiety, depression, and also improves the basic metabolic parameters like lipid profile and insulin resistance (IR). Recommended for both adolescent as well as adult PCOS.
- *Conventional physical activity/steady state cardiovascular workouts:* Aerobic exercise like brisk walking, jogging, swimming, dancing, cycling, etc. In these workouts the heart pumps to around 70% of the maximum cardiac rate. Exercise of moderate intensity has a definite impact on the pattern of ovulation and whether the frequency, type, or length of exercise duration has variable impacts and needs to be further established with larger randomized control trials.
- *Resistance training:* Exercises that improves muscle strength and endurance are sit ups, push-ups, leg squats, lunges, jumping jacks, bicep curls, crunches, and weight lifting. Moderate exercise 30 minutes a day improves reproductive and metabolic symptoms.

- *Interval training*: Exercise in this pattern is done at different intensity without reaching the maximum heart rate.
- *High-intensity interval training (HIIT)*:[4] Vigorous exercise has the maximum impact when it comes to body mass index (BMI), recommended 120 minutes of vigorous intensity exercise including balancing intense exercise burst with rest intervals. Exercise in this category includes burpees, tuck jumps, and mountain climbers. This is usually recommended for obese adult PCOS.

Whatever be the exercise pattern,[5] it is at times very difficult to burn the stubborn fat in PCOS clients. For this, it is well established that even a negligible around 7–10% of weight[6] loss is significant in improving the symptom profile. Now, even if this negligible percentage is not attained, it is worth mentioning that exercise still has a positive impact on the pathophysiology of PCOS.

Best exercise is the one that is done daily.
- When to start what:
  - If someone is sedentary, start gradually.
  - If someone has started exercising, doing it for three times a week at least improves symptoms.
  - If someone is exercising regularly, following a certified physical trainer from an accredited organization is recommended.

STUDIES SUPPORTING LIFESTYLE MODIFICATION FOR POLYCYSTIC OVARY SYNDROME

Studies supporting LSM for PCOS are as follows:
- *Cochrane database:* Lifestyle changes in women with polycystic ovary syndrome—siew selim Samantha k Hutchison and Cochrane gynecology and fertility group[7]
- *LSM and PCOS:* The role of lifestyle modification in polycystic ovary syndrome—front endocrinology 13 Aug 2022, sec reproduction[8]
- *LSM and PCOS:* Lifestyle modification programs in polycystic ovary syndrome: systematic review and meta-analysis, journal of clinical endocrinology and metabolism.[9]

EFFECTS OF LIFESTYLE MODIFICATION ON MENSES, INSULIN RESISTANCE AND ANTHROPOMETRY

Effects of LSM on menses, IR, and anthropometry are as follows:
- LSM has long-term impact on all aspects of PCOS worth mentioning menstrual cycle length, glycemic index, and insulin sensitivity as well as BMI.[10]
- Although sudden start of vigorous exercise in an otherwise sedentary woman causes amenorrhea but sustainable form of moderate physical activity has a great deal of positive impact ranging from return of ovulation and regular menstrual cycle pattern with better reproductive[11] outcome.
- Insulin sensitivity improves with diet and lifestyle changes with positive effect on all metabolic parameters including lipid profile.

CONCLUSION

Obesity being a global pandemic now, the best possible results can be obtained by a composite and holistic approach with nutritious diet as discussed earlier and regular physical activity[12] of any form. Body composition especially the fat mass has been associated with worst functional parameters of PCOS. Anthropometric measurement hence give us a fairly reliable idea of the effect of LSM on PCOS and the variability of the symptoms presented with as well as the response behaviour.[13] LSM helps in better anthropometric measurements by reducing the fat mass percentage of these women.

■ REFERENCES

1. Kite C, Lahart IM, Afzal I, Broom DR, Randeva H, Kyrou I, et al. Exercise, or exercise and diet for the management of polycystic ovary syndrome: A systematic review and meta-analysis. Syst Rev. 2019;8(1):51.
2. Dan brennan web Md, editorial contribution, June 08, 2021.
3. Journal of physical exercise for human health.
4. Hiam D, Patten R, Gibson-Helm M, Moreno-Asso A, McIlvenna L, Levinger I, et al. The effectiveness of high intensity intermittent training on metabolic, reproductive and mental health in women with polycystic ovary syndrome: Study protocol for the iHIT-randomised controlled trial. 2019;20:221.
5. Journal of sports medicine.
6. Best practice and research clinical obs and gynae.
7. Lim SS, Hutchison SK, Van Ryswyk E, Norman RJ, Teede HJ, Moran LJ. Lifestyle changes in women with polycystic ovary syndrome. Cochrane Database Syst Rev. 2019;(3):CD007506.
8. Norman RJ, Davies MJ, Lord J, Moran LJ. The role of lifestyle modification in polycystic ovary syndrome. Trends Endocrinol Metab. 2002;13(6):251-7.
9. Domecq JP, Prutsky G, Mullan RJ, Hazem A, Sundaresh V, Elamin MB, et al. Lifestyle modification programs in polycystic ovary syndrome: Systematic review and meta-analysis. J Clin Endocrinol Metab. 2013; 98(12):4655-63.
10. Journal of frontiers of physiology.
11. Ha almenn kiele et al BMJ open 2020.
12. Martin A, Booth JN, Laird Y, Sproule J, Reilly JJ, Saunders DH. Physical activity, diet and other behavioural interventions for improving cognition and school achievement in children and adolescents with obesity or overweight. Cochrane Database Syst Rev. 2018;1(1):CD009728.
13. Woodward A, Klonizakis M, Broom D. Exercise and polycystic ovary syndrome. Adv Exp Med Biol. 2020;1228:123-36.

CHAPTER 20

Medical Management of PCOS

Mousumi Das Ghosh

■ INTRODUCTION

Polycystic ovary syndrome (PCOS) is the most common endocrine disorder in women of reproductive age. It is a life-long condition where lifestyle optimization and pharmacologic measures are used to improve the metabolic and endocrine status and reduce long-term complications. Though the management is based on specific symptoms, a holistic approach should be targeted.

Multidisciplinary team of health professionals cares for women with PCOS which includes endocrinologists, general physicians, psychologists, dieticians, and gynecologists.

The goals of management are:
- To minimize the physical stigmata of hyperandrogenism like acne and hirsutism
- To regularize menstrual cycle to protect against endometrial hyperplasia or carcinoma
- To optimize blood sugar levels and improve metabolic derangements
- To maintain body mass index within reference range
- To improve over-all quality of life and encouraging positive self-image
- To induce ovulation (if anovulation is a cause of subfertility)
- To protect from cardiovascular risks.

For most components of disease, primary treatment is weight loss. This includes healthy and mindful eating, physical activity, and positive mindset. Weight loss improves metabolic parameters, clinical manifestations of androgen excess, and ovulatory dysfunction. Reducing insulin resistance through weight loss is important for reducing long-term cardiovascular risks.

■ MENSTRUAL CYCLES

Hormonal Contraceptives—First-line Pharmacologic Therapy

Menstrual cycle abnormalities require management as oligoovulation, anovulation, and reduced progesterone exposure can all increase the risk of endometrial hyperplasia and malignancy.[1] Hormonal contraceptives are recommended for patients with irregular menstrual cycles and not keen to conceive.[2]

Apart from regulating menstrual cycle, combined oral contraceptive pills (OCPs) also improve features of hyperandrogenism and provide endometrial protection through withdrawal bleeding. These pills also improve menorrhagia and dysmenorrhea, and relieve premenstrual syndrome and pelvic pain related to endometriosis.[3] Long-term use protects against endometrial and ovarian cancer.

Selection of Oral Contraceptive

There is no optimal combined OCP in PCOS. Studies show almost similar efficacy among various oral contraceptives for regulating menstrual cycle or treating hyperandrogenism. The advantages of contraceptive pills outweigh the risks in most patients with PCOS and fertility is restored after discontinuing.[4]

Estrogen component [ethinylestradiol (EE)]:[3,5,6] Actions—suppression of follicle-stimulating hormone (FSH), endometrial stabilization, potentiation of progestin action, suppression of dominant follicle formation, increase in sex hormone-binding globulin, and decrease in free androgen.

Low-dose contraceptive pills (<50 µg) contain EE in doses ranging from 15 to 35 µg.[7] World Health Organization (WHO) also recommends the use of preparations with low dose and natural estrogens and low thromboembolic risk.[1]

Progestin component: Actions—minimize the frequency of gonadotropin-releasing hormone (GnRH) pulses, luteinizing hormone (LH) suppression, inhibition of LH surge, unreceptive endometrium, hostile cervical mucus, decrease in ovarian androgen and estrogen secretion, and increased SHBG concentration.

In menorrhagia, contraceptive pills with first and second generation progestin are preferred. After a few cycles when bleeding is controlled, we can switch over to third and fourth generation OCP.[3] Newer OCPs contain fewer androgenic progestins (such as norethindrone, desogestrel, and norgestimate), and two progestins (cyproterone acetate and drospirenone) function as androgen receptor antagonists. Drospirenone is a spironolactone analog with mineralocorticoid activity; as a result, it has some diuretic property. However, it should not be prescribed to those predisposed to hyperkalemia.[8,9] Drospirenone and dienogest are considered progestins with minimal androgenicity.

Most clinically important risk of oral contraceptive use is venous thromboembolism, especially in obese women. The new third-generation oral contraceptives have approximately twofold increased risk of venous thromboembolism compared with second-generation options. However, absolute risk of venous thrombosis is very small.

It takes a minimum time of 6 months for clinical improvement in acne and hirsutism. After a 6-month trial of oral contraceptive, an antiandrogen drug can be added in combination if there is suboptimal response.

The patients who cannot take estrogen-containing pills can take only progesterone, like:
- Progestin-only pill (smokers, hypertension)
- Progestin-eluting intrauterine device (Mirena)
- To induce withdrawal bleeding (medroxyprogesterone acetate 10 mg daily for 10–14 days, micronized progesterone 400 mg daily for 10–14 days).

Monitoring of Oral Contraceptive Effects

Measure blood pressure 3 months after start of oral contraceptives, then annually thereafter. Measure glucose and lipid profile annually while oral contraceptives are used.

Insulin-sensitizing Medications

Metformin

Metformin increases insulin sensitivity in the liver to reduce gluconeogenesis and hyperinsulinemia. Clinical studies have shown that administration of metformin to PCOS women resulted in decreased androgen levels, increased rates of spontaneous ovulation, and enhanced ovulatory responses to clomiphene. It is used primarily to improve metabolic status in patients whose condition does not respond adequately to lifestyle measures.[10]

Metformin has some efficacy in normalizing ovulatory cyclicity but minimal impact on hirsutism. It does not provide endometrial protection unless normal ovulatory function is restored.

Metformin alone is less effective than clomiphene for ovulation induction, clinical pregnancy, and live birth.

Dosing: Metformin hydrochloride oral tablet can be started 500 mg once in the evening, with a meal, for 1 week. Increase 500 mg a week if tolerates to goal of 1,500 mg or 2,000 mg/day.

Results: Normal menstruation returns in 4–6 months. It also improves lipid profile. When added to clomiphene for infertility, ovulation and clinical pregnancy rates are markedly high compared to clomiphene alone. Weight loss and diet control is recommended to prevent metformin failure in severely obese patients.

Side effects of metformin include gastrointestinal symptoms, which are dose related and tend to resolve after several weeks. A rare adverse effect of metformin therapy is lactic acidosis, which may occur in individuals with systemic and debilitating diseases. Therefore metformin should not be prescribed to patients with renal, hepatic, or major cardiovascular disease.[2]

Monitoring of metformin: Obtain serum creatinine level and estimated glomerular filtration rate (GFR) at least annually in all patients.

Thiazolidinediones—Rosiglitazone and Pioglitazone

This group of drugs improves insulin sensitivity and also decrease androgen levels in women with PCOS. Studies have shown resumption of ovulation following long-term treatment. It should be avoided in patients with liver disease. As fetal safety is not well studied, the medicines should be discontinued in pregnancy.[8]

TREATMENT OPTIONS FOR ACNE AND HIRSUTISM

This depends on patient's request and her degree of distress caused by hirsutism, rather than clinician's quantitative or qualitative assessments.

Hormonal contraceptives are a first-line pharmacologic therapy. The Food and Drug Administration (FDA) approves EE/norgestimate, EE/norethindrone, and EE/drospirenone for the treatment of acne.[3] If these drugs are not effective, we can add antiandrogen drugs (e.g., spironolactone) after 6 months, preferably in combination with an oral contraceptive.

A comprehensive treatment strategy is successful in these women.

Antiandrogens

Primarily used to treat hirsutism (clinical hyperandrogenism), often in combination with an oral contraceptive.[11] With antiandrogens, concurrent contraception is crucial to limit risk of adverse pregnancy outcomes. This group of drugs can cross placenta and disrupt male sexual differentiation in a developing fetus resulting in genital ambiguity.[1,5]

Spironolactone (First-line Antiandrogen for Hirsutism and Acne)

Spironolactone is an aldosterone antagonist that, along with its major metabolite, canrenone, competes for T-binding sites, thereby exerting a direct antiandrogenic effect at the pilosebaceous unit. In addition, spironolactone appears to interfere with cytochrome P450, thereby inhibiting steroid enzyme action and resultant androgen production.[2] It is effective in decreasing degree of hirsutism and, to a lesser extent, acne.

It is a potassium-sparing diuretic. Serum potassium level has to be checked at 2 weeks after starting treatment. It has to be used cautiously if the patient is on any other medications or has a medical condition that may increase potassium.

Spironolactone oral tablet: 50–200 mg/day PO in 1 or 2 divided doses.

Finasteride (Second-line Antiandrogen for Hirsutism)

Finasteride acts by inhibiting 5α-reductase. It decreases local dihydrotestosterone (DHT) levels in hair follicles with comparable effects to other antiandrogens. The effect of finasteride is dose-dependent.[5]

Finasteride oral tablet 2.5–5 mg PO once daily either alone or in combination with oral contraceptives shown to reduce hirsutism in women with mild hirsutism. It has minimal adverse reactions compared to other antiandrogens.

Cyproterone Acetate

Cyproterone acetate is a 17-hydroxyprogesterone acetate derivative with strong progestogenic properties. It is a competitive inhibitor at the androgen receptor.[12] It is available in combination with EE in the form of combined OCPs. At a dose of 2 mg, its effect is equivalent to 50 mg of spironolactone. It has a high risk of venous thromboembolism.

Flutamide

This competes for the androgen receptor and is effective for the treatment of hirsutism. It has many side effects like abdominal discomfort and diarrhea; and methemoglobinemia in those who are susceptible to aniline toxicity or who are smokers. It is of limited value because of its dose-dependent hepatotoxicity.[4]

Monitoring of Antiandrogen Therapy

Monitoring response to treatment can be done objectively using Ferriman–Gallwey system, scoring at baseline and, if possible, at each visit.

Treatment can be continued as long as patient desires and should be discontinued if planning for pregnancy.

Monitoring testosterone levels after instituting pharmacologic therapy is generally unnecessary because hirsutism scores correlate poorly with serum androgen levels.

Other useful pharmacologic therapies can be advised based on symptoms related to hyperandrogenism, like:
- Antibiotics, topical retinoids, or isotretinoin for acne
- Minoxidil topical solution to be applied on area of desired hair growth. Maximum: 2 mL/day
- *Eflornithine for hirsutism*: Topical eflornithine slows growth of unwanted facial hair in 4–8 weeks. Inhibits hair growth (potentially by inhibiting ornithine decarboxylase)
- *Bicalutamide (≤50 mg daily)*: There is emerging data to support the use with oral contraceptives in PCOS.[8]

Nonpharmacologic cosmetic therapies for hirsutism include shaving, depilating, hair bleaching, electrolysis, and laser hair removal.

TREATMENT OPTIONS FOR ANOVULATORY INFERTILITY

Preconception counseling for ideal body weight and blood sugar optimization is crucial. This improves ovulation and live birth rates.

Pharmacotherapy options include clomiphene, aromatase inhibitors, gonadotropins, and metformin. Ovulation induction can be done using either letrozole or clomiphene. Letrozole is superior to clomiphene for achieving pregnancy and live births. Clomiphene is also a first-line drug for ovulation induction because more safety data is available. The live birth rate following 6 months of clomiphene varies from 20% to 40%.[8] Letrozole may be preferred in overweight or obese patients.

Second-line pharmacologic option for infertility is usually ovarian stimulation using low-dose urinary or recombinant gonadotropins. Cumulative 1- and 2-year singleton live birth rates are approximately 50% and 70%, respectively. A low-dose, step-up protocol is generally favored aiming for mono-ovulation, with the ovary very sensitive to exogenous stimulation once a threshold dose has been reached.

For the purpose of treating infertility, metformin alone increases ovulation rate, and use of metformin with clomiphene may offer better responses.

In vitro fertilization (IVF) for women with PCOS alone is recommended as third-line infertility therapy.[1]

Aromatase Inhibitors

Letrozole

Off-label letrozole is a first-line therapy used to achieve pregnancy with live birth for subfertile women with PCOS.[13] Letrozole diminishes hypothalamic estrogen negative feedback and is thought to transiently increase FSH release without depleting estrogen receptors (ERs).[10]

Letrozole oral tablet: 2.5 mg, 5 mg, or 7.5 mg PO once daily on days 3 through 7 of the menstrual cycle may be effective; alternatively, a 20-mg single dose on day 3 of the menstrual cycle has also been studied.

Anastrozole, which is a potent and highly selective aromatase inhibitor, is ineffective for ovulation induction.

Selective Estrogen Receptor Modulators

Clomiphene

Clomiphene citrate is a nonsteroidal, ovulation-inducing ER ligand with mixed agonistic-antagonistic properties. It blocks estrogen negative feedback and cause a prolonged increase in FSH secretion.[12]

Clomiphene citrate oral tablet: Initially 50 mg PO once daily for 5 days. If ovulation does not occur with this dosing regimen, increase to 100 mg PO once daily for 5 days with the next cycle. The incidence rate of multiple pregnancy is 6–10%. If ovulation has not occurred after three courses of treatment, the patient needs reevaluation. If pregnancy does not occur within a total of 6 cycles, discontinue. Prolonged administration of the drug is not recommended.

Gonadotropin Therapy

Typically used for ovulation induction after clomiphene or letrozole. Low-dose gonadotropin therapy aims to achieve a singleton live birth by creating a transient increase in FSH above a threshold dose for selecting a limited number of developing follicles, recognizing that PCOS women are prone to excessive follicle development.[2] Options include urinary gonadotropins or recombinant FSH.

DRUGS TO AID WEIGHT LOSS IN PCOS[14]

Orlistat

It assists in weight loss by inhibiting intestinal fat absorption (inhibits gastric and pancreatic lipases). There are various studies in PCOS obese patients with good results.

Bupropion/Naltrexone

It is a new antiobesity medication which suppresses appetite. Use and safety in PCOS need further studies.

Glucagon-like Peptide-1 (GLP-1) Receptor Agonists

This new group of medication promotes weight loss in PCOS. Liraglutide has been shown to be superior to placebo, as well as to metformin and orlistat in head-to-head comparisons. The efficacy of liraglutide in promoting weight loss in PCOS patients is proven.

Medical management may be needed for other associated problems in PCOS.[15]

- *Dyslipidemia:* Approximately 70% of patients with newly diagnosed disease have abnormal lipid levels, including increased total cholesterol level, high triglyceride levels, high LDL-C level, and decreased HDL-C level.
- *Hypertension:* Women with PCOS have risk of developing hypertension which if untreated may accelerate atherosclerotic cardiovascular disease.
- Nonalcoholic fatty liver disease is frequently seen in patients with PCOS, likely as a result of insulin resistance as well as obesity.
- *Depression and anxiety:* Increased incidence and prevalence over lifetime.

■ SPECIAL POPULATIONS

Adolescents

Diagnosis can be difficult in adolescents owing to overlap between normal pubertal development and characteristic features of PCOS. Suggested criteria include demonstration of chemical and/or biochemical hyperandrogenism and presence of persistent oligomenorrhea for at least 2 years after menarche.[16]

Hormonal Contraceptives

In early adolescence, using hormonal contraceptives is controversial. Ideal hormonal contraceptive regimen and appropriate duration of therapy for adolescents are uncertain. The standard practice is to wait for 2 years after menarche to prevent reduction in peak bone mass.[3]

Metformin Therapy

Small, short-term studies have found that metformin restores menstrual regularity and improves hyperandrogenemia, insulin resistance, and glucose intolerance in obese and nonobese adolescents with PCOS.

Postmenopausal Women

After menopause, two of the key diagnostic criteria of PCOS (irregular menses and polycystic ovaries on transvaginal ultrasonography) are no longer applicable.

Most women who had PCOS during their reproductive years continue to manifest both metabolic phenotype and unfavorable cardiovascular risk factors. Androgen levels are still higher than in postmenopausal women without history of PCOS.

It is advisable to maintain vigilance for monitoring lipid levels, blood pressure, and glycemia in accordance with standards of care in this population of women.

■ CONCLUSION

Polycystic ovary syndrome is a common condition affecting the reproductive, metabolic, and psychological health of a woman. First-line intervention is weight loss. OCPs form the first line of medical management, especially effective in restoring menstrual cycles and hirsutism. Insulin-sensitizing agents like metformin and thiazolidinediones enhance metabolic response and fertility. Antiandrogens are used for hirsutism and acne along with contraceptive pills. For anovulatory infertility, ovulation induction with clomiphene or letrozole forms the mainstay of treatment. Drugs to aid in weight loss are also used in extreme obesity when lifestyle modification fails.

■ REFERENCES

1. Joham AE, Norman RJ, Stener-Victorin E, Legro R, Franks S, Moran L, et al. Review polycystic ovary syndrome. Lancet Diabetes Endocrinol. 2022;10:668-80.
2. Chang RJ, Dumesic DA. Polycystic Ovary Syndrome and Hyperandrogenic States. In: Strauss J, Barbieri R (Eds). Yen and Jaffe's Reproductive Endocrinology. Elsevier; 2018. pp. 520-55.
3. Shah D, Patil M; On behalf of the National PCOS Working Group. Consensus statement on the use of oral contraceptive pills in polycystic ovarian syndrome women in India. J Hum Reprod Sci. 2018;11:96-118.
4. Bates GW, Propst AM. Polycystic ovarian syndrome management options. Obstet Gynecol Clin N Am. 2012;39(4):495-506.
5. Sharma A, Welt CK. Practical approach to hyperandrogenism in women. Med Clin N Am. 2021;105:1099-16.
6. Nader S, Diamanti-Kandarakis E. Polycystic ovary syndrome, oral contraceptives and metabolic issues: New perspectives and a unifying hypothesis. Hum Reprod. 2007; 22:317-22.
7. Shinkai K, Abudu B. Treatment of skin diseases; Polycystic ovary syndrome. 195-96.
8. Wu CQ, Grandi SM, Filion KB, Abenhaim HA, Joseph L, Eisenberg MJ, et al. Drospirenone-containing oral contraceptive pills and the risk of venous and arterial thrombosis: A systematic review. BJOG. 2013;120:801-10.
9. Badawy A, Elnashar A. Treatment options for polycystic ovary syndrome review. Int J Women's Health. 2011;3:25-35.
10. Harborne L, Fleming R, Lyall H, Sattar N, Norman J. Metformin or antiandrogen in the treatment of hirsutism in polycystic ovary syndrome. J Clin Endocrinol Metab. 2003;88:4116-23.
11. Benjamins LJ, Barratt MS. Practice Guidelines Evaluation and Management of Polycystic Ovary Syndrome. J Pediatr Health Care. 2009; 23:337-43.
12. Bulun SE. Physiology and pathology of the female reproductive axis. In: Polonsky KS, Larsen PR, Kronenberg HM (Eds). Williams Textbook of Endocrinology, 12th edition. Philadelphia: Elsevier/Saunders; 2011 pp.581-660.
13. Ali SS, Rehman R. Subfertility: recent advances in management and prevention; Polycystic ovary syndrome and subfertility. 115-34.
14. Markantes GK, Tsichlia G, Georgopoulos NA. Diet and exercise in the management of PCOS: Starting from the basics. In: Diamanti-Kandarakis E (Ed). Polycystic Ovary Syndrome Challenging Issues in the Modern Era of Individualized Medicine. Elsevier; 2022. pp. 97-115.
15. Armeni E, Lambrinoudaki I. Long-term health in women of age more than 40 years with polycystic ovary syndrome. In: Diamanti-Kandarakis E (Ed). Polycystic Ovary Syndrome Challenging Issues in the Modern Era of Individualized Medicine. Elsevier; 2022. pp. 245-85.
16. Makaya T, Basu S, Poole R. Symposium: Endocrinology. Management of teenagers with polycystic ovarian syndrome. Paediatrics Child Health. 2019;29(7):303-8.

CHAPTER 21

Surgery in PCOS

Sunita Tandulwadkar, Swapnil Langde, Rashmika Gandhi

■ INTRODUCTION

Laparoscopic ovarian drilling (LOD) is a fertility-enhancing surgical method of treatment for infertility in patients with the polycystic ovarian syndrome (PCOS). Problems in inducing ovulation are well-recognized in women suffering from PCOS. It is the second-line therapy in clomiphene citrate/letrozole-resistant anovulatory patients. LOD maximizes the chances of successful conception either spontaneously or in an assisted reproductive technique (ART) cycle. Laparoscopic ovarian drilling may induce overall spontaneous ovulation and pregnancy rates of 30–90% and 13–88%, respectively.[1]

Polycystic ovarian syndrome is a frequent metabolic disorder, characterized by chronic anovulation, hyperandrogenism, and polycystic ovaries in ultrasonography. It affects approximately 8–13% of reproductive-aged women and is the most common cause of anovulation according to WHO.[2] The prevalence of PCOS depends upon the diagnostic criteria used.

Rotterdam criteria:
- Oligo or anovulation
- Clinical or biochemical signs of hyperandrogenism
- Polycystic ovaries on imaging, followed by androgen excess society criteria

■ HISTORY

Stein and Leventhal in 1935 published data stating that several women undergoing wedge resection (biopsy from the bilaterally enlarged ovaries) resumed ovulation. This was attributed to the reduction in the hyperplastic central stroma. Surgical ovarian wedge resection by laparotomy was thus the first established treatment for women with anovulatory PCOS (Stein 1939). In the coming years, a boom in the practice of surgical biopsy in PCOS patients was seen making ovarian wedge resection the primary treatment for the initiation of ovulation in infertile cases. Over the time, ovarian resection was replaced by medical ovulation induction. With the advent of oral ovulatory agents, their popularity gradually waned owing to their multiple advantages specifically their noninvasive nature among others. Laparotomy was largely abandoned because of the risk of post-surgical adhesion formation, which resulted in the conversion of endocrinological subfertility to mechanical subfertility due to scar formation. However, with advancement into laparoscopic surgery, ovarian drilling came once again come into spotlight. In 1984, it was Gjönnaess who reported that in women with PCOS, electrocautery of the ovarian capsule during laparoscopy resulted in a high rate of ovulation and pregnancy. He used 200–300 watt current for 2–4 s and made three to eight punctures on each ovary.

He reported a pregnancy rate of 69% and an abortion rate of 15%.[3] This revolutionized the treatment algorithm for anovulatory patients and set the ball rolling for further research and innovation.

INDICATIONS FOR LAPAROSCOPIC OVARIAN DRILLING (FIGS. 1A TO C)

- Women who fail to ovulate on ovulation inducing medicines
- CC resistant cases
- High LH levels
- PCOS

MECHANISM OF ACTION AND ENDOCRINOLOGICAL ASPECTS OF LAPAROSCOPIC OVARIAN DRILLING

- The exact mechanism by which minimal perforations using heat or laser result in follicular growth and ovulation is yet to be elucidated and it is not known whether a prevalent effect is exerted through a direct action on the ovary or through a systemic endocrine flow mechanism (**Fig. 2**).
- The most plausible mechanism is that the thermal destruction of ovarian follicles and a part of the ovarian androgen-producing stroma results in the reduction of both local and systemic androgens,

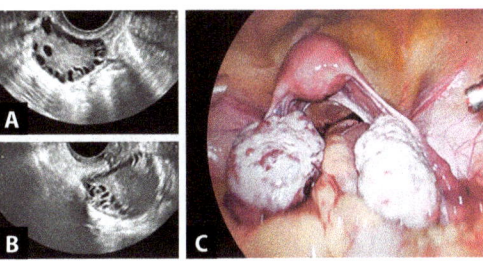

Figs. 1A to C: Surgical treatment of PCOS.

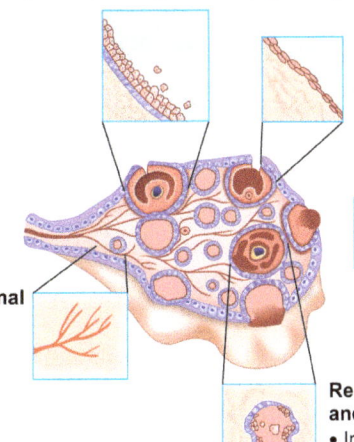

Fig. 2: Several plausible mechanisms of LOD were proposed in the amelioration of ovulation and pregnancy in women with PCOS.

re-establishment of an intrafollicular environment more convenient for normal follicular maturation and ovulation, and a secondary rise in FSH levels.[3]
- In addition, following a surgery-mediated increase in ovarian blood, the release of a cascade of local growth factors such as insulin-like growth factors interacting with FSH, in response to thermal injury, has been suggested to allow follicular growth and subsequent ovulation.[3]
- Further possible mechanisms are the decrease in AMH concentrations and the production of "holes" in the very thick cortical wall of the polycystic ovary.[3] LOD-mediated electrocauterization may loosen the hard and condensed cortical layers, which is increased by one-third and fivefold in the subcortical stroma.
- Another possible basis is the removal of the intraovarian follicular fluid that accumulates and destroys the stromal tissue of the polycystic ovary. Some factors such as CD45RO+ and IL-6 are often involved in an increased chronic low-grade proinflammatory reaction, metabolism, and oxidation process are often increased in the follicular fluid of PCOS women. At the same time, IL-13, IL-15, IL-22, macrophage inhibitory factor (MIF), C-C Motif Chemokine Ligand 2 (CCL2), innate lymphoid cells, regulatory T cells, dendritic cells, and cytotoxic T cells (CD8+ T cell counts) involved in anti-inflammatory responses or anti-oxidation/gluconeogenesis in the follicular fluid in PCOS women are significantly decreased. LOD may thus reverse these apparent poor quality small follicles containing inflammatory molecules by leakages, boiling, or aspiration. This effect, however, seems transient.[4]

The efficacy of ovarian drilling is widely variable throughout literature: in a comprehensive review, ovarian drilling is deemed to restore fertility in 20–64% of women with PCOS previously suffering from anovulatory infertility who did not respond to CC treatment; 70% of pregnancies occurred in the first 6 postoperative months.[5]

EFFECTS OF LAPAROSCOPIC OVARIAN DRILLING

Ovulation and Pregnancy Rate

Laparoscopic ovarian drilling may induce overall spontaneous ovulation and pregnancy rates of 30–90% and 13–88%.[1]

The overall miscarriage rate following LOD varies from 0 to 36.5%[6]. Amer et al. reported that LOD significantly reduced the miscarriage rates from 54 to 17%. The advantages of LOD compared to other medical ovulation induction methods have been previously demonstrated, including a statistically significantly decreased risk of OHSS and multiple pregnancies.[7]

A comparison of reproductive performance in women with clomiphene citrate-resistant polycystic ovary syndrome treated with laparoscopic ovarian drilling and non-laparoscopic ovarian drilling is shown in **Table 1**.[8]

Metabolic Effects

There are multiple molecular mechanisms that can explain the metabolic and hormonal changes in PCOS women after LOD.
- AMH is often used to evaluate the ovarian reproductive potential in women who need ART or to investigate the traumatic effects of various agents or procedures. After the LOD procedure, many studies have found a significant decline in the serum level of AMH.[9] It is also well-known that the overheating or excessive

TABLE 1: A comparison of reproductive performance in women with clomiphene citrate-resistant polycystic ovary syndrome treated with laparoscopic ovarian drilling and non-laparoscopic ovarian drilling.

Author	Article	Comparison	Outcomes
Bordewijk (2020)	Review	LOD with or without medical ovulation induction versus medical ovulation induction alone	Live birth: Slightly ameliorated by LOD (OR 0.71, 95% CI 0.54–0.92)
Yu (2019)	Review	Letrozole versus LOD	No difference in ovulation rate (RR1.12; 95% CI 0.93–1.34), and live birth rate (RR 1.27; 95% CI 0.96–1.68)
Debras (2019)	Multicenter study	LOD alone, long term effect	Mean follow-up period was 28.4 months (25.3–31.5). At least 47.4% women got pregnancy after a drilling
Abu Hashim (2018)	Review	BLOD versus ULOD	No significant differences in ovulation (OR 0.73; 95% CI 0.47–1.11) and live birth (OR 0.77; 95% CI 0.28–2.10)
Franik (2018)	Review	AI ± adjuvants versus LOD	Live birth: OR 1.38, 95% CI 0.95–2.02
Abu Hashim (2015)	Review	CC+M versus LOD	Live birth: OR 2.27, 95% CI 1.22–4.17
Kaur (2013)	Observational study	LOD alone	Clinical pregnancy rate: 47.3%; live birth rate: 40.5%
Nasr (2012)	RCT	Electrocautery versus harmonic scalpel	Similar ovulation rate (89% vs. 92.9%) and pregnancy rate (50% vs. 57%)
Farquhar (2012)	Review	LOD versus medical treatments	Live birth: 34% versus 38%. No significant difference
Abu Hashim (2011)	RCT	CC+M versus LOD	Similar ovulation rate (67% vs. 68.4%) and pregnancy rate (15.4% vs. 17%)
Abdullah (2011)	RCT	Letrozole versus LOD	*Ovulation rate:* Significantly higher in the letrozole than LOD (59.0% vs. 47.5%). Similar live birth rate
Roy (2010)	RCT	Rosiglitazone + CC versus LOD + CC	Similar ovulation (80.8 vs. 81.5%) and pregnancy rate (50 vs. 42.8%)

(CC: clomiphene citrate; M: metformin; LOD: laparoscopic ovarian drilling; ULOD: unilateral laparoscopic ovarian drilling; BLOD: bilateral laparoscopic ovarian drilling; AI: aromatase inhibitor; RCT: randomized controlled trial; OR: odds ratio; CI: confidence interval; NS: no significance)

electrocauterization of polycystic ovaries may further lead to a continuous decline in AMH. However, it is yet debatable whether this result reflects real damage to the ovarian reserve or only provides normalization from high serum AMH in POCS women before LOD.

- A decrease in androgen production is one of the most commonly detectable changes after LOD.[10]
- Saleh et al. reported that LOD reduces serum glucose levels and improved insulin sensitivity in insulin-resistant (IR) PCOS women. There was a significant

difference in insulin and glucose levels before and after LOD. The evidence also suggests that LOD can successfully reduce serum insulin-like growth factor-1 (IGF-1) levels, which may contribute to the improved IR status of PCOS women.[11]

Effect on Endometrial Homeobox Gene Expression

There is a receptivity defect in the endometrium of women with PCOS that affects fertility regardless of other causes of infertility. LOD increases endometrial HOXA-10 and HOXA-11 mRNA expressions and improves receptivity in patients with clomiphene-resistant PCOS.[12]

TECHNIQUE AND POSSIBLE COMPLICATIONS

With the advances in technology for minimally invasive surgery, laparoscopic surgeries using fewer port wounds, single incisions, or the natural orifice have become increasingly popular. Therefore, the fewer-port laparoscopic technique is also feasible for LOD.
- Careful patient selection
- For better cosmetic results and quick recovery, best is to use 5 mm laparoscope with 3 mm ancillary ports.
- Prior to the application of any form of energy, the ovary should be carefully lifted and moved away from the intestine and ureters.
- The most accredited technique universally consists of performing four punctures bilaterally, for a depth of 3–4 m, each for 4 s at 40 W *(Rule of 4)* delivering 640 J of energy per ovary **(Figs. 3A and B)**.[11]
- There is still a lack of consensus regarding the amount of electrosurgical energy and the optimal number of puncture holes to achieve maximum efficacy: reducing the thermal energy (<300 J/ovary) decreases the chances of ovulation and pregnancy, while higher thermal doses (>1,000 J/ovary) may result in extensive tissue destruction without additional improvement in outcomes. Ovarian atrophy has also been reported following high-energy drilling (eight coagulation points at 400 W for 5 s). Thus, the number of drills and amount of diathermy should be reduced to the lowest effective dose.[13]
- The use of the harmonic scalpel was found in a randomized study to be just as effective as the Nd-YAG laser, although the latter has been found to be more prone to preventing adhesion owing to lower

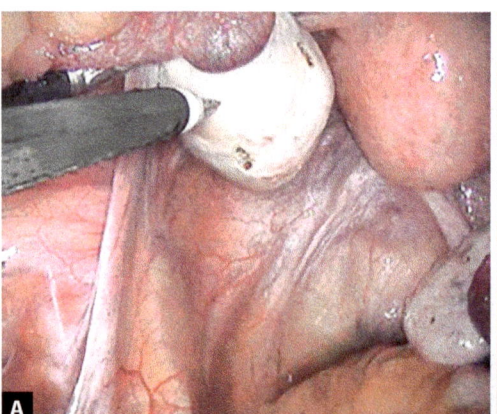
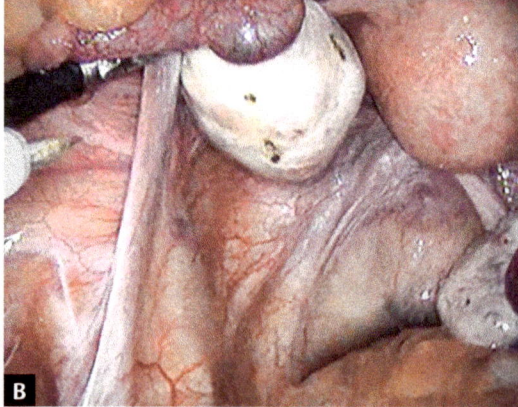

Figs. 3A and B: Technique of laparoscopic ovarian drilling (Rule of 4s).

thermal penetration by the cone-shaped lesions of laser drilling.[13]
- Peritoneal cavity and ovaries must be cooled using up to 1,000 mL of the isotonic solution to heat lesions and reduce the risk of postoperative adhesion formation. Adhesion barriers can also be used.

Among the possible adverse effects, surgical morbidity of this procedure should always be considered in high regard since it is frequently performed in obese women. In addition, specific concerns exist regarding the occurrence of iatrogenic adnexal adhesions and the possible decrease in ovarian reserve. The rate of adnexal adhesions differs widely in various studies ranging from 19 to 60%, mostly consisting of mild to moderate severity that seems to not affect pregnancy.[13] Premature ovarian failure (POF), especially if the ovarian blood supply is damaged inadvertently or if a large number of punctures are made can also occur, leading to excessive destruction of the ovarian follicular pool or production of anti-ovarian antibodies.

Predictors of a Positive Outcome[13]

- *Normal body mass index (BMI):* Patients with BMI values >35 kg/m^2 obtain lower ovulation rates (13%) compared to patients with BMI between 29 and 34 kg/m^2 (46%) and those with BMI <29 kg/m^2 (57%).
- High LH concentration (>10 UI/L)
- Short infertility duration.
- Age <35 years

Predictors of Poor Outcomes[13]

- Hyperinsulinemia
- Elevated AMH levels (>7.7 ng/mL)
- High testosterone serum levels (biochemical hyperandrogenism)

ALTERNATIVE OPTIONS TO TRADITIONAL SURGICAL OVARIAN DRILLING

- Unilateral ovarian drilling (ULOD) as modification of current procedure—promising results but paucity of studies available[13]
- Adjustment of energy applied has been tested but there is a lack of consensus due decrease in effectiveness after 6 months
- Transvaginal hydrolaparoscopy (THL) under general anesthesia using bipolar electrosurgery. This procedure has its limitations due to complications such as bleeding, bowel perforations-no access to pouch of Douglas and ovaries but results in form of ovulation and pregnancy in PCOS patients were comparable to laparoscopy.
- Ultrasound-guided transvaginal ovarian needle drilling (UTND) as a novel surgical method. A long sharp needle (35 cm—16 gauge) is connected to continuous manual vacuum pressure and used to puncture each ovary from different angles to aspirate all visible small follicles, under the guidance of the ultrasound.

POSTOPERATIVE CONSIDERATIONS AFTER LAPAROSCOPIC OVARIAN DRILLING

Laparoscopic ovarian drilling improves the responsiveness of the polycystic ovaries to subsequent ovulatory agents, and reintroduction of drug treatments can be considered in those who do not spontaneously become pregnant within 6 months.

The effectiveness of a second LOD, also called redrilling in women with PCOS has been investigated briefly. Overall, ovulation and pregnancy rates with better outcomes are observed in LOD-sensitive than LOD-resistant cases. Hence, repeated application of LOD should not be encouraged.

CURRENT RECOMMENDATIONS

- *SOGC 2010:* Laparoscopic ovarian drilling may be considered in women with clomiphene-resistant PCOS, particularly when there are other indications for laparoscopy. Surgical risks need to be considered in these patients.
- *NICE 2013:* For women with WHO Group II ovulation disorders who are known to be resistant to clomiphene citrate, consider one of the following second-line treatments, depending on clinical circumstances and the woman's preference: laparoscopic ovarian drilling or combined treatment with clomiphene citrate and metformin if not already offered as first-line treatment or gonadotropins.
- *ESHRE 2018:* Laparoscopic ovarian surgery could be second line therapy for women with PCOS, who are clomiphene citrate resistant, with anovulatory infertility and no other infertility factors. Laparoscopic ovarian surgery could potentially be offered as first-line treatment if laparoscopy is indicated for another reason in women with PCOS with anovulatory infertility and no other infertility factors.

PATIENT EDUCATION

Patient counseling along with diet modification and exercise and weight loss will also help in achieving better results. Diet with low glycemic index and lifestyle changes are very important parts of the treatment.

CONCLUSION

Laparoscopic ovarian drilling regularizes the hormonal environment, provides long-term benefits, and might improve the ovarian response to hormonal treatment. It is the requirement of invasive surgical approach, and the expertise needed along with risks involved is a disadvantage. Patients with poor responses to hormonal stimulation might benefit from the surgical approach.

REFERENCES

1. Costello MF, Misso ML, Balen A, Boyle J, Devoto L, Garad RM, et al. Evidence summaries and recommendations from the international evidence-based guideline for the assessment and management of polycystic ovary syndrome: Assessment and treatment of infertility. Hum. Reprod Open, 2019: z2019:hoy021.
2. Azziz R, Carmina E, Dewailly D, Diamanti-Kandarakis E, Escobar-Morreale HF, Futterweit W, et al. Position statement: criteria for defining polycystic ovary syndrome as a predominantly hyperandrogenic syndrome: an Androgen Excess Society guideline. J Clin Endocrinol Metab. 2006;91(11):4237-45.
3. Seow KM, Juan CC, Hwang JL, Ho LT. Laparoscopic surgery in polycystic ovary syndrome: Reproductive and metabolic effects. Semin Reprod. Med. 2008;26:101-10.
4. Wu R, Fujii S, Ryan NK, Van der Hoek KH, Jasper MJ, Sini I, et al. Ovarian leukocyte distribution and cytokine/chemokine mRNA expression in follicular fluid cells in women with polycystic ovary syndrome. Hum Reprod. 2007;22:527-35.
5. Gadalla MA, Norman RJ, Tay CT, Hiam DS, Melder A, Pundir J, et al. Medical and surgical treatment of reproductive outcomes in polycystic ovary syndrome: An overview of systematic reviews. Int J Fertil Steril. 2020;13:257-70.
6. Palomba S, Falbo A, Battista L, Russo T, Venturella R, Tolino A, t al. Laparoscopic ovarian diathermy vs clomiphene citrate plus metformin as second-line strategy for infertile anovulatory patients with polycystic ovary syndrome: a randomized controlled trial. Am J Obstet Gynecol. 2010;202:577.e1-577.e8.

7. Amer SA, Li TC, Cooke ID. A prospective dose-finding study of the amount of thermal energy required for laparoscopic ovarian diathermy. Hum Reprod. 2003;18:1693-8.
8. Seow KM, Chang YW, Chen KH, Juan CC, Huang CY, Lin LT, al. Molecular Mechanisms of Laparoscopic Ovarian Drilling and Its Therapeutic Effects in Polycystic Ovary Syndrome. Int J Mol Sci. 2020;21:8147.
9. Abu Hashim H, Foda O, El Rakhawy M. Unilateral or bilateral laparoscopic ovarian drilling in polycystic ovary syndrome: a meta-analysis of randomized trials. Arch Gynecol Obstet. 2018;297:859-70.
10. Seow KM, Lee WL, Wang PH. A challenge in the management of women with polycystic ovary syndrome. Taiwan J Obstet Gynecol. 2016;55:157-8.
11. Saleh A, Morris D, Tan SL, Tulandi T. Effects of laparoscopic ovarian drilling on adrenal steroids in polycystic ovary syndrome patients with and without hyperinsulinemia. Fertil Steril. 2001;75:501-4.
12. Senturk S, Celik O, Dalkilic S, Hatirnaz S, Celik N, Unlu C, et al. Laparoscopic Ovarian Drilling Improves Endometrial Homeobox Gene Expression in PCOS. Reprod Sci. 2020;27(2):675-80.
13. Mercorio A, Della Corte L, De Angelis MC, Buonfantino C, Ronsini C, Bifulco G, et al. Ovarian Drilling: Back to the Future. Medicina (Kaunas). 2022;58(8):1002.

CHAPTER 22

Infertility in PCOS

Kundan Ingale, S Ashok Kumar

INTRODUCTION

Polycystic ovarian syndrome (PCOS) is a medical condition characterized by chronic anovulation and hyperandrogenemia. Definition of PCOS is evolved over last three decades. Rotterdam's criteria have been recently used to identify PCOS patients. Any two of following criteria should be present: (1) polycystic ovaries, (2) anovulation and (3) clinical or biochemical evidence of hyperandrogenemia. Polycystic ovaries show two important changes on ultrasound: increase in thickness of ovarian stroma and accumulation of functionally active antral follicles typically located near subscapular region. PCOS is most common cause of anovulatory infertility. Endocrine disturbances with genetic inheritance of insulin resistance are the most common pathophysiological changes seen in creating anovulatory cycles. Ovulation induction has established as most rewarding treatment in management of PCOS infertile patient.

ENDOCRINE DYSFUNCTION IN POLYCYSTIC OVARIAN SYNDROME

Ovulatory dysfunction is the most common cause of infertility in PCOS infertile patient. Though the research to find the cause of anovulation has evolved from one hypothesis to another since last few decades, there are five proposed mechanisms causing anovulatory cycles.

1. Hyperandrogenemia
2. Overproduction of luteinizing hormone (LH)
3. Underproduction of follicle-stimulating hormone (FSH)
4. Insulin resistance
5. Higher concentration of anti-Müllerian hormone (AMH)

Hyperinsulinemia and insulin resistance are the important pathologies in creating hyperandrogenemia. Insulin resistance results into hyperinsulinemia which in turn causes decrease in sex hormone-binding globulin (SHBG) production, so ultimately free unbound circulatory testosterone levels are increased **(Flowchart 1)**. Hyperinsulinemia also produces increase in LH pulse frequency leading increase production of testosterone. Due to repeated stimulation by LH, theca cells overproduce testosterone, which is proposed possible cause of ovulatory disturbance.

The raised serum LH levels in early follicular phase leads to premature luteinization of antral and preantral follicles. Premature luteinization causes cessation of division of granulosa cells within the follicles leading to failure of follicular growth. It has been shown that LH receptor mRNA is overexpressed in granulosa cells from polycystic ovaries, supporting the theory that high LH levels can be the cause of ovulatory disturbance.

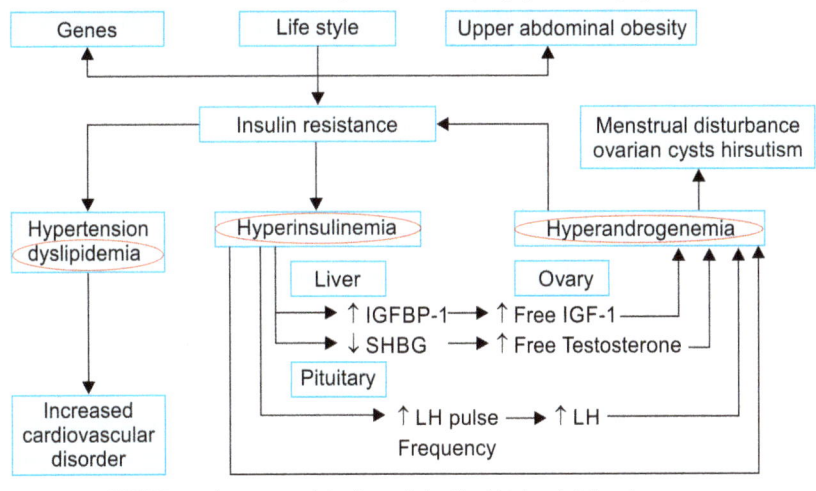

Flowchart 1: Metabolic dysfunction in polycystic ovary syndrome.

(SHBG: sex hormone-binding globulin; LH: luteinizing hormone; IGFBP: Insulin-like growth factor-binding protein)

Selection of preantral and antral follicles is dependent on FSH. So, disordered FSH production is also postulated as one of the causes of anovulation in PCOS patients. Suppression of FSH below 5 mIU/mL has been found in many but not in all PCOS patients, especially on day 2 of menses. PCOS patients do not show intercycle rise in FSH levels.

Insulin resistance is the key metabolic defect seen in PCOS patients. As discussed earlier, insulin resistance causes premature luteinization of antral and preantral follicles and causes arrested folliculogenesis in PCOS (**Box 1**). It is seen that insulin resistance is seen mainly in obese PCOS patients and weight loss in these patients also leads to spontaneous follicular growth and even spontaneous conception. The prevalence of insulin resistance among women with PCOS is 22%, 45% and 50% at the ages <20, 20–29 and 30–39 years, respectively.[1] If obesity is present with PCOS, the incidence of insulin resistance rises to 75%.[1] It is recommended to screen each PCOS patient for insulin resistance.

Anti-Müllerian hormone is proposed to inhibit the initiation of follicular growth of the primordial pool in AMH Knockout model, but it has been demonstrated that AMH was expressed in a lower percentage of preantral follicles in PCOS. This mechanism permits an accelerated follicular initiation. In AMH knockout model, the reproductive lifespan is reduced which is not the case in PCOS. So the theory of causative effect of high AMH in anovulation is not accepted so well by many.[2,3]

Dysfunctional Steroidogenesis

There is elevated production of estrogen at all stages of follicular maturation due to availability of excess androgens for aromatase activity along with over-response of follicular growth and estradiol secretion to FSH (**Flowchart 2**).[4]

BOX 1: Causes of insulin resistance.
- Peripheral target tissue resistance
  - Decreased insulin receptor number
  - Decreased insulin binding
  - Postreceptor failure
- Decreased hepatic clearance
- Increased pancreatic sensitivity

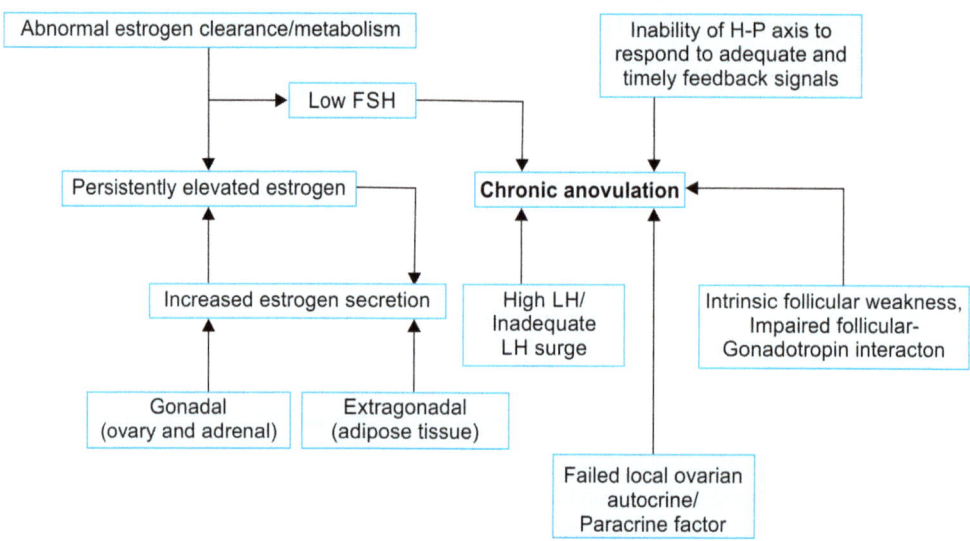

Flowchart 2: Effects of chronic anovulation.

Inhibin is FSH inducible factor. Inhibin B interferes in downregulation of steroidogenesis. Women with PCOS have elevated inhibin levels.[5] Inhibin B stimulates androgen production which in turn produces more Inhibin B. This vicious cycle in ovary inhibits follicular growth.

Dysregulation of androgen synthesis in PCOS leads to ovarian hyperresponse to gonadotropins.
- Theca cells hyperresponse to LH: Excess androgen
- Granulosa cell hyperresponse to FSH: Excess estrogen.

DEFECTIVE OOCYTES IN POLYCYSTIC OVARY SYNDROME

Reduced Energy Uptake by Oocytes (Flowchart 3)

The multiplying granulosa cells use glucose via glycolytic pathway. This in turn allows production of ATP and metabolite such as pyruvate and lactate. These are directly produced in follicular fluid or reached to oocytes via gap junctions. This glucose uptake is mediated via GLUTs (glucose transport proteins) which forms aqueous pores through which glucose can move. The translocation of GLUT-4 from intracellular to the cell surface is also insulin dependent.

In PCOS, insulin stimulated glucose uptake and metabolism pathways are impaired.[6] This results into impaired growth and proliferation of granulosa cells due to inadequate energy availability. It has adverse effects on both oocyte development and follicle growth.

Abnormal Gene Expression in Oocytes

The impact of intrafollicular high androgen and abnormal levels of insulin on oocyte gene expression was studied on oocytes in women with PCOS by microarray analysis. These oocytes from women with PCOS showed consistently different gene expression profiles. These genes are generally involved in mitotic cell cycle and maternal effect genes (required around activation of zygotic genome at the time of resumption of mitosis).[7]

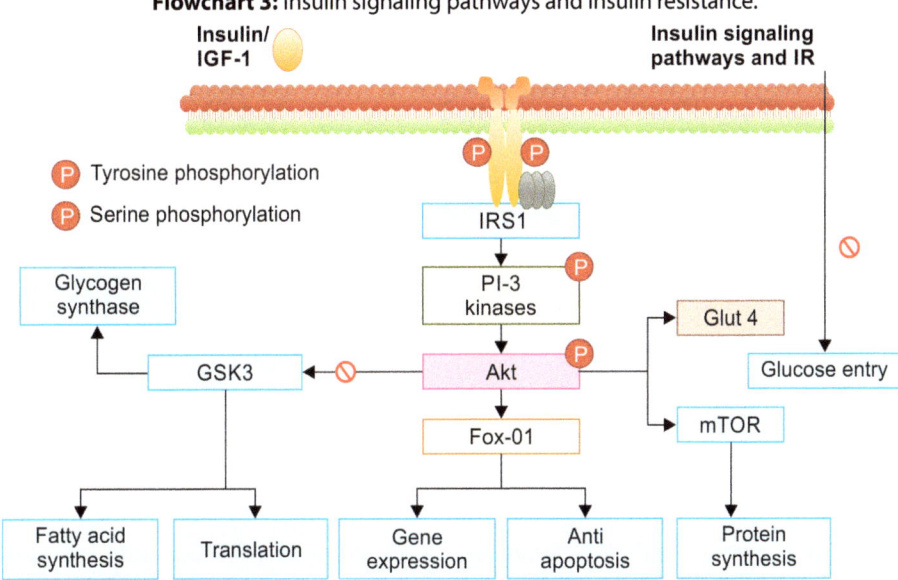

Flowchart 3: Insulin signaling pathways and insulin resistance.

NEUROENDOCRINE ABNORMALITIES IN POLYCYSTIC OVARY SYNDROME

In PCOD, the LH amplitude response to exogenous GnRH is exaggerated in women with PCOS. Additionally, the GnRH pulse frequency is increased in PCOS to one pulse per 50–60 min. There is an increase in overall amount of GnRH secreted. This pattern secretes more LH than FSH. All this suggests neuroendocrine dysfunction may be primary event in the pathogenesis in PCOS.[8]

ROLE OF OBESITY

Obesity is common association seen in women with PCOS. It is prevalent in 30–60%. Effect of obesity on gonadotropin dynamics is not at hypothalamic level but at pituitary level. Obesity causes decrease in LH responsiveness to GnRH and increase in clearance of LH. This effect is mediated at pituitary level via insulin and leptin.

Obesity both independently and by PCOS exacerbation increases hyperandrogenemia, hirsutism, infertility, and pregnancy complications. Obesity increases risk of impaired glucose tolerance and type 2 diabetes, increases cardiovascular risk, and reduces effectiveness of interventions for PCOS **(Box 2)**.

WORK UP FOR PCOS DIAGNOSIS

- Transvaginal ultrasound
- Day 2 FSH and LH
- Glucose tolerance test or HbA1c
- TSH
- Prolactin
- Androgens: DHEAS, Testosterone (Total and Free)
- 17-OH progesterone

TREATMENT IN INFERTILE WOMAN WITH PCOS

Lifestyle modification with caloric restriction and physical exercise is considered as first-line management when managing obese PCOS women.

Metformin as insulin sensitizing agent plays a very important role in reducing insulin

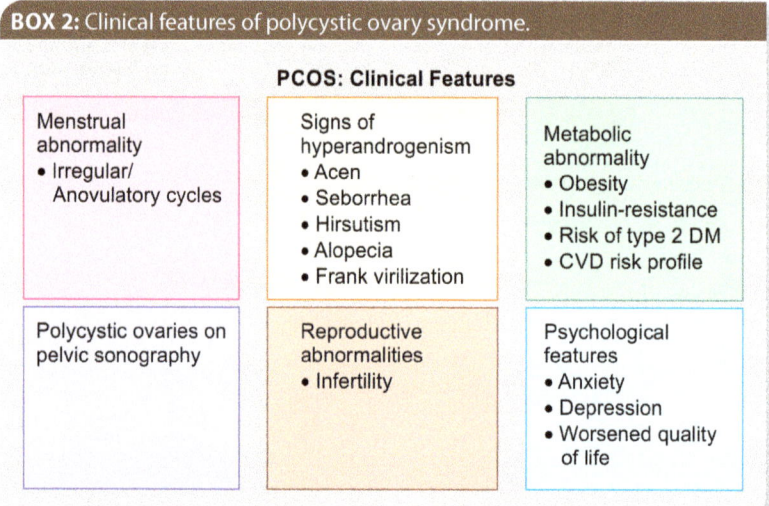

BOX 2: Clinical features of polycystic ovary syndrome.

resistance for 2 months prior to ovulation induction.

Oral ovulogens such as clomiphene citrate and aromatase inhibitors such as Letrozole are the first-line treatments for ovulation induction in anovulatory women with PCOS. In comparison with Clomiphene, Letrozole is the first choice for ovulation induction as it is associated with lowest risk of ovarian hyperstimulation syndrome (OHSS) and much better clinical pregnancy rates and lower miscarriage rates.

Use of gonadotropins as ovulation induction agent remains the second-line treatment option, especially used in CC resistant and CC failure patients. Caution regarding ovarian hyperstimulation (OHSS) and increase risk of multiple pregnancy need to be explained to patients undergoing ovarian stimulation with gonadotropins.

In vitro fertilization (IVF) is the third-line treatment option for women with PCOS who has other factors for infertility such as tubal or sperm factor in male partner or for those who have failed prior treatment with Letrozole or gonadotropins.

Laparoscopic ovarian drilling is definitely not the first choice of treatment in the management of infertility women with PCOS. It has only demonstrated advantage of reducing OHSS rates.

Each treatment option is given in detail in subsequent chapters.

■ CONCLUSION

Genetic factors play an important role in the initiation of abnormalities in development of PCOS in adult life. Insulin resistance and hyperinsulinemia cause androgen excess and LH overproduction, which lead to anovulatory infertility. Androgen excess also causes abnormal gene expression in oocytes, contributing to poor reproductive outcomes. Insulin mediated increased LH pulsatility leads to premature follicular growth arrest. The insulin stimulated glucose uptake pathway is resistant to insulin action in the follicular somatic cells of PCOS. The resulting impaired energy availability is an additional pathophysiologic mechanism causing ovarian dysfunction in PCOS. PCOS is still an enigmatic disease, further research into different aspects of PCOS will keep giving us more information on research in infertility management.

REFERENCES

1. Asuncion R, Calvo RM, San Millan JL, Sancho J, Avila S, Escobar-Morreale HF. A prospective study of the prevalence of the polycyatic ovarian syndrome in unselected Caucasian women from Spain. J Clin Endocrinol Metab. 2000;85:2434-8.
2. Durlinger AL, Visser JA, Themmen AP. Regulation of ovarian function: the role of AMH. Repruction. 2002;124(5):601-9.
3. Durlinger AL, Gruijter MJ, Kramer P, Karels B, Kumar TR, Matzuk MM et al. Anti-Mullerian hormone attenuates the effects of FSH on follicle development in the mouse ovary. Endocrinology. 2001;142(11);4891-9.
4. Erickson GF, Magoffin DA, Garza VG, Cheung AP, Chang RJ. Granulosa cells of polycystic ovaries: are they normal or abnormal? Hum Reprod. 1992;7:293-9.
5. Anderson R, Groome N, Baird D. Inhibin A and Inhibin B in women with PCOS during treatment with FSH to induce mono-ovulation. Clin Endocrinol (Oxf). 1998;48:577-84.
6. Fedorcsak P, Storeng R, Dale PO, Tanbo T, Abyholm T. Impaired insulin action on granulosa lutein cells in women with PCOS and IR. Gynecol Endocrinol. 2000;14(5): 327-36.
7. Wood JR, Dumesic DA, Abbott DH, Strauss III JH. Molecular abnormalities in oocytes from women with PCOS revealed by micro-array analysis. J Clin Endocrinol Metab. 2007;92(2);705-13.
8. Pagan YL, Srouji SS, Jimenez Y, Emerson A, Gill S, Hall JE. Inverse relationship between LH and BMI in PCOS: Investigations of hypothalamic and pituitary contributions. J Clin Endocrinol Metab. 2004;89;4343-50.

CHAPTER 23

Ovulation Induction in PCOS

Nandita Palshetkar, Tanushree Pandey Padgaonkar, Rohan Palshetkar

■ INTRODUCTION

Anovulatory infertility is a common problem faced in infertility practice. The causes of anovulation have been classified by the World Health Organization (WHO) into three categories based on the gonadotropin profile:
- *WHO type 1 (hypogonadotropic hypogonadism) (10%):* This is caused by any lesion affecting the pituitary or hypothalamus and affecting gonadotropin production including idiopathic, weight-related amenorrhea, Sheehan syndrome, extreme stress and strenuous exercise, Kallmann's syndrome, craniopharyngiomas, etc.
- *WHO type 2 (normogonadotropic hypogonadism):* This is the most common cause of anovulation accounting for 85% of cases and is most commonly caused by polycystic ovary syndrome (PCOS). Hyperprolactinemic amenorrhea is another cause, where in addition to amenorrhea and infertility, women may have galactorrhea.
- *WHO type 3 (hypergonadotropic hypogonadism) (5%):* This is usually an indication of ovarian failure.

■ TREATMENT STRATEGIES AND GOALS

In anovulatory women, the purpose of treatment in ovulation induction is the development of at least one follicle, whereas in other causes of infertility, ovarian stimulation is used to increase the number of follicles, known as super ovulation or controlled ovarian hyperstimulation. Induction of ovulation is possible in the first two types. However, in the third type, ovulation induction is usually unsuccessful due to follicular depletion and the only way to achieve a pregnancy may be through oocyte donation.

■ CLOMIPHENE CITRATE

Clomiphene is being used for over five decades for ovulation induction. It is similar in structure to estrogen and thus bindings to estrogen receptors.[1] While most modern fertility physicians have now shifted to aromatase inhibitors (AIs) as a first-line agent for oral ovulation induction, the role of clomiphene citrate (CC) and the significant body of evidence on this molecule built up over several decades need to be discussed.

As a selective estrogen receptor modulator (SERM), clomiphene acts both as an agonist and as an antagonist. For ovulation induction, the agonist feature of CC is most vital to us.[2] Clomiphene binds to estrogen receptors and provides a false sensation of low estrogen state to the hypothalamus. This causes the hypothalamic-pituitary-ovarian (HPO) axis to increase gonadotropin-releasing hormone (GnRH) secretion which in turn increases the release of gonadotropins.[1]

Treatment Regimen

Clomiphene citrate is generally started from day 2 to day 5 after the onset of menses. The rate of ovulation and pregnancy is similar irrespective of the day of menses on which clomiphene is started. Treatment with CC is associated with a higher rate of pregnancy if started early (days 1 through 5 than 5 through 9) in the menstrual cycle.[3] Ideally, clomiphene is started at a dose of 50 mg/day for 5 days. Ovulation generally occurs 5–10 days after the last CC dose. If a patient remains anovulatory, then the dose should be increased by 50 mg/day. Generally, a patient should ovulate with a dose of 50–150 mg/day.

In women who ovulate, 52% do so on taking 50 mg, 22% on taking 100 mg, and fewer with subsequent increases.[4] The Food and Drug Administration (FDA) does not approve a dose more than 100 mg/day while the American College of Obstetricians and Gynecologists gives approval for dose up to 150 mg/day. This higher dose is generally required for women with slightly higher body mass index (BMI).[5]

Indications

Anovulatory Infertility

Traditionally, the first-line treatment for anovulatory and oligoovulatory women, though recent guidance has now advocated the use of AIs as the first line of therapy, especially in polycystic ovary syndrome (PCOS) as per the new European Society of Human Reproduction and Embryology/American Society for Reproductive Medicine (ESHRE/ASRM) joint PCOS guideline.

Unexplained Infertility

In unexplained infertility, clomiphene is used rampantly. However, there is no evidence which supports significant benefit over a placebo in planned relations cycle. CC when combined with intrauterine insemination (IUI) has shown benefit over a placebo.[6]

Clomiphene citrate is an efficient, inexpensive, and well-tolerated drug with a well-known safety profile when used correctly.[7] A recent review by Birch Petersen et al. from 2014 supports the use of CC as first-line treatment for ovulation induction in PCOS.[8] The continuation of treatment for another six cycles of CC before switching to, for example, gonadotropins may be cost-effective theoretically.[9]

■ TAMOXIFEN

Tamoxifen is another SERM which is similar to CC and has proven successfully as an ovulation induction agent.[10] Traditionally, it has been used in the medical management of breast cancer. However, the lack of data and prevalence of side effect, such as hot flashes, have limited its use in clinical practice.

■ AROMATASE INHIBITORS

Aromatase inhibitors, such as anastrozole and letrozole, have been used for ovulation inductions. They prevent aromatization which prevents androgens from being converted to estrogen. This causes a low estrogenic state and therefore acts on the HPO axis and pituitary. This causes a compensatory increase in the pulsatile GnRH secretion and thereby causes follicular growth.[11]

Post letrozole supplementation, estrogen levels increase immediately, which causes an abrupt decrease in follicle-stimulating hormone (FSH) levels. This ensures monofollicular growth, and the increase in estrogen helps in endometrial preparation and production of cervical mucus.

Therapy Regimen and Efficacy

Letrozole doses can be started from 2.5 to 7.5 mg/day. Anastrozole is given as 1 mg daily. Both medications are started as per the CC protocol. Extended regimens (10 days) and single-dose regimens (20 mg on day 3) have also been used with studies suggesting positive results.[12,13]

Letrozole can be combined with planned relations or IUI. In anovulatory women, AI have shown almost a 60% ovulation rate with pregnancy rates varying from 12 to 40%.[14,15]

Indications

Letrozole is indicated in women who are resistant to CC or those women in which CC is contraindicated due to undesirable side effects.[16] AI can also be implemented in cases where the endometrium is thin (<7 mm) where CC was used as oral ovulogen.[17,18]

In a recent Cochrane review, PCOS patients seem to have better pregnancy as well as live birth rate when letrozole was used.[19] This differs from a previous review, which did not detect a difference.[20]

■ ADJUVANT REGIMENS

Adjuvant regimens have traditionally been described in textbooks of reproductive endocrinology (especially glucocorticoids and bromocriptine) and are mentioned here for completeness; their utility is restricted in day-to-day practice.

Clomiphene and Glucocorticoids

With normal and elevated levels of dehydroepiandrosterone (DHEA) in CC-resistant patients, addition of dexamethasone (0.5–2 mg) or prednisolone (5 mg) has shown increase in ovulation and pregnancy rates. The mechanism of action is not clearly known, but there is a hypothesis that suggests that the androgen suppression has direct effects on the oocyte and indirect effects on cytokines and intrafollicular growth factors.[15]

Clomiphene and Human Chorionic Gonadotropin

Human chorionic gonadotropin (hCG) injection may benefit as surrogate luteinizing hormone (LH) surge to trigger ovulation in patients where CC is used especially in cases of unexplained infertility or coexisting male factor.

Clomiphene and Metformin

Metformin should be considered in combination with CC in patients who are CC-resistant. It is usually given in a dose of 1,500–2,000 mg/day. The starting dose of 500 mg/day should be given after which the dose should be increased to the required dose. A liver function test should always be carried out prior to starting metformin.

A meta-analysis has suggested that metformin may improve success in weight management.[21] Otherwise, the role of metformin in ovulation induction is controversial. Interestingly, metformin may have a role as pretreatment before standard assisted reproduction techniques. A recent randomized controlled trial (RCT) demonstrated improved pregnancy rates after 3–9 months of metformin before assisted reproduction techniques.[22]

Exogenous Gonadotropins

Gonadotropins were first obtained by purifying urine; nowadays, many commercially available preparations are from highly purified urinary source medications or are the product of recombinant technology. The major boon of recombinant gonadotropins is that they provide a more consistent supply;

there is barely any variation in the activity of the molecule and the biggest advantage is that there is antigenic urinary protein present.[2,23]

INDICATIONS

Hypogonadotropic Hypogonadism

WHO group 1 patients, oral ovulogens are generally not effective, especially those patients who do not have an intact HPO axis. In such patients, exogenous FSH and LH restore ovulation in these patients.[24]

Clomiphene Citrate-resistant Anovulation

WHO group 2 patients who do not respond to oral ovulogens should be subjected to exogenous FSH and LH. Exogenous gonadotropins should be used as second line of treatment for ovulation induction.[25]

Unexplained Infertility

Superovulation is often the goal of using gonadotropins in this population attempting to optimize cycle fecundity.

Therapy Regimen and Efficacy

As a prerequisite, extensive counseling is essential. The couple must understand the expected expenditure and time that needs to be committed for monitoring the effects of the medicine. Serum estradiol levels as well as follicular number and growth must be monitored to prevent ovarian hyperstimulation syndrome (OHSS). The dose and duration of gonadotropins depend on age, BMI, and ovarian reserve of the patients.

The *"step-up"* protocol is aimed at crossing the FSH threshold and reducing the risk of complications. The drawback of this protocol is that it increases the duration of the cycle and can result in multifollicular growth.

The *"step-down"* protocol overcomes these problems by replicating the hormonal cycle. FSH is started at a higher dose so that the dominant follicle develops faster. Once the dominant follicle is established, the FSH levels can be reduced slowly to ensure monofollicular growth.[11]

It is important to monitor the patients, because the FSH window needs to be managed to ensure either mono- or multifollicular growth. The cycle can be cancelled if there are more than three dominant follicles. The biggest concern of the step-down protocol is starting the patient with a high initial dose of FSH whose threshold is low.

A low dose or chronic low-dose step-up regimen may be considered in the first cycle to gauge a response for an individual patient. Eventually, the other cycles can be done depending on the response in the first cycle.

GnRH Agonists and Antagonists

Among the various GnRH agonist protocols, namely ultrashort, short, and long, the long GnRH agonist protocol has been used as the gold standard in in vitro fertilization (IVF) since its discovery in the 1980s. GnRH antagonists have recently offered an alternative approach in IVF treatment.

The long GnRH agonist protocol involves administration of 0.1 mg GnRH agonist (e.g., triptorelin/leuprolide) starting on preceding cycle-day 21 followed by administration of gonadotropin at 150–225 international units (IU) daily starting on cycle-day 2. The adjustment of dose is based on follicular development and administration of GnRH agonist and gonadotropin lasts until the hCG trigger injection, which is around 14 days post GnRH agonist regimen or when follicles reach 16–18 mm in size.

For the GnRH antagonist protocol, administration of gonadotropin is initiated after monitoring of patients' follicle sizes on cycle-day 2/3. Gonadotropin dosage varies according to the follicular response. Approximately after the 6th day of gonadotropin injection or when the follicular size reaches ≥14 mm, subcutaneous administration of the GnRH antagonist (e.g., cetrorelix 0.25 mg/d) begins.

■ MYO-INOSITOL

It has been found in recent studies that insulin sensitizers like myo-inositol improved the ovulation and pregnancy rate in insulin-resistant patients with PCOS when given alone or in combination with CC.[26]

Pundir et al. conducted a systematic review and meta-analysis on inositol treatment in women with PCOS, published in the British Journal of Obstetrics and Gynaecology (BJOG) in 2017.[27] 10 trials and a total of 362 women were on inositol (257 on myo-inositol; 105 on di-chiro-inositol), 179 were on placebo, and 60 were on metformin. Inositol was associated with significantly improved ovulation rate [relative risk (RR) 2.3; 95% confidence interval (CI) 1.1–4.7; I2 = 75%] and increased frequency of menstrual cycles (RR 6.8; 95% CI 2.8–16.6; I2 = 0%) compared with placebo. One study reported on the clinical pregnancy rate with inositol compared with placebo (RR 3.3; 95% CI 0.4–27.1), and one study compared with metformin (RR 1.5; 95% CI 0.7–3.1). No studies evaluated live birth and miscarriage rates.[27]

They concluded that inositol appears to regulate menstrual cycles, improve ovulation, and induce metabolic changes in PCOS; however, evidence is lacking for pregnancy, miscarriage, or live birth. A further, well-designed multicentric trial to address this issue to provide robust evidence of benefit is warranted.

■ COCHRANE META-ANALYSIS

Forty-two RCTs and 7,935 women were analyzed in a Cochrane meta-analysis in 2018.[19] Letrozole had higher live birth rates compared to clomiphene (with timed intercourse) [odds ratio (OR) 1.68, 95% CI 1.42–1.99; 2,954 participants; 13 studies; I2 = 0%; number needed to treat for an additional beneficial outcome (NNTB) = 10].

There is evidence for a higher pregnancy rate in favor of letrozole (OR 1.56, 95% CI 1.37–1.78; 4,629 participants; 25 studies; I2 = 1%; NNTB = 10; moderate-quality evidence). There is little or no difference between treatment groups in the rate of miscarriage by pregnancy (20% with CC vs. 19% with letrozole; OR 0.94, 95% CI 0.70–1.26; 1,210 participants; 18 studies; I2 = 0%) and multiple pregnancy rate (1.7% with CC vs. 1.3% with letrozole; OR 0.69, 95% CI 0.41–1.16; 3,579 participants; 17 studies; I2 = 0%).

There is low-quality evidence that live birth rates are similar with letrozole or laparoscopic ovarian drilling (OR 1.38, 95% CI 0.95–2.02; 548 participants; 3 studies; I2 = 23%). There is low-quality evidence that pregnancy rates are similar (OR 1.28, 95% CI 0.94–1.74; 774 participants; 5 studies; I2 = 0%). There is insufficient evidence for a difference in miscarriage rate (OR 0.66, 95% CI 0.30–1.43; 240 participants; 5 studies; I2 = 0%) or multiple pregnancies (OR 3.00, 95% CI 0.12–74.90; 548 participants; 3 studies; I2 = 0%).

Additional comparisons were made for letrozole versus placebo, SERMs followed by IUI, FSH, anastrozole, and dosage and administration protocols. There is insufficient evidence for a difference in either group of treatment due to a limited number of studies. Hence, the reviewers concluded that more research is necessary.[19]

CONCLUSION

Although CC as a treatment modality has existed for more than 50 years, an increased awareness of the effect of obesity and different PCOS phenotypes has emerged. Accordingly, ovulation induction in women suffering from oligo- and anovulation seeking fertility treatment has to be individualized according to weight, treatment efficacy, and patient compliance, with the aim of achieving monofollicular growth, mono-ovulation, and subsequently the birth of a singleton baby.

REFERENCES

1. Practice Committee of the American Society for Reproductive Medicine. Use of clomiphene citrate in infertile women: a committee opinion. Fertil Steril. 2013;100(2):341-8.
2. Fritz MA, Speroff L. Clinical Gynecologic Endocrinology and Infertility, 8th edition. Philadelphia: Wolters Kluwer Health/Lippincott Williams & Wilkins; 2011. p. x, 1439.
3. Dehbashi S, Vafaei H, Parsanezhad MD, Alborzi S. Time of initiation of clomiphene citrate and pregnancy rate in polycystic ovarian syndrome. Int J Gynaecol Obstet. 2006;93(1):44-8.
4. Von Hofe J, Bates GW. Ovulation induction. Obstet Gynecol Clin North Am. 2015;42(1):27-37.
5. American College of Obstetricians and Gynecologists. ACOG practice bulletin. Management of infertility caused by ovulatory dysfunction. Number 34, February 2002. American College of Obstetricians and Gynecologists. Int J Gynaecol Obstet. 2002;77(2):177-88.
6. Deaton JL, Gibson M, Blackmer KM, Nakajima ST, Badger GJ, Brumsted JR. A randomized, controlled trial of clomiphene citrate and intrauterine insemination in couples with unexplained infertility or surgically corrected endometriosis. Fertil Steril. 1990;54(6):1083-8.
7. Palomba, S., 2015. Aromatase inhibitors for ovulation induction. J Clin Endocrinol Metab. 2015;100(5):1742-7.
8. Birch Petersen K, Pedersen NG, Pedersen AT, Lauritsen MP, la Cour Freiesleben N. Mono-ovulation in women with polycystic ovary syndrome: a clinical review on ovulation induction. Reprod Biomed Online. 2016;32(6):563-83.
9. Moolenaar LM, Nahuis MJ, Hompes PG, van der Veen F, Mol BW. Cost-effectiveness of treatment strategies in women with PCOS who do not conceive after six cycles of clomiphene citrate. Reprod Biomed Online. 2014;28(5):606-13.
10. Dhaliwal LK, Suri V, Gupta KR, Sahdev S. Tamoxifen: An alternative to clomiphene in women with polycystic ovary syndrome. J Hum Reprod Sci. 2011;4(2):76-9.
11. van Santbrink EJ, Donderwinkel PF, van Dessel TJ, Fauser BC. Gonadotropin induction of ovulation using a step-down dose regimen: single-centre clinical experience in 82 patients. Hum Reprod. 1995;10(5):1048-53.
12. Mitwally MF, Casper RF. Single-dose administration of an aromatase inhibitor for ovarian stimulation. Fertil Steril. 2005;83(1):229-31.
13. Atay V, Cam C, Muhcu M, Cam M, Karateke A. Comparison of letrozole and clomiphene citrate in women with polycystic ovaries undergoing ovarian stimulation. J Int Med Res. 2006;34(1):73-6.
14. Badawy A, Mosbah A, Tharwat A, Eid M. Extended letrozole therapy for ovulation induction in clomiphene-resistant women with polycystic ovary syndrome: a novel protocol. Fertil Steril. 2009;92(1):236-9.
15. Keay SD, Jenkins JM. Adjunctive use of dexamethasome in Clomid resistant patients. Fertil Steril. 2003;80(1):230-1.
16. Nahid L, Sirous K. Comparison of the effects of letrozole and clomiphene citrate for ovulation induction in infertile women with polycystic ovary syndrome. Minerva Ginecol. 2012;64(3):253-8.
17. Mitwally MF, Casper RF. Use of an aromatase inhibitor for induction of ovulation in patients

with an inadequate response to clomiphene citrate. Fertil Steril. 2001;75(2):305-9.
18. Begum MR, Ferdous J, Begum A, Quadir E. Comparison of efficacy of aromatase inhibitor and clomiphene citrate in induction of ovulation in polycystic ovarian syndrome. Fertil Steril. 2009;92(3):853-7.
19. Franik S, Eltrop SM, Kremer JA, Kiesel L, Farquhar C. Aromatase inhibitors (letrozole) for subfertile women with polycystic ovary syndrome. Cochrane Database of Syst Rev. 2018; 5(5):CD010287.
20. Misso ML, Wong JL, Teede HJ, Hart R, Rombauts L, Melder AM. Aromatase inhibitors for PCOS: a systematic review and meta-analysis. Hum Reprod Update. 2012; 18(3):301-12.
21. Naderpoor N, Shorakae S, de Courten B, Misso ML, Moran LJ, Teede HJ. Metformin and lifestyle modification in polycystic ovary syndrome: systematic review and meta-analysis. Hum Reprod Update. 2015;21(5):560-74.
22. Morin-Papunen L, Rantala AS, Unkila-Kallio L, Tiitinen A, Hippeläinen M, Perheentupa A, et al. Metformin improves pregnancy and live-birth rates in women with polycystic ovary syndrome (PCOS): a multicenter, double-blind, placebo-controlled randomized trial. J Clin Endocrinol Metab. 2012;97(5):1492-500.
23. Lathi RB, Milki AA. Recombinant gonadotropins. Curr Womens Health Rep. 2001; 1(2):157-63.
24. World Health Organization. Agents stimulating gonadal function in the human. Report of a WHO scientific group. World Health Organ Tech Rep Ser. 1973;514:1-30.
25. Thessaloniki. ESHRE/ASRM-Sponsored PCOS Consensus Workshop Group. Consensus on infertility treatment related to polycystic ovary syndrome. Fertil Steril. 2008; 89(3):505-22.
26. Kamenov Z, Kolarov G, Gateva A, Carlomagno G, Genazzani AD. Ovulation induction with myo-inositol alone and in combination with clomiphene citrate in polycystic ovarian syndrome patients with insulin resistance. Gynecol Endocrinol. 2015;31(2):131-5.
27. Pundir J, Psaroudakis D, Savnur P, Bhide P, Sabatini L, Teede H, et al. Inositol treatment of anovulation in women with polycystic ovary syndrome: a meta-analysis of randomised trials. BJOG. 2017;125(3):299-308.

CHAPTER 24

Role of Adjuvants in PCOS

Bhavna Mittal, Chandana Bhatt, Poonam Goyal

INTRODUCTION

Polycystic ovary syndrome (PCOS) is a lifestyle disorder and has no definite etiopathology and therefore, no definitive treatment or cure and there is a need of additional therapies which can supplement the role of the main treatment **(Flowchart 1)**. Adjuvants are agents, procedures, or tools which are used in addition to the mainline therapy in treatment of any disorder.

ROLE OF ADJUVANTS IN THE MANAGEMENT OF REPRODUCTIVE OUTCOME IN POLYCYSTIC OVARY SYNDROME

Role of adjuvants in the management of reproductive outcome in PCOS is:
- To improve ovulation
- To improve in vitro fertilization (IVF) outcome

ADJUVANTS (TABLES 1 AND 2)

- *Metformin:* The women who have proven to be resistant to clomiphene alone, the use of metformin in combination with clomiphene is a logical next step. Women with PCOS undergoing in vitro fertilization should be offered metformin to reduce their risk of ovarian hyperstimulation syndrome.[1] It can be continued through the first trimester once pregnancy has been diagnosed. Metformin may be a suitable alternative to the combined oral contraceptive pill for treating hyperandrogenic symptoms of PCOS including hirsutism and acne. More research is required to define whether metformin has a role in improving long-term health outcomes for women

TABLE 1: Adjuvants in PCOS.

Drugs	Alternate options
• Metformin	Acupuncture
• Myoinositol	
• Glucocorticoids	
• Chromium polynicotinate	
• Vitamin D	
• N-acetyl cysteine	
• Melatonin	
• Selenium	
Procedure	
LOD	

(LOD: laparoscopic ovarian drilling)

Flowchart 1: PCOS spectrum.

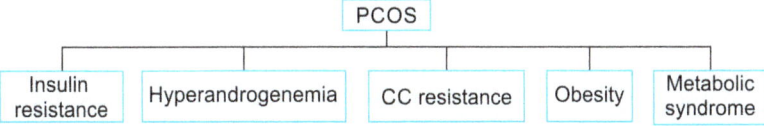

TABLE 2: Details of adjuvants used in PCOS.

Adjuvant	Mechanism of action	Dose	Indications	Side effect	Evidence
Metformin	Biguanide increases insulin sensitivity in peripheral tissues at the postreceptor level	1,500–2,550 mg/day (500 or 850 mg three times daily)	• CC resistance • IGT/T2DM • Increased waist-hip ratio • In long agonist protocol to decrease the risk of OHSS	• Nausea and diarrhea • Lactic acidosis in women with renal impairment, congestive heart failure, and sepsis	In CC resistance metformin and CC significantly improved ovulation and pregnancy rates when compared with CC alone but did not improve the odds of live birth
Myoinositol	• Act as second messengers and enhance the tyrosine kinase mediate the metabolic actions of insulin • Insulinomimetic and have an activating/sensitizing effect	2–4 g/day orally	Intolerant/when metformin is contraindicated	Mild GI disturbances, although its rare	Favorable effects on metabolic, endocrine, and ovulation parameters
Glucocorticoids	Reduce adrenal androgen production by negative feedback inhibition of ACTH	0.5–2 mg	Adjuvant in CC and gonadotropin ovulation induction, CC resistance	Weight gain, glucose intolerance, and osteoporosis	In clomiphene-resistant anovulatory infertile women, over 80% of those receiving combined treatment with clomiphene, and dexamethasone (2 mg daily, cycle days 5–14) ovulated
Chromium polynicotinate	Improves insulin sensitivity at the insulin receptor level and active glucose transport is enhanced through tyrosine kinase phosphorylation	1,000 mg/day	In adolescent and adult PCOS to improve the hormonal and metabolic profile	No adverse effects are reported with intake of chromium picolinate	–

Contd...

Contd...

Adjuvant	Mechanism of action	Dose	Indications	Side effect	Evidence
Vitamin D	Promotes insulin receptor expression and suppression of proinflammatory cytokines	800–1,000 IU/day	• To improve the menstrual regularity, follicular development, and pregnancy rate • Known to have favorable impact on hormonal and metabolic profile	High serum levels can cause vitamin D toxicity	Improves total testosterone, hs-CRP, and total antioxidant capacity
N-acetyl cysteine	Increases the cellular levels of antioxidants and effect on glutathione	1,200–1,800 mg/day, orally divided in three doses for 4–6 months	Impact on hormonal and metabolic profile	Mild GI disturbances	Favorable effect on hormonal and metabolic profile with improvement in the fasting glucose levels and reduction in BMI
Melatonin	Potent-free radical scavenger	3 mg/day oral	Metabolic and reproductive profile	--	Enhances the quality of the oocyte and embryo, increase the number of mature oocytes
Selenium	Antioxidant and insulinomimmetic	200 µg/day	Metabolic profile	–	–

(ACTH: adrenocorticotropic hormone; BMI: body mass index; CC: clomiphene citrate; GI: gastrointestinal; hs-CRP: high sensitivity C-reactive protein; IGT: impaired glucose tolerance; OHSS: ovarian hyperstimulation syndrome; PCOS: polycystic ovary syndrome; T2DM: type 2 diabetes mellitus)

with PCOS, including the prevention of diabetes, cardiovascular disease, and endometrial cancer.
- *Myoinositol:* Myoinositol and D-chiro-inositol are credited to act as second messengers, which have shown to exert a variable although significant effect in improving both symptoms and outcomes in PCOS patients.[2]
- *Glucocorticoids:* Numerous studies have examined the efficacy of adjuvant treatment with glucocorticoids in clomiphene-resistant anovulatory women, and all have found that combined treatment with clomiphene and a glucocorticoid can successfully induce ovulation in many who fail to respond to clomiphene alone. It is found to be useful in women with both normal and elevated dehydroepiandrosterone sulfate (DHEA-S). The mechanism of glucocorticoid action remains unclear but appears to involve

more than simple androgen suppression including direct effects on the developing oocyte and indirect effects on intrafollicular growth factors and cytokines, which may act synergistically with follicle-stimulating hormone (FSH).[3]

- *Chromium polynicotinate:* It improves insulin sensitivity at the insulin receptor level, which helps with the insulin resistance and the obesity seen in PCOS. It is seen that doses of 1,000 μg/day, for 2 months, led to an improvement in insulin resistance in PCOS patients.[4]
- *Vitamin D:* Its deficiency can aggravate hyperandrogenism and insulin resistance, the prevalence rate being as high as 75%. Vitamin D supplementation with a daily dose supplementation appeared to be more conducive in improving hormone, inflammation, and oxidative stress in patients with PCOS.[5]
- *N-acetyl cysteine:* It has insulin-sensitizing, androgen-reducing effects, antiapoptotic and antioxidant effects, inhibition of phospholipid metabolism, proinflammatory cytokine release, and protease activity, may lead to better folliculogenesis and ovulation rate in PCOS patients. The antioxidant effects of N-acetylcysteine and its protective characteristics against focal ischemia have positive impact on endometrial thickness.[6]
- *Melatonin:* It is a potent-free radical scavenger that exerts protective effects in female reproductive organ and is involved in the protection of the oocyte against oxidative stress, particularly at the time of ovulation. Melatonin treatment in PCOS patients can enhance the quality of the oocyte and embryo, increase the number of mature oocytes, reduce obesity, and ameliorate the proinflammatory state, which underlies the development of insulin resistance.[7]
- *Selenium:* It is an indispensable trace element because of its antioxidant and anti-inflammatory properties. It is a trace element which operates as an integral part of selenoproteins assisting redox processes as an effective antioxidant. The supplementation with selenium in improving reproductive outcomes, inflammatory biomarkers, and oxidative stress may be linked to its inhibitory effects on proinflammatory cytokines and reactive oxygen and nitrogen species. However, the available data are currently insufficient to support the protective effects of selenium on PCOS.[8]

PROCEDURES TO IMPROVE OVULATION

Laparoscopic ovarian drilling: It is the surgical option for clomiphene citrate (CC)-resistant PCOS cases. It is as effective as gonadotropins in terms of clinical pregnancy rates and live birth rates with the obvious advantages of spontaneous mono-ovulation, thereby minimizing the need for intensive monitoring and eliminating the risks of ovarian hyperstimulation syndrome and multiple pregnancies.[9]

Adverse effects: Iatrogenic adhesions and decreased ovarian reserve.

Alternate Therapies

Acupuncture: It refers to using the needle inserted into the patient's specific area of the body at a certain angle to cure diseases through the manipulations, such as twisting, lifting, and thrusting. In PCOS, it is known to regulate the function of the hypothalamus-pituitary-ovarian axis and the metabolism, promote ovulation, and improve insulin resistance and endometrial receptivity. As per the current evidence use of acupuncture for improving ovulation and menstruation rates and other hormonal changes in women with PCOS is weak.[10]

REFERENCES

1. Johnson NP. Metformin use in women with polycystic ovary syndrome. Ann Transl Med. 2014;2(6):56.
2. Unfer V, Facchinetti F, Orrù B, Giordani B, Nestler J. Myo-inositol effects in women with PCOS: A meta-analysis of randomized controlled trials. Endocr Connect. 2017;6(8):647-58.
3. Speroff L, Fritz MA. Clinical Gynecologic Endocrinology and Infertility, 9th edition. Philadelphia: Lippincott Williams & Wilkins; 2019. pp. 2810-1.
4. Ashoush S, Abou-Gamrah A, Bayoumy H, Othman N. Chromium picolinate reduces insulin resistance in polycystic ovary syndrome: Randomized controlled trial. J Obstet Gynaecol Res. 2016;42(3):279-85.
5. Davis EM, Peck JD, Hansen KR, Neas BR, Craig LB. Associations between vitamin D levels and polycystic ovary syndrome phenotypes. Minerva Endocrinol. 2019;44(2):17684.
6. Nemati M, Nemati S, Taheri AM, Heidari B. Comparison of metformin and N-acetyl cysteine, as an adjuvant to clomiphene citrate, in clomiphene-resistant women with polycystic ovary syndrome. J Gynecol Obstet Hum Reprod. 2017;46(7):579-85.
7. Mojaverrostami S, Asghari N, Khamisabadi M, Khoei HH. The role of melatonin in polycystic ovary syndrome: A review. Int J Reprod Biomed. 2019;17(12):865-82.
8. Hajizadeh-Sharafabad F, Moludi J, Tutunchi H, Taheri E, Izadi A, Maleki V. Selenium and polycystic ovary syndrome; current knowledge and future directions: A systematic review. Horm Metab Res. 2019; 51(5):279-87.
9. Mitra S, Nayak PK, Agrawal S. Laparoscopic ovarian drilling: An alternative but not the ultimate in the management of polycystic ovary syndrome. J Nat Sci Biol Med. 2015;6(1):40-8.
10. Jo J, Lee YJ, Lee H. Acupuncture for polycystic ovarian syndrome: A systematic review and meta-analysis. Medicine (Baltimore). 2017; 96(23):e7066.

ART in PCOS

Rohan Palshetkar, Nandita Palshetkar, Mayuri More

■ INTRODUCTION

According to ethnicity and the criteria used for diagnosis, polycystic ovary syndrome (PCOS) affects between 2% and 13% of women in reproductive age.[1-4] According to the World Health Organization,[5] PCOS is the most common cause of anovulatory infertility and eugonadotropic hypogonadism, with 55–91% of these women considered to have signs and/or symptoms of the disease.[6] Women with PCOS are more likely to be subfertile, with 26% struggling to conceive compared with 17% of women without signs of PCOS.[7] However, population studies have shown that while women with PCOS may take longer than expected to conceive, their lifetime fertility does not appear to be significantly impaired.[5,7]

The primary management of PCOS-related infertility includes lifestyle medication (weight loss) and the use of drugs to induce monofollicular ovulation. Drugs treatments typically begin with the use of letrozole followed by the administration of gonadotropins, with planned relations or intrauterine insemination. Assisted reproductive techniques (ART) mainly in vitro fertilization (IVF) and intracytoplasmic sperm injection (ICSI) represent the third line of treatment.

Multiple pregnancy and ovarian hyperstimulation syndrome (OHSS) remain the major complications of ovulation induction and occur despite ultrasound monitoring.[8,9] Women with PCOS are typically more difficult to stimulate in a controlled manner, whether the intention is to induce a monofollicular or multifollicular response, are more likely to demonstrate resistance to stimulation and/or exaggerated response, and experience higher cycle cancellation rate than women without PCOS. While a high number of oocytes may be obtained during ART, there are concerns that the quality and maturity of these oocytes may be compromised.[10-17] Despite all this, live birth rates after ART in women with PCOS seem to be comparable with those of women with other diagnoses, such as endometriosis, unexplained infertility, or male factor infertility.[18,19]

To avoid the risks of OHSS and cycle cancellation and to improve oocyte quality various measures have been introduced. These include, priming with metformin, use of gonadotropin-releasing hormone (GnRH) antagonist cycles as compared to the conventional long GnRH agonist (GnRHa) protocol, administration of dopamine agonist, and oocyte retrieval without controlled ovarian stimulation through in vitro maturation (IVM) of oocytes.[10,20-26]

■ OVULATION INDUCTION

The first ovulation-inducing drug of choice for women with PCOS was clomiphene citrate. However, the Pregnancy in Polycystic

Ovary Syndrome II (PPCOS II) randomized controlled trial established superiority of letrozole (an aromatase inhibitor) over clomiphene in achieving significantly higher live birth and ovulation rates among infertile women with PCOS.[27,28] The incidence of clomiphene resistance (i.e., failure to ovulate) was as high as 25%, underscoring a need to explore alternative treatment options to achieve successful ovulation in women with PCOS. In PPCOS II trial, women with PCOS were randomized to treatment with starting doses of 50 mg of clomiphene or 2.5 mg of letrozole, with increased doses as needed for each group (not to exceed the maximum dose of 150 or 7.5 mg, respectively). Significantly higher cumulative live birth rate of 27.5% was observed in subjects randomized to receive letrozole compared to 19.1% in women receiving clomiphene in a rate ratio of 1.44 [95% confidence interval (CI) 1.10–1.87].[27,28]

Treatment with insulin-sensitizing agents (metformin, thiazolidinediones, D-chiro-inositol, and myo-inositol) has been used in attempts to increase/improve ovulation rates. Metformin has been widely used for this purpose, yet studies have not demonstrated superiority to other agents/ovulation induction regimens.[29-32]

Induction of ovulation with exogenous gonadotropins is highly effective, but requires careful monitoring to avoid the intrinsic risks of multiple pregnancy and OHSS. Many women are highly sensitive to low doses of medication and exhibit a relatively narrow therapeutic range.[33-38]

IN VITRO FERTILIZATION IN POLYCYSTIC OVARY SYNDROME

Women with PCO produced more follicles, oocytes, and embryos. Fertilization, cleavage, and spontaneous abortion rates were similar in the two groups. However, when adjusted for age the cumulative conception rate after three cycles of IVF was higher in women with PCO compared with women with normal ovaries. It appears that ovaries with polycystic morphology confer a benefit regarding the outcome of IVF treatment.[39]

Elevated luteinizing hormone (LH) concentrations commonly associated with the syndrome have been blamed for increased incidence of OHSS and spontaneous abortions. Due to the above concerns, gonadotropin preparations devoid of LH were advocated. Although there are no comparative data regarding the outcome of IVF in PCOS patients stimulated with different gonadotropin preparations, data from ovulation induction cycles suggest that there are no outcome differences in the gonadotropin preparations studied.[40]

Recombinant follicle-stimulating hormone (rec-FSH) was found to yield higher pregnancy rates and the total gonadotropin dose required was lower.[41] In this meta-analysis, the study also concluded that for every 19 patients treated one additional patient would conceive when treated with rec-FSH. Spontaneous abortion, multiple pregnancy, and OHSS rates were similar for both gonadotropins. As women with PCOS have elevated LH concentrations, gonadotropin preparations devoid of LH may in theory be more physiological. It has been shown that in women with polycystic ovaries suppression of LH concentrations with GnRHa prior to stimulation may reduce the incidence of spontaneous abortions.[42]

The recent introduction of GnRH antagonists provides a new and exciting means to ovarian stimulation. Both the duration and cost of treatment appear to be decreased with antagonist use.

The dose of gonadotropin used in the PCO/PCOS patient should be selected very carefully. These patients are particularly prone to ovarian hyperstimulation. Mild hyperstimulation is encountered in almost all patients with PCOS. However, severe forms of the disease should be avoidable in most cases.

Administration of oral contraceptives prior to initiation of GnRHa has been shown to decrease the rate of OHSS and increase the rates of fertilization, embryo implantation, and clinical pregnancy.[43] Whether administration of insulin-sensitizing agents prior to and during ovarian stimulation in women with PCOS improves the treatment outcome is also controversial.

The dose of gonadotropin should initially be as low as possible. It is current practice to start the treatment at a dose of 150 IU/day considering the body mass index (BMI). Conditions for starting gonadotropins are the same as in women with normal ovaries. A lower dose protocol with a starting dose of 75 IU of rec-FSH has yielded impressive results in women with PCOS undergoing ovarian stimulation for IVF.[44]

Protocols utilizing GnRH antagonists can also be used for women with PCOS undergoing ovarian stimulation for IVF.

Oral contraceptive pretreatment and maintaining or increasing the dose of gonadotropins once the antagonist is initiated should yield better results.

The later may, however, render cycle management in the brittle PCOS patient more difficult, as coasting is often necessary in these patients as a measure to prevent overstimulation. GnRH antagonists during coasting have been successfully used in a patient at risk of hyperstimulation during ovulation induction with a low-dose step-up protocol.[45]

IN VITRO MATURATION IN POLYCYSTIC OVARY SYNDROME

The technique of IVM has been used in veterinary practice for a long time.[46,47] However, the first pregnancy resulting from IVM in humans was reported in 1991 using donor oocytes from unstimulated ovaries from women undergoing gynecological surgery.[48] The use of IVM for infertility treatment has several perceived advantages over conventional IVF for women with a high antral follicle count, such as women with PCOS. These include a shorter duration of stimulation and the use of less gonadotropins. Additionally, there is the avoidance of the suprapyhsiologic levels of estradiol, with its symptomatic benefits, and the opportunity to minimize exposure to high estradiol concentrations for a woman undergoing ovarian stimulation for fertility preservation with breast cancer, or a woman with a thrombophilia, and the elimination of the risk of OHSS.

In vitro maturation can be used in patients with ovarian resistance to FSH,[49] fertility preservation of cancer patients (particularly women with leukemia and estrogen-sensitive tumors), and endometriosis patients undergoing extensive endometrioma excision.[49] It can also be used as a fertility-preserving option for women at risk of premature ovarian failure.[50] It has also been used in normal responders with history of poor oocyte/embryo quality as well as for oocyte donation cycles to avoid the discomfort of the stimulation for a donor.

The effect of various IVM protocols using no priming, FSH only, human chorionic gonadotropin (hCG) only, and FSH with hCG had been studied by Fadini et al. in normoovulatory women[51] and reviewed by Siristatidis et al.[52] Their data demonstrate the use of FSH with hCG improved clinical pregnancy rates and implantation rates in a randomized trial.[51] The effects of FSH priming in the follicular phase are due to the recruitment of greater number of follicles, whereas hCG priming causes maturation of some follicles in vivo leading to recruitment of oocytes at different stages.[53,54] Hence, in IVM cycles with hCG priming, it is possible to collect oocytes in various stages of maturity from follicles from 2 to 13 mm in size.

Tannus et al. have reported clinical pregnancy rates of 44.7% and live birth rate of 34.6%, for women undergoing IVM treatment, with the majority of transfers being single.[55]

The IVM approach offers an excellent treatment option for women with PCOS, who are required to undergo assisted reproduction, as many subfertile women with PCOS will conceive with ovulation induction therapy alone. IVM offers several advantages over standard IVF, particularly the elimination of the risk of OHSS; it is cheaper and with a lower side effect profile than IVF, and offers a "patient friendly" approach to assisted reproduction.

■ REFERENCES

1. Asunción M, Calvo RM, San Millán JL, Sancho J, Avila S, Escobar-Morreale HF. A prospective study of the prevalence of the polycystic ovary syndrome in unselected Caucasian women from Spain. J Clin Endocrinol Metab. 2000;85:2434-38.
2. Azziz R, Carmina E, Dewailly D, Diamanti-Kandarakis E, Escobar-Morreale HF, Futterweit W, et al.; Task Force on the Phenotype of the Polycystic Ovary Syndrome of The Androgen Excess and PCOS Society. The Androgen Excess and PCOS Society criteria for the polycystic ovary syndrome: the complete task force report. Fertil Steril. 2009;91:456-88.
3. Rotterdam ESHRE/ASRM-Sponsored PCOS consensus workshop group. Revised 2003 consensus on diagnostic criteria and long-term health risks related to polycystic ovary syndrome (PCOS). Hum Reprod. 2004;19:41-7.
4. Wang S, Alvero R. Racial and ethnic differences in physiology and clinical symptoms of polycystic ovary syndrome. Semin Reprod Med. 2013;31:365-9.
5. ESHRE Capri Workshop Group. Health and fertility in World Health Organization group 2 anovulatory women. Hum Reprod Update. 2012;18:586-99.
6. Broekmans FJ, Knauff EA, Valkenburg O, Laven JS, Eijkemans MJ, Fauser BC. PCOS according to the Rotterdam consensus criteria: Change in prevalence among WHO-II anovulation and association with metabolic factors. BJOG. 2006;113:1210-7.
7. Koivunen R, Pouta A, Franks S, Martikainen H, Sovio U, Hartikainen AL, et al.; Northern Finland Birth Cohort 1966 Study. Fecundability and spontaneous abortions in women with self-reported oligo-amenorrhea and/or hirsutism: Northern Finland Birth Cohort 1966 Study. Hum Reprod. 2008;23: 2134-9.
8. Brown J, Farquhar C, Beck J, Boothroyd C, Hughes E. Clomiphene and anti-oestrogens for ovulation induction in PCOS. Cochrane Database Syst Rev. 2009;CD002249.
9. Nastri CO, Ferriani RA, Rocha IA, Martins WP. Ovarian hyperstimulation syndrome: pathophysiology and prevention. J Assist Reprod Genet. 2010;27:121-8.
10. Baumgarten M, Polanski L, Campbell B, Raine-Fenning N. Do dopamine agonists prevent or reduce the severity of ovarian hyperstimulation syndrome in women undergoing assisted reproduction? A systematic review and meta-analysis. Hum Fertil. 2013;16:168-74.
11. Kumar P, Nawani N, Malhotra N, Malhotra J, Patil M, Jayakrishnan K, et al. Assisted reproduction in polycystic ovarian disease: A multicentric trial in India. J Hum Reprod Sci. 2013;6:49-53.
12. Siristatidis CS, Vrachnis N, Creatsa M, Maheshwari A, Bhattacharya S. In vitro maturation in subfertile women with

polycystic ovarian syndrome undergoing assisted reproduction. Cochrane Database Syst Rev. 2013;10:CD006606.
13. Coffler MS, Patel K, Dahan MH, Malcom PJ, Kawashima T, Deutsch R, et al. Evidence for abnormal granulosa cell responsiveness to follicle-stimulating hormone in women with polycystic ovary syndrome. J Clin Endocrinol Metab. 2003;88:1742-7.
14. Coffler MS, Patel K, Dahan MH, Yoo RY, Malcom PJ, Chang RJ. Enhanced granulosa cell responsiveness to follicle-stimulating hormone during insulin infusion in women with polycystic ovary syndrome treated with pioglitazone. J Clin Endocrinol Metab. 2003;88:5624-31.
15. Doronzo G, Russo I, Mattiello L, Anfossi G, Bosia A, Trovati M. Insulin activates vascular endothelial growth factor in vascular smooth muscle cells: influence of nitric oxide and of insulin resistance. Eur J Clin Invest. 2004;34:664-73.
16. Jayaprakasan K, Chan Y, Islam R, Haoula Z, Hopkisson J, Coomarasamy A, et al. Prediction of in vitro fertilization outcome at different antral follicle count thresholds in a prospective cohort of 1,012 women. Fertil Steril. 2012;98:657-63.
17. Ocal P, Sahmay S, Cetin M, Irez T, Guralp O, Cepni I. Serum anti-Müllerian hormone and antral follicle count as predictive markers of OHSS in ART cycles. J Assist Reprod Genet. 2011;28:1197-203.
18. Sigala J, Sifer C, Dewailly D, Robin G, Bruyneel A, Ramdane N, et al. Is polycystic ovarian morphology related to a poor oocyte quality after controlled ovarian hyperstimulation for intracytoplasmic sperm injection? Results from a prospective, comparative study. Fertil Steril. 2015;103:112-8.
19. Stern JE, Brown MB, Wantman E, Kalra SK, Luke B. Live birth rates and birth outcomes by diagnosis using linked cycles from the SART CORS database. J Assist Reprod Genet. 2013;30:1445-50.
20. Al-Inany HG, Youssef MA, Aboulghar M, Broekmans F, Sterrenburg M, Smit J, et al. GnRH antagonists are safer than agonists: an update of a Cochrane review. Hum Reprod Update. 2011;17:435.
21. Nardo LG, Bosch E, Lambalk CB, Gelbaya TA. Controlled ovarian hyperstimulation regimens: a review of the available evidence for clinical practice. Produced on behalf of the BFS Policy and Practice Committee. Hum Fertil. 2013;16:144-50.
22. Ortega-Hrepich C, Stoop D, Guzmán L, Van Landuyt L, Tournaye H, Smitz J, et al. A "freeze-all" embryo strategy after in vitro maturation: a novel approach in women with polycystic ovary syndrome? Fertil Steril. 2013;100:1002-7.
23. Tang H, Hunter T, Hu Y, Zhai SD, Sheng X, Hart RJ. Cabergoline for preventing ovarian hyperstimulation syndrome. Cochrane Database Syst Rev. 2012;2:CD008605.
24. Tso LO, Costello MF, Albuquerque LE, Andriolo RB, Freitas V. Metformin treatment before and during IVF or ICSI in women with polycystic ovary syndrome. Cochrane Database Syst Rev. 2009;(2):CD006105.
25. Tso LO, Costello MF, Albuquerque LE, Andriolo RB, Macedo CR. Metformin treatment before and during IVF or ICSI in women with polycystic ovary syndrome. Cochrane Database Syst Rev. 2014;2014(11):CD006105.
26. Nastri CO, Teixeira DM, Moroni RM, Leitao VM, Martins WP. Ovarian hyperstimulation syndrome: pathophysiology, staging, prediction and prevention. Ultrasound Obstet Gynecol. 2015;45:377-93.
27. Legro RS, Kunselman AR, Brzyski RG, Casson PR, Diamond MP, Schlaff WD, et al. The pregnancy in polycystic ovary syndrome II (PPCOS II) trial: rationale and design of a double-blind randomized trial of clomiphene citrate and letrozole for the treatment of infertility in women with polycystic ovary syndrome. Contemp Clin Trials. 2012;33(3):470-81.
28. Legro RS, Brzyski RG, Diamond MP, Coutifaris C, Schlaff WD, Casson P, et al. Letrozole versus clomiphene for infertility in the polycystic ovary syndrome. N Engl J Med. 2014;371(2):119-29.

29. Morley LC, Tang T, Yasmin E, Norman RJ, Balen AH. Insulin-sensitising drugs (metformin, rosiglitazone, pioglitazone, D-chiro-inositol) for women with polycystic ovary syndrome, oligo amenorrhoea and subfertility. Cochrane Database Syst Rev. 2017;11(11):CD003053.
30. Practice Committee of the American Society for Reproductive Medicine, Practice Committee of the American Society for Reproductive Medicine. Role of metformin for ovulation induction in infertile patients with polycystic ovary syndrome (PCOS): a guideline. Fertil Steril. 2017;108:426.
31. Moll E, Bossuyt PM, Korevaar JC, Lambalk CB, van der Veen F. Effect of clomifene citrate plus metformin and clomifene citrate plus placebo on induction of ovulation in women with newly diagnosed polycystic ovary syndrome: randomised double blind clinical trial. BMJ. 2006;332:1485.
32. Legro RS, Barnhart HX, Schlaff WD, Carr BR, Diamond MP, Carson SA, et al. Clomiphene, metformin, or both for infertility in the polycystic ovary syndrome. N Engl J Med. 2007;356:551.
33. van Santbrink EJ, Fauser BC. Ovulation induction in normogonadotropic anovulation (PCOS). Best Pract Res Clin Endocrinol Metab. 2006;20:261.
34. López E, Joanne G, Daya S, Parrilla JJ, Abad L, Balasch J. Ovulation induction in women with polycystic ovary syndrome: randomized trial of clomiphene citrate versus low-dose recombinant FSH as first line therapy. Reprod Biomed Online. 2004;9(4):382-90.
35. Christin-Maitre S. A comparative randomized multicentric study comparing the step-up versus step-down protocol in polycystic ovary syndrome. Hum Reprod. 2003;18:1626.
36. Mulders AG, Eijkemans MJ, Imani B, Fauser BC. Prediction of chances for success or complications in gonadotrophin ovulation induction in normogonadotrophic anovulatory infertility. Reprod Biomed Online. 2003;7:170.
37. Tummon I, Gavrilova-Jordan L, Allemand MC, Session D. Polycystic ovaries and ovarian hyperstimulation syndrome: a systematic review. Acta Obstet Gynecol Scand. 2005;84:611.
38. Navot D, Goldstein N, Mor-Josef S, Simon A, Relou A, Birkenfeld A. Multiple pregnancies: risk factors and prognostic variables during induction of ovulation with human menopausal gonadotrophins. Hum Reprod. 1991;6:1152.
39. Engmann L, Maconochie N, Sladkevicius P, Bekir J, Campbell S, Tan SL. The outcome of in-vitro fertilization treatment in women with sonographic evidence of polycystic ovarian morphology. Hum Reprod. 1999;14(1):167-71.
40. Nugent D, Vanderkerckhove P, Hughes E, Arnot M, Lilford R. Gonadotrophin therapy for ovulation induction in subfertility associated with polycystic ovary syndrome. Cochrane Database Syst Rev. 2000;(4):CD000410.
41. Daya S. Updated meta-analyses of recombinant follicle stimulating hormone (FSH) versus urinary FSH for ovarian stimulation in assisted reproduction. Fertil Steril. 2002;77(4):711-4.
42. Balen AH. Hypersecretion of luteinizing hormone and the polycystic ovary syndrome. Hum Reprod. 1993;8 (suppl 2):123-8.
43. Damario MA, Barmat L, Liu HC, Davis OK, Rosenwaks Z. Dual suppression with oral contraceptives and gonadotropin releasing-hormone agonists improves in-vitro fertilization outcome in high responder patients. Hum Reprod. 1997;12(11):2359-65.
44. Marci R, Senn A, Dessole S, Chanson A, Loumaye E, De Grandi P, et al. A low-dose stimulation protocol using highly purified follicle-stimulating hormone can lead to high pregnancy rates in in-vitro fertilization patients with polycystic ovaries who are at risk of a high ovarian response to gonadotropins. Fertil Steril. 2001;75(6):1131-5.
45. Fatemi HM, Platteau P, Albano C, Van Steirteghem A, Devroey P. Rescue IVF and coasting with the use of a GnRH antagonist after ovulation induction. Reprod Biomed Online. 2002;5(3):273-5.
46. Lu KH, Gordon I, Gallagher M, McGovern H. Pregnancy established in cattle by transfer

of embryos derived from in vitro fertilisation of oocytes matured in vitro. Vet Rec. 1987; 121(11):259-60.
47. Goto K, Kajihara Y, Kosaka S, Koba M, Nakanishi Y, Ogawa K. "Pregnancies after co-culture of cumulus cells with bovine embryos derived from in-vitro fertilization of in-vitro matured follicular oocytes." J Reprod Fertil. 1988l;83(2):753-8.
48. Cha KY, Koo JJ, Ko JJ, Choi DH, Han SY, Yoon TK. Pregnancy after in vitro fertilization of human follicular oocytes collected from nonstimulated cycles, their culture in vitro and their transfer in a donor oocyte program. Fertil Steril. 1991;55(1):109-13.
49. Grynberg M, El Hachem H, de Bantel A, Benard J, le Parco S, Fanchin R. In vitro maturation of oocytes: uncommon indications. Fertil Steril. 2013;99(5):1182-8.
50. Fadini R, Mignini Renzini M, Dal Canto M, Epis A, Crippa M, Caliari I, et al. Oocyte in vitro maturation in normo-ovulatory women. Fertil Steril. 2013;99(5):1162-9.
51. Fadini R, Dal Canto MB, Mignini Renzini M, Brambillasca F, Comi R, Fumagalli D, et al. Effect of different gonadotrophin priming on IVM of oocytes from women with normal ovaries: a prospective randomized study. Reprod Biomed Online. 2009;19(3):343-51.
52. Siristatidis C, Sergentanis TN, Vogiatzi P, Kanavidis P, Chrelias C, Papantoniou N, et al. In vitro maturation in women with vs. without polycystic ovarian syndrome: a systematic review and meta-analysis. PloS One. 2015;10(8):e0134696.
53. Junk SM, Yeap D. Improved implantation and ongoing pregnancy rates after single-embryo transfer with an optimized protocol for in vitro oocyte maturation in women with polycystic ovaries and polycystic ovary syndrome. Fertil Steril. 2012;98(4):888-92.
54. De Vos M, Ortega-Hrepich C, Albuz FK, Guzman L, Polyzos NP, Smitz J, et al. Clinical outcome of non–hCG-primed oocyte in vitro maturation treatment in patients with polycystic ovaries and polycystic ovary syndrome. Fertil Steril. 2011;96(4):860-4.
55. Tannus S, Hatirnaz S, Tan J, Ata B, Tan SL, Hatirnaz E, et al. Predictive factors for live birth after in vitro maturation of oocytes in women with polycystic ovary syndrome. Arch Gynecol Obstet. 2018;297(1):199-204.

CHAPTER 26

Pregnancy in PCOS

Jaideep Malhotra, Parul Sinha, Asha Baxi

■ INTRODUCTION

- Polycystic ovary syndrome (PCOS) affects about 1 in 10 women of reproductive age of various ethnicities and races[1,2] but the heterogenous phenotypes in women with PCOS have variable pregnancy outcomes.
- PCOS women usually face challenges in conception due to the effects of obesity, metabolic dysfunction which includes insulin resistance (IR), inflammation, and/or endocrine abnormalities influencing ovulatory function, endometrial receptivity, and quality of oocytes.[3]
- This phenotypic variability along with different diagnostic criteria from adolescence to adulthood has led to various researches, interventions, and clinical management challenges.[1,4]
- Pregnancy in PCOS women causes various adverse pregnancy outcomes, independent of subfertility and use of assisted reproductive technology (ART).[5]
- Adverse perinatal outcomes include early pregnancy loss, gestational diabetes mellitus (GDM), hypertensive spectrum disorder [i.e., gestational hypertension (HTN) and preeclampsia], small for gestational age (SGA) and large for gestational age (LGA) infants, preterm births (PTB), and cesarean deliveries.[6-8]
- Although PCOS causes such high rates of adverse pregnancy outcomes, still some specific consensus on perinatal guidelines for the management of PCOS in pregnancy is lacking.[9,10]

■ PERINATAL OUTCOMES

Polycystic ovary syndrome is a common disorder associated with an increased risk of adverse perinatal outcomes **(Fig. 1)**, but the impact of different PCOS phenotypes on these adverse effects is inconsistent.[11,12]

- PCOS women who underwent in vitro fertilization (IVF) had clinical pregnancy rates almost same as other women undergoing IVF for causes of infertility other than PCOS.
- A recent meta-analysis associated PCOS women undergoing IVF with an increased miscarriage rate [odds ratio (OR): 1.52; 95% confidence interval (CI): 1.04-2.22], ovarian hyperstimulation syndrome (OR: 4.62; 95% CI: 3.20-6.68), GDM (OR: 2.67; 95% CI: 1.43-4.98), gestational HTN (OR: 2.06; 95% CI: 1.45-2.91), LGA (OR: 2.10; 95% CI: 1.01-4.37), and PTB (OR: 1.60; 95% CI: 1.25-2.04) as compared to IVF done for other reasons.[5]
- The most frequently reported pregnancy complications in women with PCOS are GDM (OR: 2.78-3.58) and hypertensive disorders of pregnancy (OR: 2.46-3.43), which are markedly increased irrespective of age, any treatment done for infertility/subfertility, obesity index, or any other confounding demographic factors.[7,8,13,14]

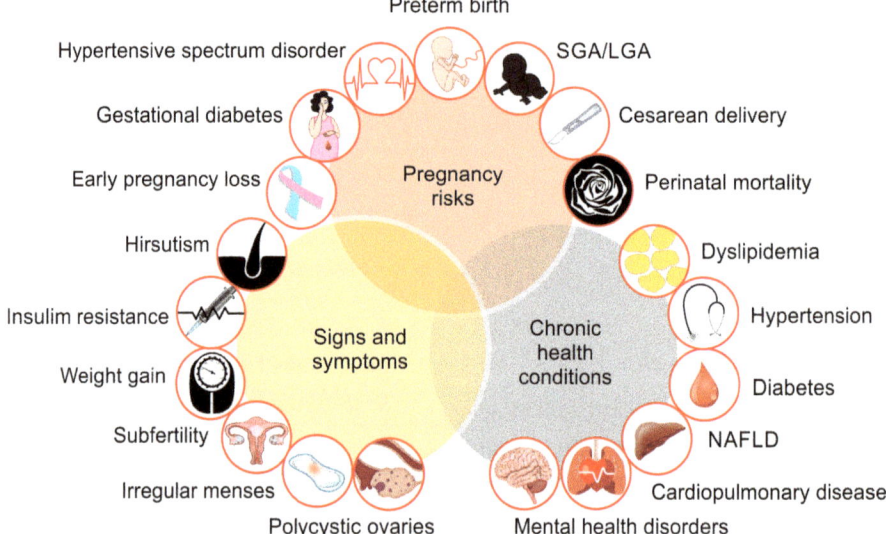

Fig. 1: Polycystic ovary syndrome (PCOS) is a pathophysiologically complex disorder with serious risks of perinatal complications and adverse chronic health conditions. (NAFLD: nonalcoholic fatty liver disease; SGA/LGA: small/large for gestational age).

- The association between PCOS and adverse neonatal outcomes is conflicting. A very recent meta-analysis associated PCOS with an increased risk of PTB (OR: 1.52–1.93).[5,7,14]
- Studies have cited a higher risk for both SGA and LGA in women with PCOS, but this holds true only in certain prospective studies and within specific population groups.[5,7]
- Newborns born to mothers with PCOS have a higher neonatal intensive care unit (NICU) admission rate (OR: 1.74–2.31) along with high perinatal mortality (OR: 1.83–3.07).[7,13,14]

PERINATAL, PRENATAL, AND POSTNATAL EVALUATION AND MANAGEMENT

Perinatal (Fig. 2)

- Several factors are associated with the increase in perinatal complications in individuals with PCOS.[15]
- This period can be utilized as a window of opportunity to discuss pregnancy-related complications, for the initiation of preventive screening and safe treatments during pregnancy.
- Oocyte quality can be improved by optimizing nutritional and lifestyle behaviors and thus leading to better pregnancy outcomes.[16,17]
- Prepregnancy body mass index (BMI) is a strong predictor of adverse perinatal outcomes, and the risk for preeclampsia, GDM, indicated preterm delivery, and macrosomia is increased in an incremental manner.[18]
- Therefore, the primary approach which helps in losing weight and improving health begins in the prepregnancy period which includes lifestyle modifications incorporating high-quality nutrition, adequate physical activity, and various other behavioral strategies.[19]
- Antiobesity medications should be avoided during pregnancy, and if the

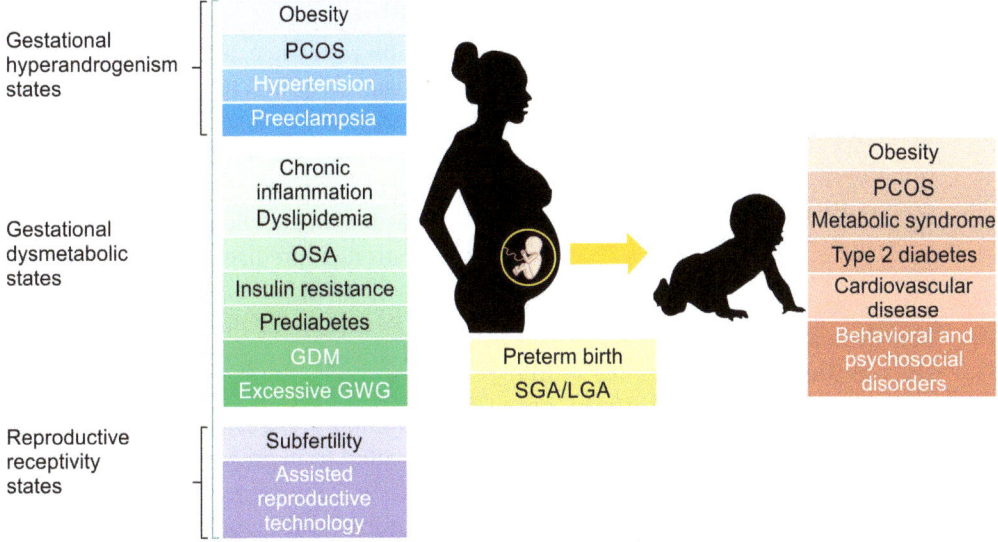

Fig. 2: Polycystic ovary syndrome (PCOS), PCOS-related conditions, and associated perinatal complications influence the intrauterine environment, leading to the developmental programming of the offspring for long-term, chronic health conditions. (GDM: gestational diabetes; GWG: gestational weight gain; OSA: obstructive sleep apnea; SGA/LGA: small/large for gestational age)
Source: Valent A, Barbour N. Management of women with polycystic ovary syndrome during pregnancy. Endocrinol Metab Clin N Am. 2021;50:57-69.

woman is using it since prepregnancy period, she should discontinue it and utilize other strategies.[20]
- Bariatric surgery has been found to reduce the rates of GDM, hypertensive disorders of pregnancy, and macrosomia, but it has potential postsurgical complications, fetal growth restriction, and numerous nutritional challenges that need to be addressed.[21]
- PCOS diagnosis should be followed by routine screening for mental health disorders such as depression and anxiety.
- If the patient is screen negative at the time of initial diagnosis, she is rescreened if she develops any of the high-risk factors such as obesity, diabetes, pregnancy, postpartum or if there is any family history of mental health disorders.[22]
- It is recommended to screen PCOS women for diabetes and cardiovascular risk factors such as obesity, disturbed lipid profile, HTN, and nicotine use before conception.[9,10]
- Overweight/obese individuals with PCOS are considered a high-risk population and should be screened using an oral glucose tolerance test (OGTT) early in gestation and retested at 24–28 weeks if early testing results are normal for prediabetes.[10,23]
- Since IR and obesity are strongly associated with sleep-breathing disorders, women with PCOS should be screened for sleep-breathing disorders preconceptionally and then throughout pregnancy.[24]

Prenatal

Since PCOS women are predisposed to more adverse pregnancy outcomes, they should have more robust surveillance during the prenatal and postnatal periods. However, there are no specific guidelines for antenatal fetal surveillance or ultrasound assessments for PCOS.

- *Metformin during pregnancy in women with PCOS:*
  - Majority of the randomized controlled trials (RCTs) have not found metformin to be useful for improving pregnancy outcomes or having any beneficial effects in preventing miscarriages, PTB, macrosomia, LGA, GDM, or preeclampsia.[25]
  - There are many studies citing concerns about potential long-term risks to the offspring because of the pleiotropic effects of metformin and its concentration in fetal mitochondria which has reduced its use in women with PCOS during pregnancy.[26]
  - The American Society for Reproductive Medicine guidelines (ASRM) on the role of metformin for ovulation induction in PCOS have also concluded that there is inadequate evidence for metformin to increase live birth rates or decrease pregnancy losses. It has been further added that discontinuing metformin on pregnancy confirmation has no effect on the rates of miscarriage.[27]
  - Current evidence also does not support using metformin in obese PCOS women for preventing GDM, preeclampsia, or LGA.
  - Metformin has many pleiotropic effects on fetoplacental tissues and it may cause potential long-term metabolic offspring consequences because it inhibits mitochondrial activity resulting in relative nutrient restriction which affects growth, function, and/or differentiation of fetal–placental tissues.
  - In special situations, it can be used beyond the first trimester keeping in mind the potential offspring risks or for promotion of research studies for examining its longitudinal, perinatal, and late childhood outcomes.

Postnatal

- Insulin resistance, effects of hyperandrogenism on prolactin, and breast tissue transformation in PCOS women commonly lead to biologically plausible physiological and psychological causes of breastfeeding challenges, but higher BMI is a stronger predisposing factor for lower breastfeeding rates than PCOS alone.[28]
- PCOS is linked with many health issues and adverse pregnancy outcomes that may have many unknown and sometimes challenging effects hampering smooth transition from pregnancy to motherhood and distress of managing long-term chronic health sequelae.
- It is imperative to focus on maternal health during this "fourth trimester" as it can help PCOS women sail through these transitions and obstacles while coordinating ongoing care of chronic conditions, decreasing maternal morbidity and mortality and optimizing long-term family health.

CONCLUSION

- PCOS women should be properly counseled and informed about their increased pregnancy risks.
- Preconceptional health optimization with screening for diabetes, mood disorders, and cardiopulmonary risk factors along with lifestyle interventions or specific targeted therapies is strongly recommended.
- More researches and evidences are needed to comprehend the genetic and epigenetic contributions of PCOS, PCOS-related comorbidities, role of placenta in nutrient availability as well as emphasis on the role of medications that may affect the long-term health of newborns.
- Metformin has not been recommended for use beyond the first trimester on the

pretext of improving perinatal outcomes, but it can be started again after delivery.
- Clinicians should recommend an individualized comprehensive care plan beginning prenatally, followed through the first year postpartum to optimize transitions to motherhood, long-term health consequences, and preconception health for future pregnancies.

■ REFERENCES

1. Fauser BC, Tarlatzis BC, Rebar RW, Legro RS, Balen AH, Lobo R, et al. Consensus on women's health aspects of polycystic ovary syndrome (PCOS): the Amsterdam ESHRE/ASRM-Sponsored 3rd PCOS Consensus Workshop Group. Fertil Steril. 2012;97(1): 28-38.e25.
2. Wolf WM, Wattick RA, Kinkade ON, Olfert MD. Geographical Prevalence of Polycystic Ovary Syndrome as Determined by Region and Race/Ethnicity. Int J Environ Res Public Health. 2018;15(11):2589.
3. He Y, Lu Y, Zhu Q, Wang Y, Lindheim SR, Qi J, et al. Influence of metabolic syndrome on female fertility and in vitro fertilization outcomes in PCOS women. Am J Obstet Gynecol. 2019;221(2):138.e1-12.
4. Balen AH, Morley LC, Misso M, Franks S, Legro RS, Wijeyaratne CN, et al. The management of anovulatory infertility in women with polycystic ovary syndrome: an analysis of the evidence to support the development of global WHO guidance. Hum Reprod Update. 2016;22(6):687-708.
5. Sha T, Wang X, Cheng W, Yan Y. A meta-analysis of pregnancy-related outcomes and complications in women with polycystic ovary syndrome undergoing IVF. Reprod Biomed Online. 2019;39(2):281-93.
6. Roos N, Kieler H, Sahlin L, Ekman-Ordeberg G, Falconer H, Stephansson O. Risk of adverse pregnancy outcomes in women with polycystic ovary syndrome: population based cohort study. BMJ. 2011;343: d6309.
7. Yu HF, Chen HS, Rao DP, Gong J. Association between polycystic ovary syndrome and the risk of pregnancy complications: A PRISMA-compliant systematic review and meta-analysis. Medicine (Baltimore). 2016;95(51):e4863.
8. Palomba S, de Wilde MA, Falbo A, Koster MP, La Sala GB, Fauser BC. Pregnancy complications in women with polycystic ovary syndrome. Hum Reprod Update. 2015;21(5):575-92.
9. Goodman NF, Cobin RH, Futterweit W, Glueck JS, Legro RS, Carmina E, et al. American Association of Clinical Endocrinologists, American College of Endocrinology, and androgen excess and PCOS society disease state clinical review: guide to the best practices in the evaluation and treatment of polycystic ovary syndrome-part 2. Endocr Pract. 2015;21(12):1415-26.
10. Teede HJ, Misso ML, Costello MF, Dokras A, Laven J, Moran L, et al. Recommendations from the international evidence-based guideline for the assessment and management of polycystic ovary syndrome. Hum Reprod. 2018;33(9): 1602-18.
11. Palomba S, Falbo A, Russo T, Tolino A, Orio F, Zullo F. Pregnancy in women with polycystic ovary syndrome: the effect of different phenotypes and features on obstetric and neonatal outcomes. Fertil Steril. 2010;94(5):1805-11.
12. Mumm H, Jensen DM, Sørensen JA, Andersen LL, Ravn P, Andersen M, et al. Hyperandrogenism and phenotypes of polycystic ovary syndrome are not associated with differences in obstetric outcomes. Acta Obstet Gynecol Scand. 2015;94(2):204-11.
13. Boomsma CM, Eijkemans MJ, Hughes EG, Visser GH, Fauser BC, Macklon NS. A meta-analysis of pregnancy outcomes in women with polycystic ovary syndrome. Hum Reprod Update. 2006;12(6):673-83.

14. Qin JZ, Pang LH, Li MJ, Fan XJ, Huang RD, Chen HY, et al. Obstetric complications in women with polycystic ovary syndrome: a systematic review and meta-analysis. Reprod Biol Endocrinol. 2013;11:56.
15. Doherty DA, Newnham JP, Bower C, Hart R. Implications of polycystic ovary syndrome for pregnancy and for the health of offspring. Obstet Gynecol. 2015;125(6):1397-406.
16. Gu L, Liu H, Gu X, Boots C, Moley KH, Wang Q. Metabolic control of oocyte development: linking maternal nutrition and reproductive outcomes. Cell Mol Life Sci. 2015;72(2):251-71.
17. Forsum E, Brantsæter AL, Olafsdottir AS, Olsen SF, Thorsdottir I. Weight loss before conception: A systematic literature review. Food Nutr Res. 2013;57.
18. Schummers L, Hutcheon JA, Bodnar LM, Lieberman E, Himes KP. Risk of adverse pregnancy outcomes by prepregnancy body mass index: a population-based study to inform prepregnancy weight loss counseling. Obstet Gynecol. 2015; 125(1):133-43.
19. Lim SS, Hutchison SK, Van Ryswyk E, Norman RJ, Teede HJ, Moran LJ. Lifestyle changes in women with polycystic ovary syndrome. Cochrane Database Syst Rev. 2019;3(3):CD007506.
20. Yanovski SZ, Yanovski JA. Long-term drug treatment for obesity: a systematic and clinical review. JAMA. 2014;311(1):74-86.
21. Falcone V, Stopp T, Feichtinger M, Kiss H, Eppel W, Husslein PW, et al. Pregnancy after bariatric surgery: a narrative literature review and discussion of impact on pregnancy management and outcome. BMC Pregnancy Childbirth. 2018;18(1):507.
22. Dokras A, Stener-Victorin E, Yildiz BO, Li R, Ottey S, Shah D, et al. Androgen Excess-Polycystic Ovary Syndrome Society: position statement on depression, anxiety, quality of life, and eating disorders in polycystic ovary syndrome. Fertil Steril. 2018;109(5):888-99.
23. American Diabetes Association. Classification and Diagnosis of Diabetes: Standards of Medical Care in Diabetes-2020. Diabetes Care. 2020; 43(Suppl 1):S14-31.
24. Kahal H, Kyrou I, Tahrani AA, Randeva HS Obstructive sleep apnoea and polycystic ovary syndrome: A comprehensive review of clinical interactions and underlying pathophysiology. Clin Endocrinol (Oxf). 2017;87(4):313-9.
25. Bidhendi Yarandi R, Behboudi-Gandevani S, Amiri M, Ramezani Tehrani F. Metformin therapy before conception versus throughout the pregnancy and risk of gestational diabetes mellitus in women with polycystic ovary syndrome: a systemic review, meta-analysis and meta-regression. Diabetol Metab Syndr. 2019;11:58.
26. Doi SAR, Furuya-Kanamori L, Toft E, Musa OAH, Islam N, Clark J, et al. Metformin in pregnancy to avert gestational diabetes in women at high risk: Meta-analysis of randomized controlled trials. Obes Rev. 2020;21(1):e12964.
27. Practice Committee of the American Society for Reproductive Medicine. Role of metformin for ovulation induction in infertile patients with polycystic ovary syndrome (PCOS): a guideline. Fertil Steril. 2017;108(3):426-41.
28. Joham AE, Nanayakkara N, Ranasinha S, Zoungas S, Boyle J, Harrison CL, et al. Obesity, polycystic ovary syndrome and breastfeeding: an observational study. Acta Obstet Gynecol Scand. 2016; 95(4):458-66.

CHAPTER 27

Bariatric Surgery in PCOS

Subash Mallya, Sonalica Suresh

INTRODUCTION

Polycystic ovary syndrome (PCOS) is the most common endocrine disorder affecting women of reproductive age group. It has a prevalence of 2.2–26% depending upon the population studied and the criteria used for diagnosis. It is a heterogeneous disorder with features of hyperandrogenism, ovulatory dysfunction, and polycystic ovaries. It mainly affects the reproductive system with health effects on metabolic, cardiovascular, and psychological functions. Patients with PCOS are at risk of developing metabolic syndrome with features of obesity, dyslipidemia, cardiovascular disease, and diabetes. The main pathophysiology in PCOS is hyperinsulinemia secondary to insulin resistance and hyperandrogenism, which is worsened by obesity.

OBESITY AND POLYCYSTIC OVARY SYNDROME

About 40–80% of women with PCOS are either overweight or obese. The World Health Organization (WHO) defines obesity according to body mass index (BMI) in kg/m^2: 18.5–24.9 normal range, 25–29.9 overweight, 30–34.9 class 1 obese, 35–39.9 class 2 obese, 40–49.9 class 3 obese/morbid obesity, and >50 super obesity. Obesity aggravates all the clinical features of PCOS. Furthermore, it leads to hyperandrogenism, and hence manifestation of hirsutism is more in obese PCOS patients when compared to lean PCOS. Obesity has an adverse effect on the reproductive outcome. It decreases the chance of natural conception and also the response to fertility treatment. Obesity causes a sevenfold increased risk of abnormal glucose tolerance when compared with women with PCOS having normal BMI. In pregnancy, it increases the chance of miscarriage, congenital anomalies such as neural tube defects, macrosomia, and still birth, and pregnancy complications such as gestational diabetes, pregnancy-induced hypertension, and thromboembolism. Moderate weight loss of 5–10% of body weight is sufficient to restore fertility and improve metabolic parameters. Lifestyle modification including diet and exercise helps to reduce weight in short term, but there could be cyclical rebound weight gain. There is no medical treatment which is safe and cost-effective on a long-term basis. When these lifestyle measures and other medical treatment have failed, bariatric surgery has a role in the management of obese women with PCOS.[1]

BARIATRIC SURGERY

Bariatric surgery involves manipulation of stomach or small intestine to aid weight loss. The history of bariatric surgery began in the 1950s with intestinal bypass. But it was only after 1965 that a lot of development was made in this field when Dr Edward E Mason (father of bariatric surgery) developed the technique of gastric bypass which had lesser complication and better outcome. Bariatric surgery leads to weight loss of 25–35% of body weight after 1 year and this is sustained at 15–25% after 20 years with proper follow-up. In addition to weight loss, bariatric surgery has additional benefits. Obesity-related diseases such as diabetes and metabolic syndrome improve with bariatric surgery; hence, now it is also termed "metabolic surgery."

Indication

According to the National Institute for Health and Care Excellence (NICE)[2] guidelines, bariatric surgery is recommended if lifestyle measures and medical management are ineffective in:
- *Morbidly obese patients:* BMI >40 kg/m^2
- BMI >35 kg/m^2 with comorbid conditions such as diabetes, hypertension, dyslipidemia, obstructive sleep apnea, gastroesophageal reflux disease (GERD), nonalcoholic fatty liver disease, and PCOS.

Polycystic ovary syndrome in itself is considered as a comorbid condition.

Absolute contraindications include pregnancy, severe psychiatric illness, eating disorders, substance misuse (alcoholism), severe coagulopathies, and end-stage liver and renal disease.

Because of the improved surgical techniques and their effectiveness, in October 2022, the International Federation for the Surgery of Obesity (IFSO) has revised the criteria and included adult patients with BMI >35 kg/m^2 and BMI >30 kg/m^2 with comorbid conditions to consider for bariatric surgery.

Bariatric surgery has to be done in a dedicated tertiary center with a multidisciplinary approach involving the bariatric surgeon, physician, dietitian, specialist nurse, exercise therapist, anesthetist, and other secondary care specialists. Women must be properly counseled before surgery about the risks and lifestyle implication of surgery and need for proper follow-up. With improved techniques, most of the surgeries are now done laparoscopically with enhanced recovery.

Types of Bariatric Surgery

Bariatric surgery is classified into restrictive, malabsorptive, and mixed types. Laparoscopic adjustable gastric banding (LAGB), sleeve gastrectomy, and Roux-en-Y gastric bypass (RYGB) are the most commonly done procedures because of less complication rates.

Restrictive Type—Gastric Banding and Sleeve Gastrectomy

The restrictive surgeries reduce food intake by reducing gastric capacity. The most commonly done procedures in this type are LAGB and sleeve gastrectomy.

Laparoscopic adjustable gastric banding: Here, a band is placed just below the esophagogastric junction, to make a small gastric pouch with a narrow stoma through the band that communicates with the rest of the stomach. The band has a rigid outer ring and an inner inflatable balloon reservoir which is connected by a tubing to the subcutaneous access port. The access port is then sutured to the fascia. The band can be adjusted by injection or aspiration of saline in the follow-up visits to regulate weight gain. It works by reducing the gastric volume and thus limiting the amount of food intake. 40–50% of extra weight is lost by this procedure. It is least invasive and reversible and has very few complications with less

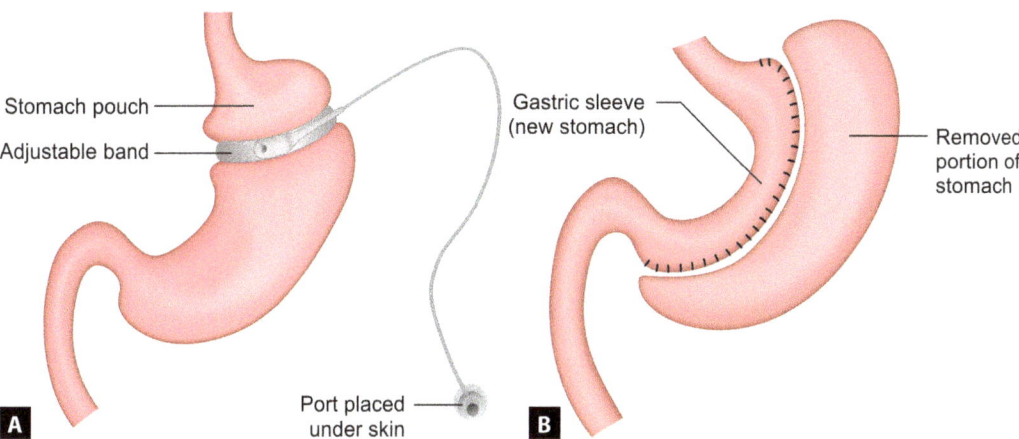

Figs. 1A and B: (A) Adjustable gastric band (lap band); (B) Vertical sleeve gastrectomy.

nutritional deficiencies. Band infection, slippage, gastric erosion, pouch dilatation, and infection at the port site are some of the potential complications with this procedure **(Fig. 1A)**.

Sleeve gastrectomy: In this procedure, 75–80% of stomach in the area of greater curvature is removed and the remaining stomach is formed into a sleeve-like structure with reduced capacity. It works by adjusting the amount of food taken and also reduces the hunger hormone—ghrelin produced by cells in the fundus of the stomach. The procedure can be performed laparoscopically. It causes a weight loss of about 60% of excess weight and diabetic remission in 50%. Sleeve gastrectomy is an irreversible procedure and has risks of stenosis, staple line leak, and GERD **(Fig. 1B)**.

Malabsorptive Type—Biliopancreatic Diversion

This includes biliopancreatic diversion and jejunoileal bypass. Biliopancreatic diversion with duodenal switch is usually done in patients with higher range of BMI—above 50 kg/m^2. Even though with these procedures 70–80% of extra weight is lost and diabetic remission of 80% is achieved, nutritional complication rates are high. Here, sleeve gastrectomy is done initially followed by division of duodenum just distal to the pylorus. Ileum is then transected at 250 cm from the ileocecal junction and a duodenoileal anastomosis is done. The ileoileal anastomosis is then created at 100 cm from the ileocecal valve with the biliary limb. The main mechanism of action is by malabsorption of calories as the food bypasses major portion of the small intestine. Iron, calcium, thiamine, fat-soluble vitamins, and vitamin B12 deficiencies can occur leading to malnutrition. These procedures produce extreme malabsorption than other procedures and have high morbidity and mortality and hence are not done commonly **(Fig. 2A)**.

Mixed Type—Roux-en-Y Gastric Bypass

Roux-en-Y gastric bypass is a hormonal procedure in addition to restriction and malabsorption properties. Here, a small pouch is created in the stomach and the newly created pouch is then connected directly into the small intestine facilitating the food to bypass major part of the stomach, duodenum, and initial 40–50 cm of jejunum.

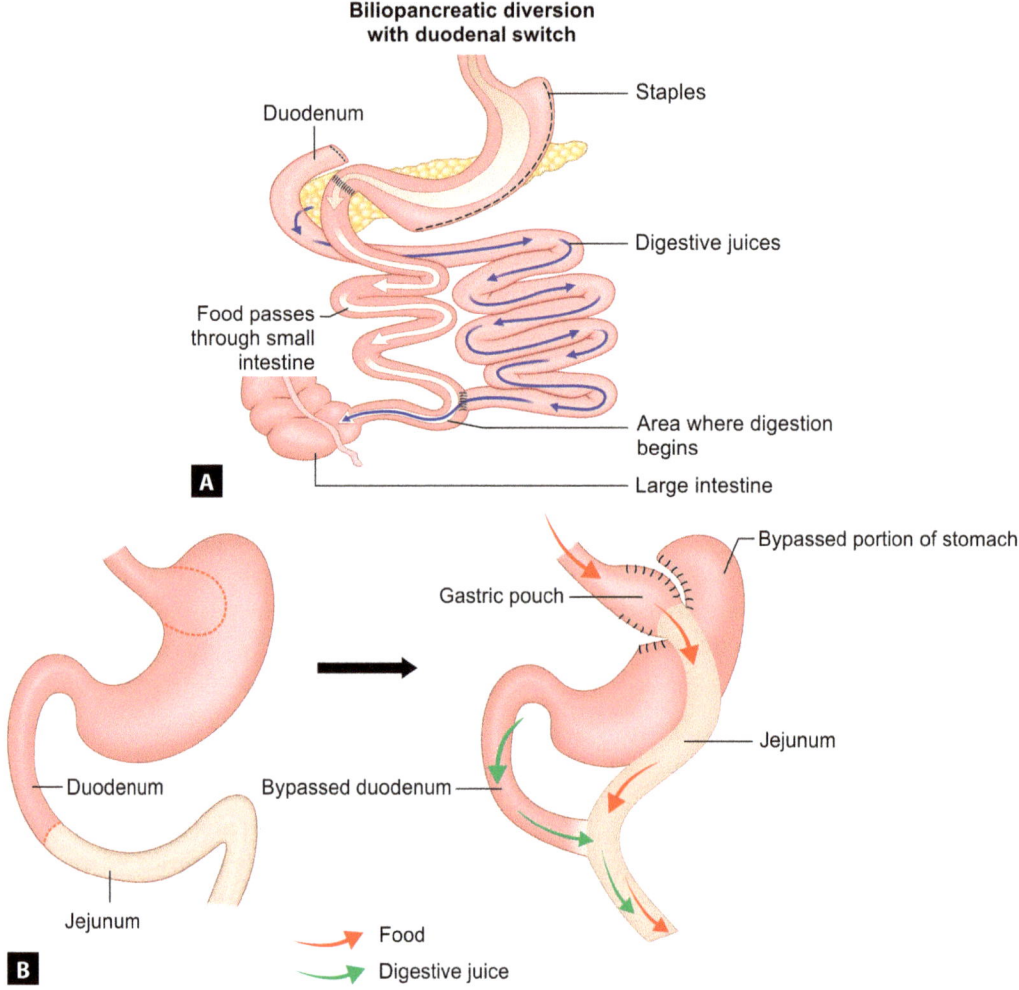

Figs. 2A and B: (A) Biliopancreatic diversion with duodenal switch; (B) Roux-en-Y gastric bypass (RYGB).

Thus, there is only a reorganization of food flow and no part is removed. The steps include: (1) Gastric pouch creation: A small pouch of about 20–30 cc is created involving the lesser curvature of stomach. (2) Creation of biliopancreatic limb: It includes the remnant stomach, duodenum, and proximal jejunum and contains the digestive enzymes from the stomach, hepatobiliary tract, and pancreas. (3) Creation of jejunojejunostomy: The biliopancreatic limb is anastomosed to the distal segment of jejunum to create side-to-side jejunojejunostomy. (4) Creation of gastrojejunostomy: The Roux limb of jejunum is brought up and side-to-side gastrojejunostomy is created. It works by restricting the amount of food intake, malabsorption of calories, and altering the hunger and anorexigenic hormones. 60–70% of extra weight is lost after the procedure and a reduction in diabetes and hypertension was also seen. Early complications include leak from the anastomotic site, small bowel obstruction, and deep vein thrombosis or pulmonary embolism. Stenosis at the anastomotic site, marginal ulcers, small bowel obstruction, intestinal hernias, nephrolithiasis, cholelithiasis, micronutrient deficiency (thiamine, vitamin B12, folate, iron, zinc, vitamin D), metabolic bone disease, and dumping syndrome are some of the late complications. Dumping syndrome presents as nausea, diarrhea, tachycardia, abdominal cramps, and postprandial malaise precipitated by ingestion of large quantities of food or carbohydrates or after glucose challenge test **(Fig. 2B)**.

Follow-up after Surgery

Constructive follow-up program has to be provided after surgery to maintain optimum results and to bring down the complications. Patients must be regularly assessed for diet, comorbidities, medication, and physical and psychological activities. Almost all the bariatric surgeries cause vitamin and mineral deficiency. Hence, all patients after surgery should undergo routine metabolic and micronutrient monitoring for lifelong. This is to be done every 3-6 monthly in the first year, 6-12 monthly in the second year, and at least annually thereafter. Multivitamins and minerals including vitamins B12, D, A, E, and K, iron, folic acid, calcium, selenium, copper, and zinc are to be supplemented according to the need.

Effect of Bariatric Surgery in Polycystic Ovary Syndrome

In PCOS, bariatric surgery results in normalization of hormones and thus improves anovulation and results in increased fertility.[3] Some studies suggest that the need for fertility treatment is low after bariatric surgery. Most of the features of PCOS are completely resolved by weight loss following surgery.[4] Bariatric surgery not only benefits weight loss, but also improves diabetes, cardiovascular risk, fatty liver disease, mental health issues, and life expectancy. The success of any type of bariatric surgery depends on the adherence to a healthy diet habit and exercise with proper follow-up after surgery.

PREGNANCY AFTER BARIATRIC SURGERY

Pregnancy after bariatric surgery is safe and has fewer complications when compared with morbidly obese women. According to the current recommendation, it is advisable to delay pregnancy for at least 1 year following bariatric surgery.[5] This is due to the rapid weight loss that occurs in the first year of surgery with nutritional deficiencies and electrolyte imbalances. Folic acid supplementation has to be given preconceptionally to women planning pregnancy to prevent neural tube defects. Pregnancy after bariatric surgery is safe and has fewer complications when compared with morbidly obese women.[5] Pregnancy must be managed in a multidisciplinary setting to have an optimum pregnancy outcome. Baseline nutritional status has to be determined and vitamins and minerals to be supplemented according to the individual needs.[6] In most of the studies, the incidence of preeclampsia, gestational diabetes mellitus (GDM), and macrosomia was on the lower side after bariatric surgery when compared with obese group and has a healthy maternal and neonatal outcome. Cesarean delivery is indicated only for obstetric reasons. After pregnancy most of the women desire to undergo a cosmetic surgery to get rid of the redundant loose and damaged skin.

CONCLUSION

Obesity has become a global epidemic and there has been a sixfold increase in bariatric surgery in the last few decades. Laparoscopic adjustable gastric banding, sleeve gastrectomy, and RYGB are the most commonly done procedures. Even though fertility improves after surgery, bariatric surgery should not be done for treating infertility. In addition to weight loss, it also improves obesity-associated comorbid conditions. Lifestyle modification with diet and exercise is the key to prevention of obesity and surgery is considered as the last alternative.

REFERENCES

1. Balen AH. Polycystic ovary syndrome (PCOS). Obstet Gynaecol. 2017;19:119-29.
2. Centre for Public Health Excellence at NICE (UK); National Collaborating Centre for Primary Care (UK). Obesity: The Prevention, Identification, Assessment and Management of Overweight and Obesity in Adults and Children [Internet]. London: National Institute for Health and Clinical Excellence (UK); 2006.
3. Shekelle PG, Newberry S, Maglione M, Li Z, Yermilov I, Hilton L, et al. Bariatric surgery in women of reproductive age: special concerns for pregnancy. Evid Rep Technol Assess (Full Rep). 2008;(169):1-51.
4. Eid GM, Cottam DR, Velcu LM, Mattar SG, Korytkowski MT, Gosman G, et al. Effective treatment of polycystic ovarian syndrome with Roux-en-Y gastric bypass. Surg Obes Relat Dis. 2005;1(2):77-80.
5. Khan R, Dawlatly B, Chappatte O. Pregnancy outcome following bariatric surgery. Obstet Gynaecol. 2013;15:37-43.
6. American College of Obstetricians and Gynecologists. ACOG Committee Opinion number 315, September 2005. Obesity in pregnancy. Obstet Gynecol. 2005;106(3):671-5.

CHAPTER 28

Aesthetics in PCOS

Ragini Agrawal, Natasha Vijayendram

■ INTRODUCTION

Cosmetic concerns of polycystic ovarian disease (PCOD) are due to cutaneous manifestations which create an unseemly appearance and can be cause of anxiety in women. This is effect of hyperandrogenism which is a cardinal feature of PCOD.

Polycystic ovary syndrome (PCOS) is a metabolic disorder which affects many systems of body and has an impact on the quality of life. A very common endocrinological disorder, which has effects across all the stages of women's life. Its prevalence in society is >15% and variable according to ethnicity and presents with different complaints in different women.

A revised definition of PCOS was proposed in 2003 at an international joint consensus meeting of the European Society for Human Reproduction and Embryology and the American Society for Reproductive Medicine. The group recommended that a PCOS diagnosis could be achieved if two of the following three criteria are present:
1. Oligo-ovulation (fewer than 8 menses per 12-month period) and/or anovulation
2. Clinical hyperandrogenism and/or biochemical signs of hyperandrogenism
3. Polycystic ovaries (≥12 follicles in each ovary measuring 2–9 mm in diameter and/or increased ovarian volume >10 mL) by ultrasonography.

Insulin resistance (IR) is considered its root cause and has potential to develop type 2 diabetes mellitus (T2DM) in the future. PCOD has long-term sequel such as metabolic syndrome and endometrial cancers so early diagnosis and prompt treatment is a necessity.

Cutaneous manifestations of PCOS occur early in the course of the disease. They are associated with obesity and are major cosmetic concerns which can lead to depression in women.

■ CUTANEOUS MANIFESTATIONS

- *Hirsutism:* Hirsutism was assessed using the modified Ferriman-Gallwey (F–G) score, in which a score >8 indicates hirsutism.
- *Acne:* The presence of and nodules and cysts, comedones, erythematous papules and pustules, on the face, neck, upper chest, upper back, and upper arms were classified as acne.
- *Androgenic alopecia:* Androgenic alopecia evaluation is done by Ludwig's classification.
- *Acanthosis nigricans (AN):* It presents with pigmented, raised, warty, velvety skin patches on the intramammary folds, nape of neck, and antecubital fossae were classified as acanthosis nigricans.
- *Striae:* Stretch marks on the breast, buttocks, thighs, and shoulder areas.

- Skin Tags
- *Seborrhea:* The presence of greasy or oily and shiny skin on the nasolabial folds, the forehead, or behind the ear and hair was defined as seborrhea or oily skin.

Hirsutism

Hirsutism is defined as presence of male pattern terminal hair on the face and/or body. 60-80% of PCOS women presents to cosmetic clinic with complaint of unwanted hairs on face, chin and body. It is considered one of major signs of hyperandrogenism.

Severity of hair growth is determined by the androgens, particularly testosterone. Hirsutism in PCOS women is due to increased circulatory levels of free testosterone and more active form of testosterone, i.e., dihydrotestosterone, formed by the activity of 5α reductase on testosterone in the hair follicles. Hirsutism is the most consistent and reliable symptom used for evaluating clinical hyperandrogenism.

Ferriman and Gallwey described a visual scoring method to clinically assess the degree of hirsutism known as the Ferriman-Gallwey (F–G) score. According to the F–G score, hair is scored in nine parts of the body, which include the upper lip, chin, chest, upper and lower back, upper and lower abdomen, and upper and lower limbs. A score of 0–4 is given on these nine body parts to determine the extent of hirsutism, with a score of 0 representing a complete absence of terminal hair and a score of 4 represents extensive hair growth. The score of all nine areas is added up to get the final score used for diagnosis. Women with an F–G score of 8 or higher are regarded as hirsutism.

Underlying serious medical problems such as androgen secreting tumor evaluation is mandatory and plan of treatment is devised. Its presence causes mental trauma in sufferer so it is very important to counsel these patients for basic education regarding this disease.

Terminal hair must be differentiated from vellus hair. Vellus hair is fine, soft, and lightly pigmented. By contrast, terminal hair is coarse, curly, and pigmented. Terminal hairs are androgen dependent but vellus hair is independent to androgen secretion **(Figs. 1A and B)**.

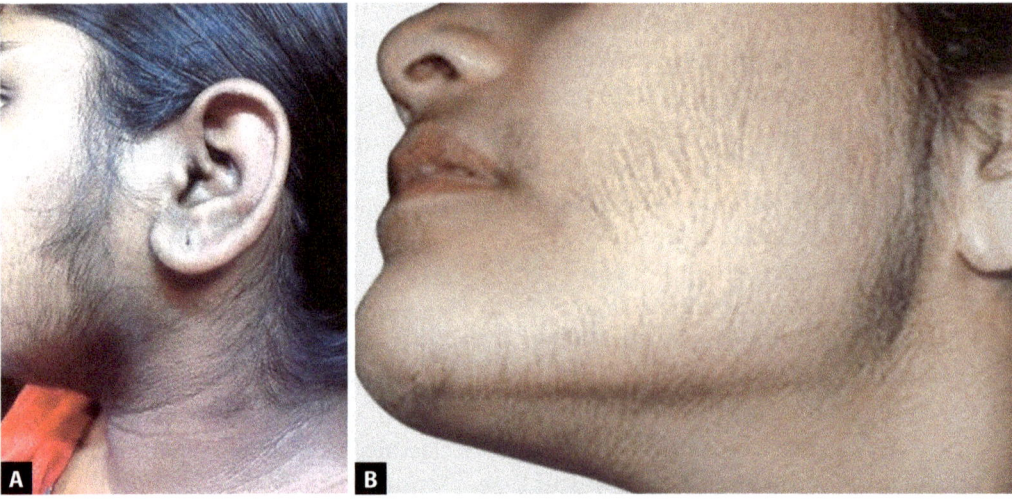

Figs. 1A and B: (A) Terminal hair; (B) Vellus hair.

After clinical evaluation and laboratory testing, perform ovarian ultrasonography to evaluate for either ovarian or adrenal sources of androgen production.

Management begins with a careful explanation about the cause of the problem and reassurance that the patient is not losing her femininity. The most effective strategy is to combine systemic therapy, which has a slow onset of effectiveness, with mechanical depilation (shaving, plucking, waxing, depilatory creams) or light-based (laser or pulsed-light) hair removal. Systemic therapies include glucocorticoids, oral contraceptives (OCs), spironolactone, flutamide, finasteride, cyproterone acetate (not available in the United States), and insulin sensitizers (metformin and rosiglitazone).

Laser therapy has been shown not only to reduce unwanted hair but also to improve depression and anxiety in women with hirsutism. In many patients, hirsutism can be controlled just with laser, without using any drugs.

Acne

Studies have estimated the prevalence of acne in PCOS at 9.8–34%. Acne mainly is a manifestation due to the increased levels of androgens affecting the sebum glands and its production, increased follicular desquamation and increased colonization on *Propionibacterium acnes*. Acne is usually mild to moderate in nature **(Figs. 2A to F)**. A premenstrual flare is common due to the

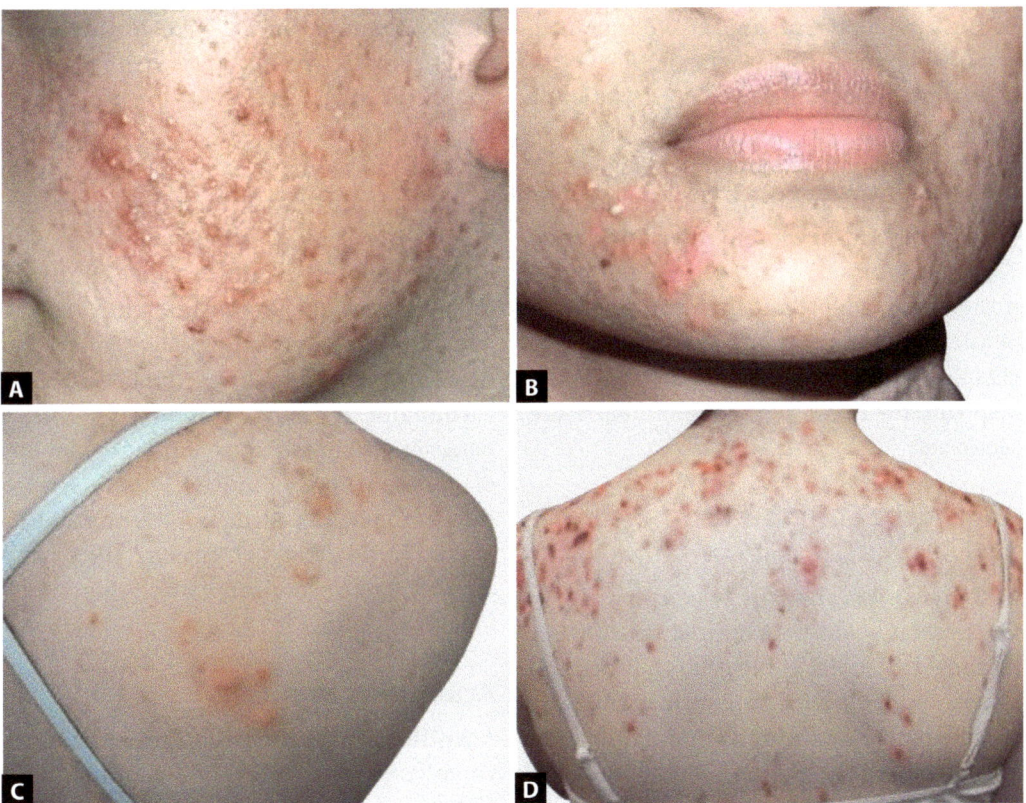

Figs. 2A to D

Contd...

Contd...

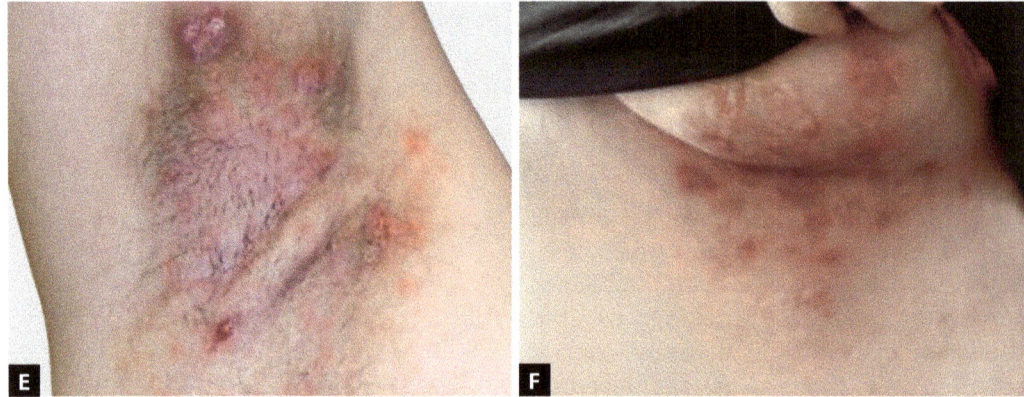

Figs. 2A to F: Different types of acne.

effects of androgens and progesterone. It affects most commonly the chin, jawline, cheeks, and trunk. Its sequelae usually having a psychological impact and leading to postinflammatory hyperpigmentation (PIH), postinflammatory erythema (PIE), atrophic scars, and hypertrophic scars.

Management includes proper counseling, low GI diet, weight reduction, metformin, doxycycline, minocycline, or isotretinoin. Topical therapies with benzoyl peroxide, nadifloxacin, adapalene, tretinoin, zinc PCA, clindamycin is used. Procedures such as chemical peels, intense pule light (IPL), lasers help with the cosmetic manifestations of the sequelae.

Androgenetic Alopecia

Androgenetic alopecia (AGA) in women is characterized by hair loss primarily on the central scalp with miniaturization of terminal hair follicles into vellus follicles and shortening of the anagen (growth) phase.

In women, AGA can be more difficult to diagnose because of the varying patterns of hair loss that have been described, the unclear relationship of the disease to androgens and heredity, and the need to exclude other conditions such as alopecia areata and telogen effluvium.

The features of hair loss are directly linked to dihydrotestosterone levels. The **Figure 3** shows the two scoring systems for female pattern hair loss.

Management includes trichoscopy to help distinguish from other hair disorders, blood investigations, supplementation with biotin, calcium pantothenate. Minoxidil remains the mainstay of treatment. It stimulates anagen or growing phase. In AGA, it helps by increasing intracellular Ca^{2+}. As a vasodilator, it opens up the ATP sensitive potassium channels, thus improving viability of hair cells **(Figs. 4A and B)**. Peptide serums such as Capixyl 5%, Redensyl 3%, procapil 3% also help. Platelet-rich plasma (PRP) and growth factor concentrate helps boost follicular health.

Acanthosis Nigricans

Acanthosis nigricans is characterized by velvety, brown, thickened plaques with accentuated skin markings. These lesions are most commonly localized to the nape

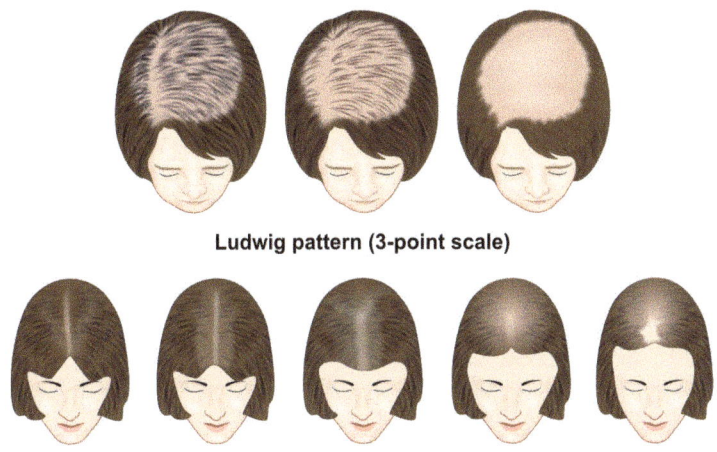

Fig. 3: Scoring systems for female pattern hair loss—Ludwig and Sinclair patterns.

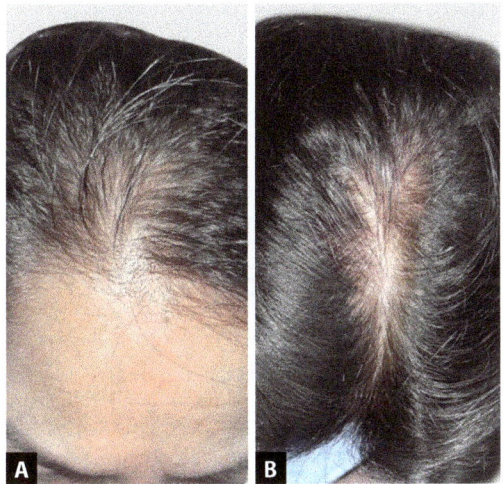

Figs. 4A and B: Male androgenetic alopecia.

and sides of the neck as well as intertriginous areas such as the axillae, groin, anogenital region, and inframammary region **(Figs. 5A to F).**

If left untreated, lesions can continue to thicken, producing a leathery, warty, or papillomatous surface.

Acanthosis nigricans is associated with diabetes mellitus, metabolic syndrome, obesity, medication, genetic sensitivity to hyperinsulinemia, HAIR-AN syndrome (hyperandrogenism, insulin resistance, acanthosis nigricans).

It represents an elevated production of insulin ± androgen or estrogen on insulin or insulin-like growth factor receptors in the skin and this hyperinsulinemia leads to increase in IGF-1 further causing aberrant keratinocyte and fibroblast proliferation.

Metabolic correction, lifestyle management and weight loss are the mainstay of treatment. Investigations such as hormonal assays, vitamin D3, B12, HbA1c, serum insulin is required. Treatment includes topical medications like moisturizers, urea based creams, tretinoin, demelanizing agents along with oral metformin. Procedures such as microdermabrasion, chemical peels, fractional and Q-switch ND:YAG lasers help with textural and pigmentation changes.

Striae

Striae are defined as the linear ridge or groove on the surface of the skin with textural changes. These are most commonly seen over the breast, buttocks, thighs, and shoulder areas. Frequent weight fluctuations and/or

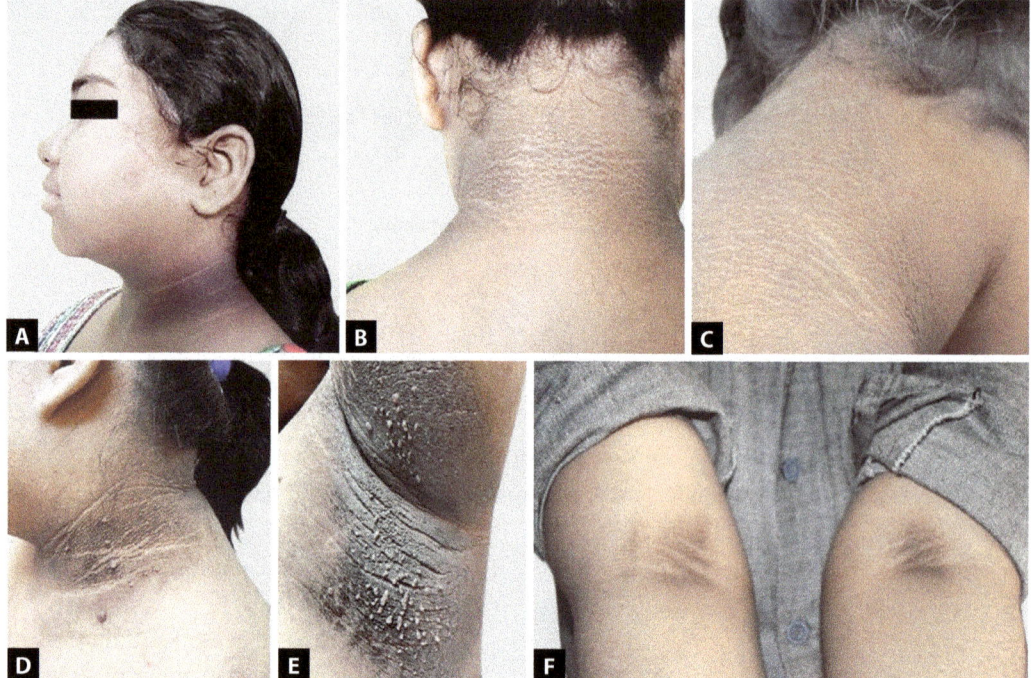

Figs. 5A to F: Examples of acanthosis nigricans.

sudden weight gain and or loss and a genetic predisposition are the main causes.

The various types include:
- *Striae rubrae:* Pink/red stretch marks
- *Striae albae:* White stretch marks
- *Striae nigrae:* Dark gray or black stretch marks (usually applicable to darker complexion skin types)
- *Striae caerulea:* Dark blue/purplish stretch marks
- *Striae atrophicans:* Thinned skin associated with stretch marks.

Management is for pure cosmetic reasons, chemical peels, fractional CO_2 laser, fraction RF and carboxytherapy are treatment modalities.

Skin Tags

Skin tags are also known as acrochordon **(Fig. 6)**. They are benign growths. Clinically,

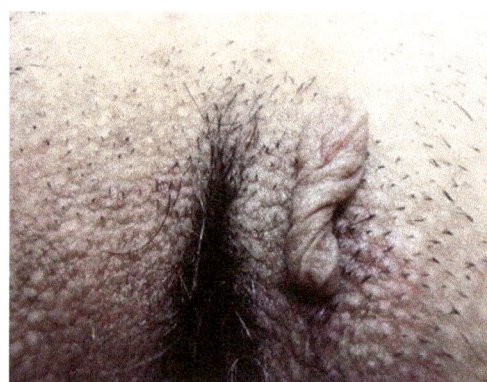

Fig. 6: Skin tags.

they are brown or beige in color and attached to the rest of the skin by a thin stalk. Treatment includes surgical removal or removal with a CO_2 laser.

Seborrhea

The presence of greasy or oily and shiny skin on the nasolabial folds, the forehead, or behind the ear and hair is defined as seborrhea or oily skin. Increased levels of androgens affect the sebum glands and leads to increased sebum production.

Treating the underlying disorder helps reduce symptoms. Topical salicylic acid, glycolic acid and antifungal lotions help.

■ CONCLUSION

Polycystic ovary syndrome is one of the most common endocrine disorders in women of reproductive age and can be associated with multiple long-term health risks and substantial psychological impact. The dermatologic manifestations of PCOS play a significant role in diagnosis and constitute a substantial portion of the symptoms experienced by women with this syndrome. Patients must be counseled regarding the long duration of treatment that includes lifestyle modifications along with systemic treatment. Success in the effective management of women with PCOS is through a synchronized effort between the dermatologist, endocrinologist, gynecologist, nutritionist, and physical trainer.

CHAPTER 29: Sequelae of PCOS

Shama Batra, Vandana Gupta

INTRODUCTION

Polycystic ovary syndrome (PCOS) is a frequent endocrine disease affecting 10–15% of women. Menstrual disorders, hyperandrogenism, and ultrasonographic aspect of ovaries are diagnostic criteria of PCOS. PCOS has been associated with numerous reproductive and metabolic dysfunction. But PCOS has long-term complications that are frequently forgotten and underestimated. While most attention has been paid to the management of the presenting complaints, it has become clear that the polycystic ovary phenotype is linked to a number of metabolic disturbances which required long-term surveillance. During pregnancy, gestational diabetes and gestational hypertensive disorders can occur.

With advancing age, there is increased risk of metabolic diseases such as:
- Glucose intolerance
- Type-2 diabetes
- Dyslipidemia
- Cardiovascular risk
- Mood disorders such as depression and anxiety
- Obstructive sleep apnea
- Nonalcoholic fatty liver diseases
- Cancer like endometrial, breast, or ovarian.

Women with PCOS have increased classical cardiovascular risks and subclinical cardiovascular risks without proven increase of cardiovascular morbidity and mortality. Endometrial cancer seems to be more frequent in women with PCOS.

Polycystic ovary syndrome has long-term health risk and long follow-up is needed for these women to detect and prevent complications.

LONG-TERM CONSEQUENCES

Obesity

Obesity clearly has a role in long-term health and may predict both reproductive and metabolic dysfunction and negatively affect the response to treatment in women with PCOS.

TABLE 1: Criteria for the metabolic syndrome in women with polycystic ovary syndrome (PCOS).

Risk factor	Cutoff
Abdominal obesity in women	>88 cm (>35 in)
Triglycerides	≥150 mg/dL
HDL-C in women	<50 mg/dL
Blood pressure	≥130/≥85 mm Hg
• Fasting and 2-hour glucose and/or from oral glucose • 2-hour glucose tolerance test	• 110–126 mg/dL • 140–199 mg/dL

Note: Three of the five symptoms qualify for the syndrome.
(HDL-C: high-density lipoprotein cholesterol)

Long-term follow-up of women with PCOS is defined by ultrasound and with few other presenting symptoms.

Diabetes

Insulin resistance and resulting hyperinsulinemia have been recognized features of PCOS for many years.

Insulin resistance is defined as reduction in the glucose response to a given amount of insulin. It has been involved in pathogenesis of many aspects of the syndrome.

It is now believed that insulin resistance is an underlying disorder of polycystic ovary/PCOS. Obese women with PCOS were 3-4 times more likely to develop diabetes than women without PCOS or obesity.[1]

The women with PCOS may be at an increased risk of developing noninsulin-dependent diabetes mellitus (NIDDM). Evidence that women with PCOS are at increased risk of NIDDM is quite common.

Besides insulin resistance, it has been seen that some of these women have alterations in pancreatic beta-cell functions. Both disorders (insulin resistance and beta-cell dysfunction) are recognized as major risk factors for the development of type 2 diabetes. The risk of glucose intolerance among PCOS subjects seems to be 5-10-fold higher than normal population.

However, other risk factors, such as obesity, a positive family history of type 2 diabetes, and hyperandrogenism may contribute to increase the diabetes risk in PCOS.

DIAGNOSIS OF INSULIN RESISTANCE (FLOWCHART 1)

Fasting glucose levels are relatively poor predictors of type 2 diabetes as determined by glucose challenge test in PCOS.

This suggests that all PCOS women should be screened for glucose intolerance

BOX 1: Summary of diagnostic recommendations.
- No test of insulin resistance is necessary to make the diagnosis of PCOS, nor is it needed to select treatments
- Obese women with PCOS should be screened for the metabolic syndrome, including circulating lipids, and glucose intolerance with an oral glucose tolerance test
- Further studies are necessary in nonobese women with PCOS to determine the utility of these tests, although they may be considered if additional risk factors for insulin resistance, such as a family history of diabetes, are present

(PCOS: polycystic ovary syndrome)

and that basal and 2-hour glucose stimulated levels rather than fasting glucose levels alone.

It combines sensitivity (95%) and specificity (84%) for insulin resistance with positive and negative predictive values of 87 and 97% in obese patients with PCOS.

Diagnostic recommendations are summarized in **Box 1**.

CARDIOVASCULAR DISEASES

Clinicians have been concerned for some time about the possibility of an increase in cardiovascular disease (CVD) in women with PCOS, due to disturbances in insulin resistance and lipid profiles that often accompany this diagnosis.

Women with PCOS may have a higher risk of cardiovascular risk factors including high blood pressure and high cholesterol. The Women's Ischemia Syndrome Evaluation (WISE) study suggested that postmenopausal women with history of menstrual irregularities and evidence of hyperandrogenemia are at an increased risk of CVD.

There is also some evidence that women with PCOS may have compromised endothelial function (the endothelium is the inner lining of blood vessels) which is an early marker of CVD.

The association of PCOS with CVD was compromised from the start. Long-term studies of well-characterized women with PCOS are lacking, and the link to primary cardiovascular events such as stroke or myocardial infarction remains more speculative than substantive.

Studies that suggest a slight increase in cardiovascular events in women with polycystic ovaries markers of premature coronary artery and cerebrovascular disease are prevalent. Women with polycystic ovaries are seen to have more extensive coronary artery disease by angiography. In control studies, women in their 40s had greater intima-media thickness of the carotid vessels and more cerebrovascular diseases are prevalent and more atherogenic lipid profiles increased total and low-density lipoprotein (LDL) cholesterol and triglyceride levels and decreased high-density lipoprotein (HDL) cholesterol.

These metabolic abnormalities are compounded by prevalence of obesity, which occur in >65% of women with PCOS. Abnormal androgen production declines as menopause approaches.

However in cohort studies, premenopausal and postmenopausal women with history of PCOS had an increased rate of type 2 diabetes, hypertension, and coronary artery disease compared with control patients.

For women with PCOS, it is important to have regular health checkups including blood pressure and cholesterol monitoring and routinely assess cardiovascular risk factors, particularly the cases diagnosed with insulin resistance or type 2 diabetes.

It is recommended that they follow a healthy balanced diet that is low in saturated fat and salt, stop smoking, and exercise regularly.

CANCER

Recent interest has focused on possible association of PCOS with endometrial, ovarian, and breast cancers.

Our understanding of cancer risk in women with PCOS comes from studies of women who have had anovulatory infertility, menstrual irregularity, or estrogen replacement therapy, as well as studies of women with clinically defined PCOS.[2]

The association between exposure to unopposed estrogen and an increased risk of endometrial cancer has been well established.

Hypersecretion of luteinizing hormone (LH), chronic hyperinsulinemia, obesity, and increased serum insulin-like growth factor (IGF)-1 levels may represent risk factors for endometrial cancer. Those with persistently thickened endometrium when measured by transvaginal ultrasound should be advised to have an endometrial biopsy and/or hysteroscopy to rule out endometrial hyperplasia.

Obesity has been shown consistently to be an important risk factor for endometrial cancer and is therefore likely to contribute to cancer risk in overweight women with PCOS.

Diagnostic criteria by Rotterdam for PCOS

The risk of breast cancer in women with PCOS appears to be no greater than for women in general population. A large prospective study was investigated to look for association between Stein–Leventhal syndrome (severe form of PCOS) and breast carcinoma. 34,835 women aged over 55 years found that woman with self-reported history of PCOS were no more likely to develop breast cancer than women without such a history, giving a relative risk estimate of 1.0 [95% confidence interval (CI) 0.6–1.9]. These results suggest that the syndrome is not associated with an

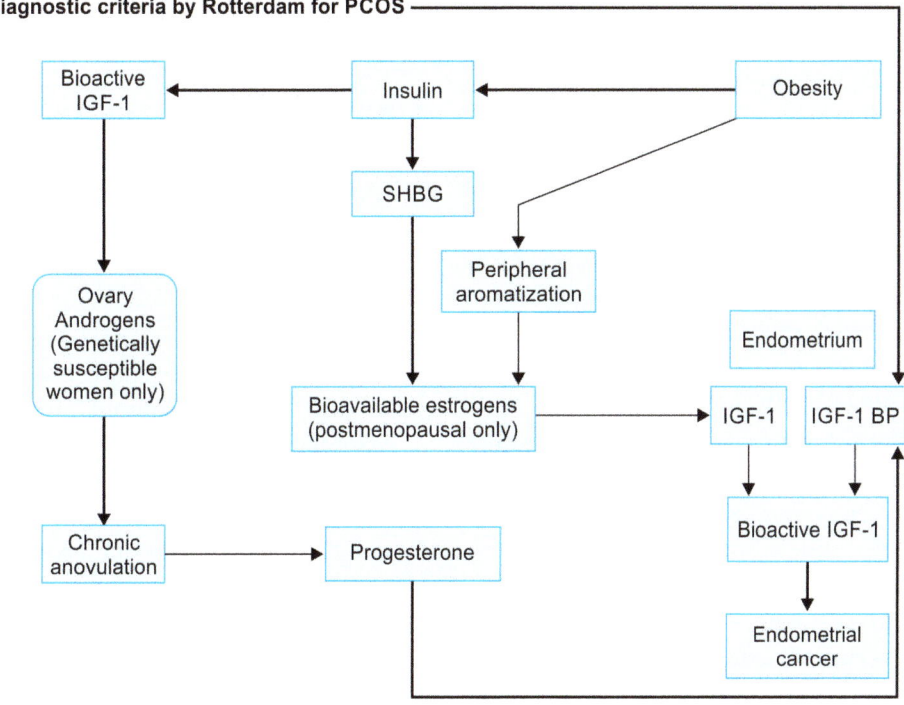

Flowchart 1: Mechanism through which hormonal factors and insulin resistance contribute to increased risk for endometrial cancer.

Source: Kaaks et al. 2022.
(BP: blood pressure; IGF: insulin-like growth factor; SHBG: sex hormone binding globulin)

increased risk of postmenopausal breast carcinoma. Ovarian cancer has been less well-studied in women with PCOS than breast and endometrial cancer. Cohort studies that have examined ovarian cancer in infertile women with progesterone deficiency have shown no significant increase in risk. Data from the cancer and steroid hormone study showed that ovarian cancer risk was found to be increased 2.5-fold among women with PCOS. This association is found to be stronger among women who never used oral contraceptive, and women who were in the first quartile of body mass index (13.3–18.5 kg/m²) at the age of 18 years appeared to have high risk. It means that oral contraceptive also results in reduction in risk of endometrial and ovarian cancer[3] with no increase in long-term metabolic risk.

A Danish case–control study showed no association between invasive ovarian cancer and history of hyperandrogenism. Ovarian cancer was not associated with a history of irregular periods in a large Australian case–control study. Agents that induce ovulation and improve the chance of pregnancy would also combat the unopposed estrogen and possibly lower the risk of endometrial hyperplasia and cancer, but expose the patient to a higher risk of ovarian cancer.

■ SLEEP APNEA

A study suggests that women with PCOS have a much higher risk of having obstructive sleep apnea than those without PCOS.[4] Sleep apnea causes interrupted breathing during sleep which leads to daytime fatigue and sleepiness and increased risk of developing high blood pressure, irregular heartbeat, and type 2 diabetes. One study even suggests that women with PCOS are 30 times more likely to suffer from sleep-disordered breathing than those who do not have PCOS and that insulin resistance is linked with sleep apnea more strongly than being overweight or obese or having high testosterone level.

■ MENTAL WELL-BEING

Symptoms of PCOS can affect your self-esteem and confidence. They can also lead to mental health problems such as depression, anxiety, and mood swings. One study claims that women with PCOS may have a significantly higher level of psychological distress than the general population. Another report suggests that women with PCOS are likely to develop eating disorder and sexual relationship problems.

■ MORBIDITY AND MORTALITY

Mortality from all causes for the group of women diagnosed with PCOS was no higher than the national rates for women of the same age. However, diabetes was mentioned as an underlying or a contributing cause of death for six of the women with PCOS. Therefore, the extent to which NIDDM contributes to premature morbidity and mortality for women with PCOS remains unclear at present.

There is a little evidence that women with PCO/PCOS are at an increased risk of CVD independent of NIDDM and there is some limited evidence that they have a lower rate of some forms of CVD than women without this diagnosis. It is speculated that the action of unopposed estrogen in anovulatory cycles might protect women with PCOS from circulatory disease, despite the presence of other CVD risk factors.

■ HOW TO REDUCE THE RISK?

- Obesity, central obesity, and insulin resistance are strongly implicated in the etiology of PCOS, and reduction of these risk factors should be a central treatment focus.
- Obesity and glucose intolerance are common but not the universal features of PCOS that compound an accurate assessment of the risk inherent in this syndrome.
- Lifestyle modifications form the foundation for treating obese women with PCOS and may reduce the incidence of diabetes, CVDs, and cancer.
- The management of PCOS also includes pharmacologic interventions, including metformin and oral contraceptives, that are targeted to the individual's disease process and treatment goals.

■ CONCLUSION

- PCOS is associated with several reproductive and metabolic abnormalities.
- Long-term metabolic abnormalities, above and beyond obesity, are related to reduced sensitivity to insulin and compensatory hyperinsulinemia in women with PCOS.
- Ethnicity may contribute independently to a worsening risk of glucose intolerance, with South Asian women being more at risk than their white Caucasian counterparts.
- The features of the insulin resistance syndrome are common in overweight women with PCOS.

- Subclinical and clinical atherosclerotic disease has been described in women with PCOS at a greater rate than in women with normal ovaries, although this is not apparent until the perimenopause.
- Women with PCOS have been reported to be at an increased risk for a number of gynecological neoplasias, including endometrial, breast, and ovarian cancer. The data supporting an increased risk are almost entirely inferential, based primarily on small cases series or shared risk factors.
- Ultrasonography has been found to be a useful screening tool for endometrial pathology in a postmenopausal symptomatic population; an endometrial thickness of <5 mm is rarely associated with endometrial carcinoma. The mean thickness of the endometrium was significantly elevated in endometrium.
- There is no consistent association reported between PCOS and breast cancer. Based on conflicting literature, it is premature to recommend either alternative screening strategies or preventative strategies for breast cancer in women with PCOS.
- An association between PCOS and ovarian cancer seems unlikely.

REFERENCES

1. Wang R, Mol BW. The Rotterdam criteria for polycystic ovary syndrome: evidence-based criteria?. Hum Reprod. 2017;32:261-4.
2. Chittenden BG, Fullerton G, Maheshwari A, Bhattacharya S. Polycystic ovary syndrome and the risk of gynaecological cancer: a systematic review. Reprod Biomed Online. 2009;19(3):398-405.
3. Cramer DW. The epidemiology of endometrial and ovarian cancer. Hematol Oncol Clin North Am. 2012;26(1):1-12.
4. Nandalike K, Agarwal C, Strauss T, Coupey SM, Isasi CR, Sin S, et al. Sleep and cardiometabolic function in obese adolescent girls with polycystic ovary syndrome. Sleep Med. 2012; 13(12):1307-12.

CHAPTER 30: PCOS in Indian Scenario

Sadhana Gupta, Shikha Sachan, Mamta

INTRODUCTION

Polycystic ovary syndrome (PCOS) is a multifaceted varied disorder with unclear genetic trait, affecting women in reproductive age as well as in menopausal and adolescent age groups with multiple etiologies. Women with PCOS often bear the stigma of subfertility and infertility, hyperandrogenism, menstrual irregularity, and metabolic dysfunction. In 1935, Irving F. Stein and Michael L. Leventhal first described a symptom complex associated with anovulation.[1] Careful histologic studies of the "Stein–Leventhal ovary" revealed that they had twice the cross-sectional area of normal ovaries, the same number of primordial follicles, double the number of developing and atretic follicles, a 50% thicker and more collagenized tunica, a fivefold thicker subcortical stroma, and a fourfold greater number of hilar cell "nests" than normal ovaries. It is one of the most common endocrinological disorders resulting from functional derangement which is contributed by many etiologies.[2] PCOS is not a discrete or specific endocrine disorder having a unique cause or pathophysiology; rather, PCOS is a heterogeneous disorder that is best approached as a diagnosis of exclusion.

The diagnostic criterion most commonly utilized in clinical practice for diagnosing PCOS is the "Rotterdam" criterion **(Table 1)**.[7]

EPIDEMIOLOGY OF POLYCYSTIC OVARY SYNDROME IN INDIA

The prevalence of PCOS in India ranges from 3.7 to 22.5% depending on the population studied and the criteria used for diagnosis.[3-7] A cross-sectional community-based study was conducted in a Mumbai to assess that the prevalence of PCOS among adolescent

TABLE 1: Insulin resistance in polycystic ovary syndrome.

Criteria	National institute of health (NIH) criteria 1990	Rotterdam criteria 2003	Androgen excess and PCOS society criteria 2006
• Irregular periods • Elevated serum androgens or 　– Hyperandrogenism 　　- Hirsutism 　　- Acne 　　- Androgenetic alopecia • Polycystic ovarian morphology (PCOM) or polycystic ovary (PCO)	1 and 2	Any 2 of 3	1 and 2 or 2 and 3

and young girls was 22.5% by Rotterdam and 10.7% by Androgen Excess Society criteria. Nonobese comprised 71.8% of PCOS diagnosed by Rotterdam criteria. Mild PCOS which was associated with oligomenorrhea and polycystic ovaries on ultrasonography (USG) was the phenotype most commonly reported (52.6%). Obese girls with PCOS were more hirsute, hypertensive, and had significantly higher mean insulin and 2 hours post 75 g glucose levels compared with nonobese PCOS.[8] A pilot cross-sectional study conducted in Tamil Nadu determined urban and rural differences in the burden of PCOS among Indian adolescent females aged 12-19 years. Close to 18% of adolescent population were confirmed of having PCOS (presence of all three elements) by recent guidelines of Rotterdam Consensus for adolescent diagnosis of PCOS. The proportion of participants diagnosed with PCOS was higher among urban participants in comparison to rural participants.[9]

A study conducted in south India using a self-administered questionnaire showed that a greater proportion of PCOS cases was seen in the age group of 23-25 years, among those with family history of PCOS, among those who were permanent residents of urban areas, and among those who were overweight or obese. About 92.3% of PCOS cases and all those at high risk had emotional problems such as feeling moody or experiencing fatigability.[10] A study conducted from Lucknow in college girls showed the calculated prevalence of PCOS of 3.7% in this population. Only 12% girls had a body mass index (BMI) ≥27.5 kg/m^2, but 44% had waist-hip ratio >0.81, again highlighting that despite low BMI, Indians have more abdominal obesity.[11] Another study conducted in Andhra Pradesh assessed that the prevalence of PCOS was 9.1% among adolescents.[12] Vidya Bharathi et al.[13] showed that the prevalence of PCOS diagnosed by the Rotterdam criteria in women from urban and rural areas of Chennai was 6% **(Fig. 1)**.

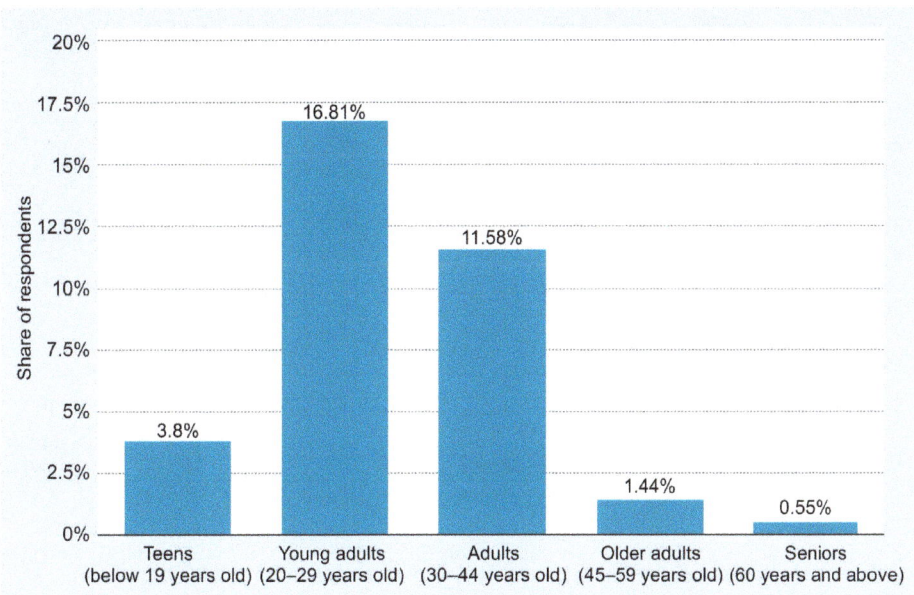

Fig. 1: Polycystic ovary syndrome issues among women across India during 2020, by age group.

PATHOPHYSIOLOGY OF POLYCYSTIC OVARY SYNDROME

Gonadotropins and sex steroid concentrations have very little variation in PCOS. There is higher than baseline increase of both androgens and estrogens. Serum estradiol levels are typically those observed in the early follicular phase and do not fluctuate much,[11-14] combined with insulin resistance (IR).[15] Genetic variants and environmental factors interact, combine, and contribute to the pathophysiology.[5] Increased luteinizing hormone (LH) pulse frequency leads to ovarian androgen excess by stimulating ovarian stroma. This also causes impaired follicle development and results in chronic anovulation. This hyperandrogenism which has resulted from ovarian androgen excess in turn leads to more IR and the resultant hyperinsulinemia[15]. A vicious cycle is thus created with insulin excess and resistance causing increased hyperandrogenism by increasing ovarian androgen production and decreasing hepatic sex hormone-binding globulin (SHBG) production.[16-19]

Gonadotropin Secretion and Action

Luteinizing hormone pulse frequency in women with PCOS does not exhibit the normal cyclic variation seen in ovulatory women and is relatively constant, at approximately one pulse per hour **(Fig. 3)**.[20-25] This pattern presumably reflects a similar increase in hypothalamic gonadotropin-releasing hormone (GnRH) pulse frequency, which favors secretion of LH more than FSH.[26,27,28]

Insulin acts synergistically with LH to perpetuate ovarian androgen production; these effects of insulin are mediated via a distinct pathway specific to insulin binding to its own receptor.[29] Hyperandrogenemia from any cause, arising during fetal life [maternal hyperandrogenism, classical congenital

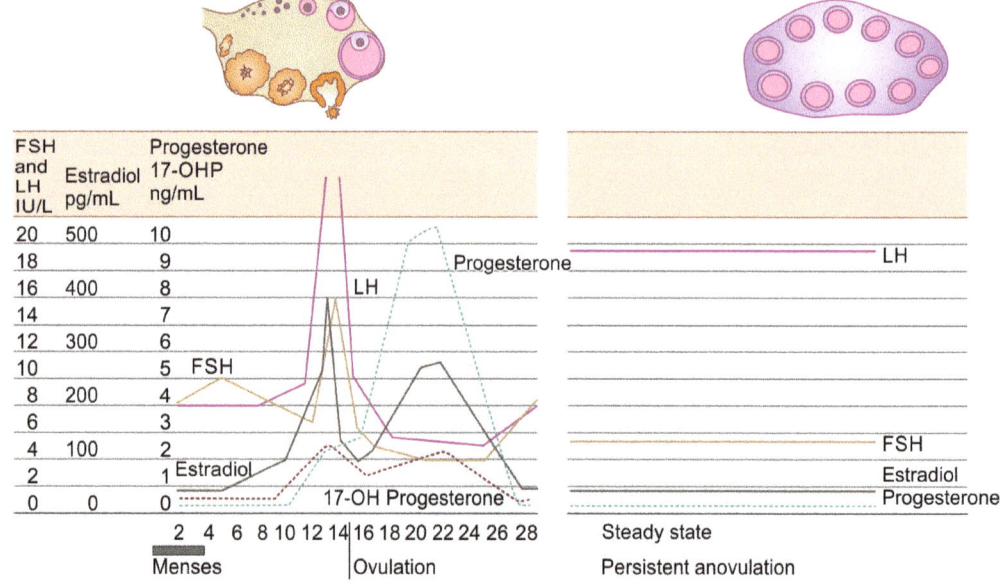

Fig. 2: Difference in hormonal changes between normal ovulating woman and PCOD woman.
Source: Speroff's clinical gynecologic endocrinology and infertility.
(FSH: follicle stimulating hormone; LH: luteinizing hormone; OHP: hydroxyprogesterone)

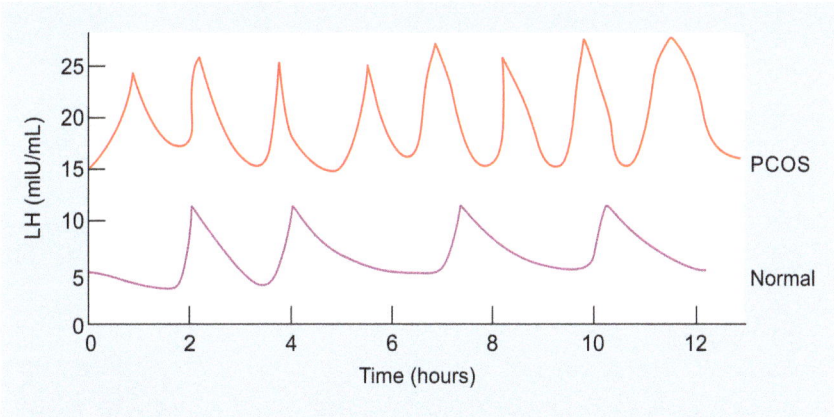

Fig. 3: LH levels in PCOS.
(LH: luteinizing hormone)

adrenal hyperplasia (CAH)], adolescence (premature adrenarche, nonclassical CAH), or in adulthood (obesity, hyperinsulinemia), induces abnormalities in the feedback control of pulsatile GnRH secretion, resulting in increased LH secretion, which stimulates increased ovarian androgen production.[30-33]

Insulin Secretion and Action

Insulin sensitivity is decreased by an average of 35–40% in women with PCOS. Up to 35% of women with PCOS exhibit impaired glucose tolerance, and 7–10% meet the criteria for type 2 diabetes mellitus.[34,35,36] Decreased glucose utilization mostly in muscles and increased gluconeogenesis in liver due to IR results in increased blood glucose concentrations and a compensatory hyperinsulinemia. Elevated fasting insulin levels are recognized as biochemical evidence of IR. Insulin response in women with PCOS is often exaggerated.[37-40]

The combined actions of insulin and androgens lower SHBG concentrations, yielding increased free androgen levels, which aggravate the underlying IR.[41-44] Ultimately, these conditions foster a self-propagating positive feedback loop that can increase in severity over time **(Fig. 4)**.

Obesity, Weight, and Energy Regulation

The risk for developing PCOS-like picture rises with increasing obesity,[45,46,47] as does the severity of IR, hyperinsulinemia, and ovulatory dysfunction and the prevalence of metabolic syndrome, glucose intolerance, risk factors for cardiovascular disease, and sleep apnea.[34,48-51] Insulin resistance is most highly correlated with intra-abdominal obesity because visceral fat is more active metabolically than subcutaneous fat and is more sensitive to lipolysis. The accumulation of free fatty acids in tissues causes lipotoxicity and IR, in part via tumor necrosis factor alpha (TNF-α), which increases serine phosphorylation and thereby inhibits insulin signaling. Obesity relates primarily to genetic and environmental factors and is a common, but not essential, feature of PCOS. Obesity contributes modestly to the risk for developing PCOS and adds to the pathophysiology in already affected women by aggravating the degree of IR and hyperinsulinemia.[52,53]

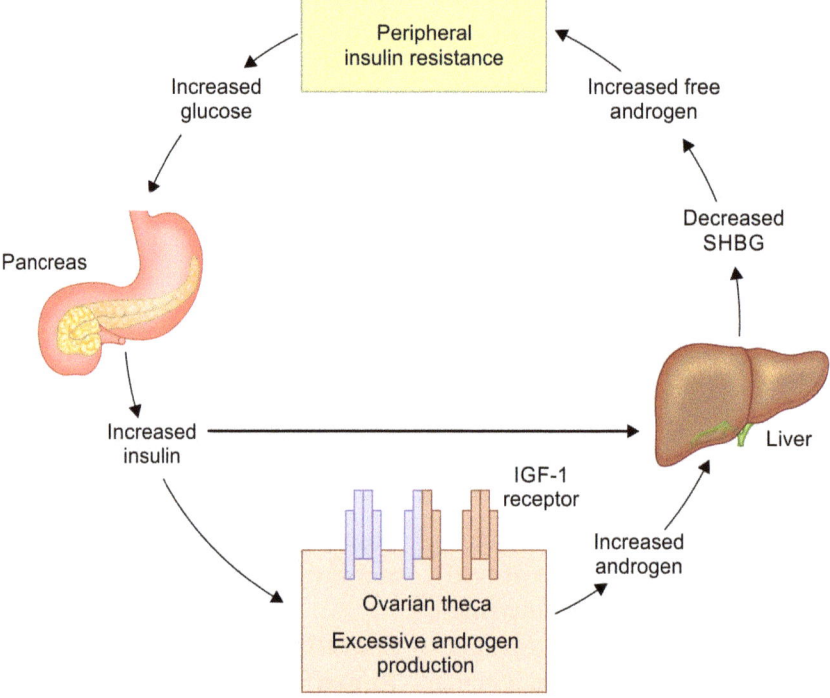

Fig. 4: Insulin resistance in PCOS.
(IGF-1: insulin-like growth factor 1; SHBG: sex hormone-binding globulin)

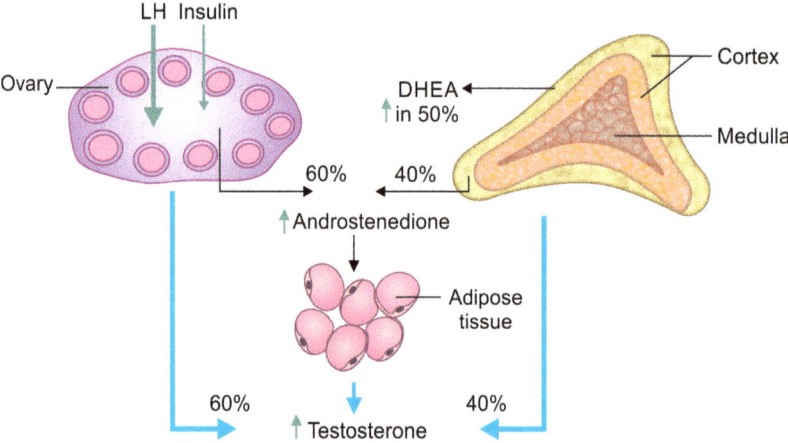

Fig. 5: Hyperandrogenism in PCOS.
(DHEA: dehydroepiandrosterone; LH: luteinizing hormone)

Androgen Synthesis and Action

Hyperandrogenism is the key feature of PCOS, resulting primarily from excess androgen production in the ovaries and, to a lesser extent, in the adrenals as well as in excess body fat **(Fig. 5)**.[54] In women with PCOS, approximately 60% of circulating androstenedione derives directly from the ovaries and the remainder from the adrenals; similarly, 60% of circulating testosterone is secreted directly by the ovaries, with most of the remainder deriving from peripheral conversion of androstenedione.[55]

There is abnormal LH secretion due to hyperinsulinemia and increased LH bioactivity, which potentiates the action of LH. This is worsened by obesity. Adrenal androgen production [androstenedione, dehydroepiandrosterone (DHEA), DHEA-S (sulfate)] is also increased in women with PCOS; over half exhibit moderately increased circulating DHEA-S levels.[56] Adrenal androgens have little or no intrinsic androgenic activity, but contribute to the pathophysiology of PCOS via conversion to testosterone in the periphery **(Fig. 6)**.

Genetic Considerations

Familial clustering of hyperandrogenism, anovulation, and polycystic ovary (PCO) suggests an underlying genetic basis or cause. Genome-wide association studies (GWAS) identified several possible candidate genes, including the *DENND1A* (differentially expressed in normal and neoplastic cell domain–containing protein 1A) and *THADA* (thyroid adenoma–associated protein) genes.[35] Further support for *DENND1A* comes from studies demonstrating increased levels of the V2 isoform of *DENND1A* in theca cells obtained from women with PCOS.[57]

GENETICS OF POLYCYSTIC OVARY SYNDROME FROM INDIA

Diabetes and metabolic syndrome-related genes: A study was conducted in Hyderabad where 15 single-nucleotide polymorphisms (SNPs) from nine type 2 diabetes-related genes (such as *TCF7L2, IGF2BP2, SLC30A8, HHEX, CDKAL1, CDKN2A, IRS1, CAPN10,* and *PPAR-γ*) were studied in PCOS women and controls; no significant association was found.[58] There was a positive association of Gly972Arg SNP of insulin receptor substrate 1 (IRS1) in PCOS women in a study done in south India.[48] Insulin receptor gene polymorphism was studied later,[59] for its association with IR in Indian women with PCOS; the study suggested that CC genotype (C1085T) might be developed as a marker for IR and metabolic complications in Indian women. Pro12Ala polymorphism of peroxisome proliferator-activated receptor gamma (PPAR-γ) showed significant association with reduced susceptibility for PCOS in a study published from Mumbai.[60] Angiotensin-converting enzyme (ACE) insertion/deletion (I/D) polymorphism was found to be associated with an early age at onset of PCOS symptoms in a case–control study from Hyderabad.[61]

Ovarian function-related gene polymorphism: Connexin37/Gap junction alpha 4 gene C1019T SNP is associated with the susceptibility to PCOS.[62] The luteinizing hormone/choriogonadotropin receptor *(LHCGR)* gene polymorphism rs-2293275 was found to be significantly associated with PCOS.[63] Vascular endothelial growth factor +405G/C polymorphism might constitute an inheritable risk factor for PCOS in south Indian women.[64] There was significant association between rs6523 polymorphism and an increased risk of PCOS.[65]

Oxidative stress and cytokine-related gene polymorphism: Two polymorphisms (L55M and Q192R) of paraoxonase 1 *(PON1)* gene were studied and one of those SNPs (L55M) was associated with reduced PCOS susceptibility only in lean women.[66] Interleukin 6 *(IL-6) 174* G/C SNP was found to be significantly associated with PCOS risk.[67]

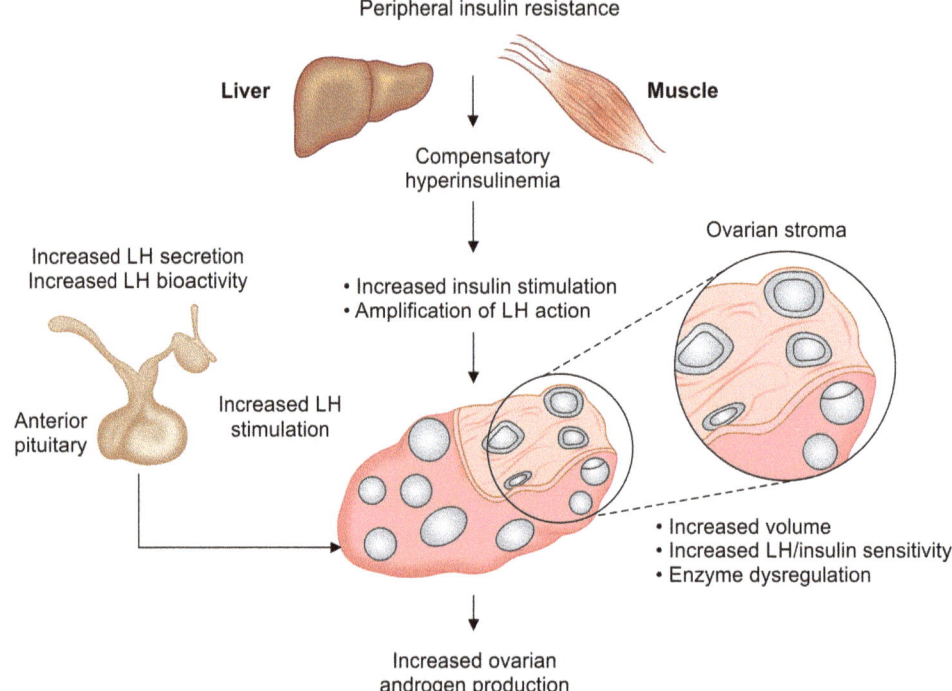

Fig. 6: Basic pathophysiology in PCOS.
(LH: luteinizing hormone)

Polymorphisms of *TNF-α* gene found that the distribution of genotypes for rs1799964 was significantly different between the groups.[68] *IL-1β, IL-1Ra* (receptor antagonist), and fatty acid binding protein 1 (*FABP1*) gene variants were found to be significantly associated with many metabolic features of PCOS.[69]

CLINICAL FEATURES OF POLYCYSTIC OVARY SYNDROME IN INDIA

The phenotype with hyperandrogenism and regular menstrual cycles had higher IR and gonadotropic hormonal abnormalities compared to the subgroup which had patients with irregular menstruation.[70] Hyperandrogenic phenotypes of PCOS were found to be more prone to metabolic complications.[70,71]

The incidence of PCOS is equal in both obese and nonobese women, but the markers of IR were more common in obese women.[72] In a study conducted in south India, the incidence of acanthosis nigricans was 50% among the women diagnosed with PCOS.[73]

The prevalence of abnormal glucose tolerance (AGT) detected by oral glucose tolerance test (OGTT) was found to be high (around 35%) in a large number of young Indian women with PCOS.[74]

MANAGEMENT OF POLYCYSTIC OVARY SYNDROME

The management approach for women with PCOS must be individualized to address the symptom burden while harnessing an individual's risks and minimizing long-term clinical consequences through tailored management and timely intervention of preventative strategies.

Long-term health risks in women with PCOS include:
- Increased risk for endometrial hyperplasia and neoplasia
- Increased risk for infertility
- Increased risk for type 2 diabetes
- Increased risk for cardiovascular disease.

Lifestyle changes are an important part of the clinical management, requiring careful education, counseling, encouragement, and follow-up.

REFERENCES

1. Stein IF, Leventhal ML. Amenorrhea associated with bilateral polycystic ovaries. Am J Obstet Gynecol. 1935;29(2):181-91.
2. Kyritsi EM, Dimitriadis GK, Kyrou I, Kaltsas G, Randeva HS. PCOS remains a diagnosis of exclusion: a concise review of key endocrinopathies to exclude. Clin Endocrinol (Oxf). 2017;86(1):1-6.
3. Rotterdam ESHRE/ASRM-Sponsored PCOS Consensus Workshop Group. Revised 2003 consensus on diagnostic criteria and long-term health risks related to polycystic ovary syndrome. Fertil Steril. 2004;81(1):19-25.
4. Rotterdam ESHRE/ASRM-Sponsored PCOS consensus workshop group. Revised 2003 consensus on diagnostic criteria and long-term health risks related to polycystic ovary syndrome (PCOS). Hum Reprod. 2004;19(1):41-7.
5. Azziz R, Carmina E, Dewailly D, Diamanti-Kandarakis E, Escobar-Morreale HF, Futterweit W, et al. Task Force on the Phenotype of the Polycystic Ovary Syndrome of The Androgen Excess and PCOS Society. The Androgen Excess and PCOS Society criteria for the polycystic ovary syndrome: the complete task force report. Fertil Steril. 2009;91(2):456-88.
6. Tal R, Seifer D, Tal R. Anti-Müllerian Hormone: Biology, Role in Ovarian Function and Clinical Significance. Obstetrics and Gynecology Advances. New York: Nova Science; 2016.
7. Abbott DH, Bacha F. Ontogeny of polycystic ovary syndrome and insulin resistance in utero and early childhood. Fertil Steril. 2013;100(1):2-11.
8. Joshi B, Mukherjee S, Patil A, Purandare A, Chauhan S, Vaidya R. A cross-sectional study of polycystic ovarian syndrome among adolescent and young girls in Mumbai, India. Indian J Endocrinol Metab. 2014;18(3):317-24.
9. Balaji S, Amadi C, Prasad S, Kasav JB, Upadhyay V, Singh AK, et al. Urban rural comparisons of polycystic ovary syndrome burden among adolescent girls in a hospital setting in India. Biomed Res Int. 2015;2015:158951.
10. Joseph N, Reddy AG, Joy D, Patel V, Santhosh P, Das S, et al. Study on the proportion and determinants of polycystic ovarian syndrome among health sciences students in South India. J Nat Sci Biol Med. 2016;7(2):166-72.
11. Gill H, Tiwari P, Dabadghao P. Prevalence of polycystic ovary syndrome in young women from North India: A Community-based study. Indian J Endocrinol Metab. 2012;16(Suppl 2):S389-92.
12. Nidhi R, Padmalatha V, Nagarathna R, Amritanshu R. Prevalence of polycystic ovarian syndrome in Indian adolescents. J Pediatr Adolesc Gynecol. 2011;24(4):223-7.
13. Vidya Bharathi R, Swetha S, Neerajaa J, Varsha Madhavica J, Janani DM, Rekha SN, et al. An epidemiological survey: Effect of predisposing factors for PCOS in Indian urban and rural population. Middle East Fertil Soc J. 2017;22:313-6.
14. Venturoli S, Porcu E, Fabbri R, Magrini O, Gammi L, Paradisi R, et al. Episodic pulsatile secretion of FSH, LH, prolactin, oestradiol, oestrone, and LH circadian variations in polycystic ovary syndrome. Clin Endocrinol (Oxf). 1988;28(1):93-107.
15. Dumesic DA, Oberfield SE, Stener-Victorin E, Marshall JC, Laven JS, Legro RS. Scientific Statement on the Diagnostic Criteria, Epidemiology, Pathophysiology, and

Molecular Genetics of Polycystic Ovary Syndrome. Endocr Rev. 2015;36(5):487-525.
16. Stein IF, Leventhal ML, Amenorrhea associated with bilateral polycystic ovaries. Am J Obstet Gynecol. 1935;29(2):181-91.
17. Taylor AE, McCourt B, Martin KA, Anderson EJ, Adams JM, Schoenfeld D, et al. Determinants of abnormal gonadotropin secretion in clinically defined women with polycystic ovary syndrome. J Clin Endocrinol Metabol. 1997;82(7):2248-56.
18. Rebar R, Judd HL, Yen SS, Rakoff J, Vandenberg G, Naftolin F. Characterization of the inappropriate gonadotropin secretion in polycystic ovary syndrome. J Clin Invest. 1976;57(5):1320-9.
19. Balen AH. Hypersecretion of luteinizing hormone and the polycystic ovary syndrome. Hum Reprod. 1993;8(Suppl 2):123-8.
20. Waldstreicher J, Santoro NF, Hall JE, Filicori M, Crowley WF Jr. Hyperfunction of the hypothalamic-pituitary axis in women with polycystic ovarian disease: indirect evidence for partial gonadotroph desensitization. J Clin Endocrinol Metab. 1988;66(1):165-72.
21. Kazer RR, Kessel B, Yen SS. Circulating luteinizing hormone pulse frequency in women with polycystic ovary syndrome. J Clin Endocrinol Metab. 1987;65(2):233-6.
22. Imse V, Holzapfel G, Hinney B, Kuhn W, Wuttke W. Comparison of luteinizing hormone pulsatility in the serum of women suffering from polycystic ovarian disease using a bioassay and five different immunoassays. J Clin Endocrinol Metab. 1992;74(5):1053-61.
23. Hayes FJ, Taylor AE, Martin KA, Hall JE. Use of a gonadotropin-releasing hormone antagonist as a physiologic probe in polycystic ovary syndrome: assessment of neuroendocrine and androgen dynamics. J Clin Endocrinol Metab. 1998;83(7):2343-9.
24. Lockwood GM, Muttukrishna S, Groome NP, Matthews DR, Ledger WL. Mid-follicular phase pulses of inhibin B are absent in polycystic ovarian syndrome and are initiated by successful laparoscopic ovarian diathermy: a possible mechanism regulating emergence of the dominant follicle. J Clin Endocrinol Metab.1998;83(5):1730-5.
25. Laven JS, Imani B, Eijkemans MJ, de Jong FH, Fauser BC. Absent biologically relevant associations between serum inhibin B concentrations and characteristics of polycystic ovary syndrome in normogonadotrophic anovulatory infertility. Hum Reprod. 2001;16(7):1359-64.
26. Wildt L, Häusler A, Marshall G, Hutchison JS, Plant TM, Belchetz PE, et al. Frequency and amplitude of gonadotropin-releasing hormone stimulation and gonadotropin secretion in the rhesus monkey. Endocrinology. 1981;109(2):376-85.
27. Gross KM, Matsumoto AM, Bremner WJ. Differential control of luteinizing hormone and follicle-stimulating hormone secretion by luteinizing hormone-releasing hormone pulse frequency in man. J Clin Endocrinol Metab. 1987;64(4):675-80.
28. Spratt DI, Finkelstein JS, Butler JP, Badger TM, Crowley WF Jr. Effects of increasing the frequency of low doses of gonadotropin-releasing hormone (GnRH) on gonadotropin secretion in GnRH-deficient men. J Clin Endocrinol Metab. 1987;64(6):1179-86.
29. Nestler JE. Insulin regulation of human ovarian androgens. Hum Reprod. 1997; 12(Suppl 1):53-62.
30. Berga SL, Yen SS. Opioidergic regulation of LH pulsatility in women with polycystic ovary syndrome. Clin Endocrinol (Oxf). 1989;30(2):177-84.
31. Carmina E, Koyama T, Chang L, Stanczyk FZ, Lobo RA. Does ethnicity influence the prevalence of adrenal hyperandrogenism and insulin resistance in polycystic ovary syndrome? Am J Obstet Gynecol. 1992;167(6):1807-12.
32. Dunaif A. Insulin resistance and the polycystic ovary syndrome: mechanism and implications for pathogenesis. Endocr Rev. 1997;18(6):774-800.
33. Legro RS, Finegood D, Dunaif A. A fasting glucose to insulin ratio is a useful measure of insulin sensitivity in women with polycystic ovary syndrome. J Clin Endocrinol Metab. 1998;83(8):2694-8.

34. Legro RS, Kunselman AR, Dodson WC, Dunaif A. Prevalence and predictors of risk for type 2 diabetes mellitus and impaired glucose tolerance in polycystic ovary syndrome: a prospective, controlled study in 254 affected women. J Clin Endocrinol Metab. 1999;84(1):165-9.
35. 35-McCartney ChR, Marshall JC. Polycystic ovary syndrome. N Engl J Med. 2016; 375(14):1398-9.
36. Ehrmann DA, Barnes RB, Rosenfield RL, Cavaghan MK, Imperial J. Prevalence of impaired glucose tolerance and diabetes in women with polycystic ovary syndrome. Diabetes Care. 1999;22(1):141-6.
37. Tok EC, Ertunc D, Evruke C, Dilek S. The androgenic profile of women with non-insulin-dependent diabetes mellitus. J Reprod Med. 2004;49(9):746-52.
38. Franks S, Gilling-Smith C, Watson H, Willis D. Insulin action in the normal and polycystic ovary. Endocrinol Metab Clin North Am. 1999;28(2):361-78.
39. Nelson-Degrave VL, Wickenheisser JK, Hendricks KL, Asano T, Fujishiro M, Legro RS, et al. Alterations in mitogen-activated protein kinase and extracellular regulated kinase signaling in theca cells contribute to excessive androgen production in polycystic ovary syndrome. Mol Endocrinol. 2005; 19(2):379-90.
40. Willis D, Mason H, Gilling-Smith C, Franks S. Modulation by insulin of follicle-stimulating hormone and luteinizing hormone actions in human granulosa cells of normal and polycystic ovaries. J Clin Endocrinol Metab. 1996;81(1):302-9.
41. Cohen JC, Hickman R. Insulin resistance and diminished glucose tolerance in powerlifters ingesting anabolic steroids. J Clin Endocrinol Metab. 1987;64(5):960-3.
42. Nestler JE, Jakubowicz DJ, de Vargas AF, Brik C, Quintero N, Medina F. Insulin stimulates testosterone biosynthesis by human thecal cells from women with polycystic ovary syndrome by activating its own receptor and using inositolglycan mediators as the signal transduction system. J Clin Endocrinol Metab. 1998;83(6):2001-5.
43. Barbieri RL, Makris A, Ryan KJ. Insulin stimulates androgen accumulation in incubations of human ovarian stroma and theca. Obstet Gynecol. 1984;64(3 Suppl): 73S-80S.
44. Book CB, Dunaif A. Selective insulin resistance in the polycystic ovary syndrome. J Clin Endocrinol Metab. 1999;84(9):3110-6.
45. Korhonen S, Hippeläinen M, Niskanen L, Vanhala M, Saarikoski S. Relationship of the metabolic syndrome and obesity to polycystic ovary syndrome: a controlled, population-based study. Am J Obstet Gynecol. 2001; 184(3):289-96.
46. Alvarez-Blasco F, Botella-Carretero JI, San Millán JL, Escobar-Morreale HF. Prevalence and characteristics of the polycystic ovary syndrome in overweight and obese women. Arch Intern Med. 2006;166(19):2081-6.
47. Yildiz BO, Yarali H, Oguz H, Bayraktar M. Glucose intolerance, insulin resistance, and hyperandrogenemia in first degree relatives of women with polycystic ovary syndrome. J Clin Endocrinol Metab. 2003;88(5):2031-6.
48. Ehrmann DA, Liljenquist DR, Kasza K, Azziz R, Legro RS, Ghazzi MN, et al. Prevalence and predictors of the metabolic syndrome in women with polycystic ovary syndrome. J Clin Endocrinol Metab. 2006;91(1):48-53.
49. Dokras A, Jagasia DH, Maifeld M, Sinkey CA, VanVoorhis BJ, Haynes WG. Obesity and insulin resistance but not hyperandrogenism mediates vascular dysfunction in women with polycystic ovary syndrome. Fertil Steril. 2006;86(6):1702-9.
50. Barber TM, McCarthy MI, Wass JAH, Franks S. Obesity and polycystic ovary syndrome. Clin Endocrinol (Oxf). 2006;65(2):137-45.
51. Boomsma CM, Eijkemans MJC, Hughes EG, Visser GHA, Fauser BC, Macklon NS. A meta-analysis of pregnancy outcomes in women with polycystic ovary syndrome. Hum Reprod Update. 2006;12(6):673-83.
52. Gambineri A, Pelusi C, Vicennati V, Pagotto U, Pasquali R. Obesity and the polycystic ovary syndrome. Int J Obes Relat Metab Disord. 2002;26(7):883-96.
53. Baillargeon JP, Nestler JE. Polycystic ovary syndrome: a syndrome of ovarian

hypersensitivity to insulin? J Clin Endocrinol Metab. 2006;91(1):22-4.
54. Kumar A, Woods KS, Bartolucci AA, Azziz R. Prevalence of adrenal androgen excess in patients with the polycystic ovary syndrome (PCOS). Clin Endocrinol (Oxf). 2005;62(6): 644-9.
55. Cedars MI, Steingold KA, de Ziegler D, Lapolt PS, Chang RJ, Judd HL. Long-term administration of gonadotropin-releasing hormone agonist and dexamethasone: assessment of the adrenal role in ovarian dysfunction. Fertil Steril. 1992;57(3): 495-500.
56. Azziz R, Black V, Hines GA, Fox LM, Boots LR. Adrenal androgen excess in the polycystic ovary syndrome: sensitivity and responsivity of the hypothalamic-pituitary-adrenal axis. J Clin Endocrinol Metab. 1998;83(7):2317-23.
57. McAllister JM, Modi B, Miller BA, Biegler J, Bruggeman R, Legro RS, et al. Overexpression of a DENND1A isoform produces a polycystic ovary syndrome theca phenotype. Proc Natl Acad Sci U S A. 2014;111(15):E1519-27.
58. Reddy BM, Kommoju UJ, Dasgupta S, Rayabarapu P. Association of type 2 diabetes mellitus genes in polycystic ovary syndrome aetiology among women from southern India. Indian J Med Res. 2016;144(3):400-8.
59. Gangopadhyay S, Agrawal N, Batra A, Kabi BC, Gupta A. Single-Nucleotide Polymorphism on Exon 17 of Insulin Receptor Gene Influences Insulin Resistance in PCOS: A Pilot Study on North Indian Women. Biochem Genet. 2016;54(2):158-68.
60. Shaikh N, Mukherjee A, Shah N, Meherji P, Mukherjee S. Peroxisome proliferator activated receptor gamma gene variants influence susceptibility and insulin related traits in Indian women with polycystic ovary syndrome. J Assist Reprod Genet. 2013;30(7): 913-21.
61. Deepika MLN, Reddy KR, Rani VU, Balakrishna N, Latha KP, Jahan P. Do ACE I/D gene polymorphism serve as a predictive marker for age at onset in PCOS? J Assist Reprod Genet. 2013;30(1):125-30.
62. Guruvaiah P, Govatati S, Reddy TV, Beeram H, Deenadayal M, Shivaji S, et al. Analysis of Connexin37 gene C1019T polymorphism and PCOS susceptibility in South Indian population: case-control study. Eur J Obstet Gynecol Reprod Biol. 2016;196:17-20.
63. Thathapudi S, Kodati V, Erukkambattu J, Addepally U, Qurratulain H. Association of luteinizing hormone chorionic gonadotropin receptor gene polymorphism (rs2293275) with polycystic ovarian syndrome. Genet Test Mol Biomarkers. 2015;19(3):128-32.
64. Guruvaiah P, Govatati S, Reddy TV, Lomada D, Deenadayal M, Shivaji S, et al. The VEGF +405 G and C 5' untranslated region polymorphism and risk of PCOS: A study in the South Indian women. J Assist Reprod Genet. 2014;31:1383-9.
65. Shaikh N, Dadachanji R, Meherji P, Shah N, Mukherjee S. Polymorphisms and haplotypes of insulin-like factor 3 gene are associated with risk of polycystic ovary syndrome in Indian women. Gene. 2016;577:180-6.
66. Dadachanji R, Shaikh N, Khavale S, Patil A, Shah N, Mukherjee S. PON1 polymorphisms are associated with polycystic ovary syndrome susceptibility, related traits, and PON1 activity in Indian women with the syndrome. Fertil Steril. 2015;104(1):207-16.
67. Tumu VR, Govatati S, Guruvaiah P, Deenadayal M, Shivaji S, Bhanoori M. An interleukin-6 gene promoter polymorphism is associated with polycystic ovary syndrome in South Indian women. J Assist Reprod Genet. 2013;30(12):1541-6.
68. Deepika MLN, Reddy KR, Yashwanth A, Rani VU, Latha KP, Jahan P. TNF-α haplotype association with polycystic ovary syndrome–A South Indian study. J Assist Reprod Genet. 2013;30(11):1493-503.
69. Rashid N, Nigam A, Saxena P, Jain SK, Wajid S. Association of IL-1β, IL-1Ra and FABP1 gene polymorphisms with the metabolic features of polycystic ovary syndrome. Inflamm Res. 2017;66(7):621-36.
70. Suri J, Suri JC, Chatterjee B, Mittal P, Adhikari T. Obesity may be the common pathway for sleep-disordered breathing in women with polycystic ovary syndrome. Sleep Med. 2016; 24:32-9.
71. Kar S. Anthropometric, clinical, and metabolic comparisons of the four Rotterdam

PCOS phenotypes: A prospective study of PCOS women. J Hum Reprod Sci. 2013;6(3): 194-200.
72. Ramanand SJ, Ghongane BB, Ramanand JB, Patwardhan MH, Ghanghas RR, Jain SS. Clinical characteristics of polycystic ovary syndrome in Indian women. Indian J Endocrinol Metab. 2013;17(1):138-45.
73. Shivaprakash G, Basu A, Kamath A, Shivaprakash P, Adhikari P, Up R, et al. Acanthosis Nigricans in PCOS Patients and its Relation with Type 2 Diabetes Mellitus and Body Mass at a Tertiary Care Hospital in Southern India. J Clin Diagn Res. 2013;7(2): 317-9.
74. Ganie MA, Dhingra A, Nisar S, Sreenivas V, Shah ZA, Rashid A, et al. Oral glucose tolerance test significantly impacts the prevalence of abnormal glucose tolerance among Indian women with polycystic ovary syndrome: lessons from a large database of two tertiary care centers on the Indian subcontinent. Fertil Steril. 2016;105(1):194-201.e1-3.

Annexure

CONSENSUS GUIDELINES ON POLYCYSTIC OVARY SYNDROME—ADOPTED FROM INTERNATIONAL EVIDENCE-BASED GUIDELINE FOR THE MANAGEMENT OF POLYCYSTIC OVARY SYNDROME 2018

— By Editorial Team

■ RECOMMENDATIONS SUMMARY
Table Notes

The recommendation number reflects the corresponding evidence section.

Clinical consensus recommendations (CCR) and clinical practice points (CCP) do not have a 'GRADE' rating.

No.	Category	recommendation	Quality and grade
1		Screening, diagnostic assessment, risk assessment, and life stage	
1.1		Irregular cycles and ovulatory dysfunction	
1.1.1	CCR	Irregular menstrual cycles are defined as: • Normal in the first year postmenarche as part of the pubertal transition • >1 to <3 years post menarche: <21 or >45 days • >3 years postmenarche to perimenopause: < 21 or >35 days or <8 cycles per year • >1 year postmenarche > 90 days for any one cycle • Primary amenorrhea by age 15 or >3 years post-thelarche (breast development) When irregular menstrual cycles are present a diagnosis of polycystic ovary syndrome (PCOS) should be considered and assessed according to the guidelines	❖❖❖❖
1.1.2	CCR	In an adolescent with irregular menstrual cycles, the value and optimal timing of assessment and diagnosis of PCOS should be discussed with the patient, considering diagnostic challenges at this life stage and psychosocial and cultural factors	❖❖❖❖
1.1.3	CPP	For adolescents who have features of PCOS but do not meet diagnostic criteria, an "increased risk" could be considered, and reassessment advised at or before full reproductive maturity, 8 years postmenarche. This includes those with PCOS features before combined oral contraceptive pill (COCP) commencement, those with persisting features and those with significant weight gain in adolescence	

Contd...

Contd…

1.1.4	CPP	Ovulatory dysfunction can still occur with regular cycles and if anovulation needs to be confirmed serum progesterone levels can be measured
1.2		Biochemical hyperandrogenism
1.2.1	EBR	Calculated free testosterone, free androgen index or calculated bioavailable testosterone should be used to assess biochemical hyperandrogenism in the diagnosis of PCOS ❖❖❖❖ ⊕⊕○○
1.2.2	EBR	High-quality assays such as liquid chromatography–mass spectrometry (LCMS)/mass spectrometry and extraction/chromatography immunoassays, should be used for the most accurate assessment of total or free testosterone in PCOS ❖❖❖❖ ⊕⊕○○
1.2.3	EBR	Androstenedione and dehydroepiandrosterone sulfate (DHEAS) could be considered if total or free testosterone is not elevated; however, these provide limited additional information in the diagnosis of PCOS ❖❖❖ ⊕⊕○○
1.2.4	CCR	Direct free testosterone assays, such as radiometric or enzyme-linked assays, preferably should not be used in assessment of biochemical hyperandrogenism in PCOS, as they demonstrate poor sensitivity, accuracy, and precision ❖❖❖❖
1.2.5	CPP	Reliable assessment of biochemical hyperandrogenism is not possible in women on hormonal contraception, due to effects on sex hormone-binding globulin and altered gonadotropin-dependent androgen production
1.2.6	CPP	Where assessment of biochemical hyperandrogenism is important in women on hormonal contraception, drug withdrawal is recommended for three months or longer before measurement, and contraception management with a nonhormonal alternative is needed during this time
1.2.7	CPP	Assessment of biochemical hyperandrogenism is most useful in establishing the diagnosis of PCOS and/or phenotype where clinical signs of hyperandrogenism (in particular hirsutism) are unclear or absent
1.2.8	CPP	Interpretation of androgen levels needs to be guided by the reference ranges of the laboratory used, acknowledging that ranges for different methods and laboratories vary widely. Normal values are ideally based on levels from a well phenotyped healthy control population or by cluster analysis of a large general population considering age and pubertal specific stages
1.2.9	CPP	Where androgen levels are markedly above laboratory reference ranges, other causes of biochemical hyperandrogenism need to be considered. History of symptom onset and progression is critical in assessing for neoplasia, however, some androgen-secreting neoplasms may only induce mild-to-moderate increases in biochemical hyperandrogenism
1.3		Clinical hyperandrogenism
1.3.1	CCR	A comprehensive history and physical examination should be completed for symptoms and signs of clinical hyperandrogenism, including acne, alopecia and hirsutism and, in adolescents, severe acne, and hirsutism ❖❖❖❖
1.3.2	CCR	Health professionals should be aware of the potential negative psychosocial impact of clinical hyperandrogenism. Reported unwanted excess hair growth and/or alopecia should be considered important, regardless of apparent clinical severity ❖❖❖❖

Contd…

Contd...

1.3.3	CCR	Standardized visual scales are preferred when assessing hirsutism, such as the modified Ferriman–Gallwey score (mFG) with a level ≥ 4–6 indicating hirsutism, depending on ethnicity, acknowledging that self-treatment is common and can limit clinical assessment ❖❖❖❖
1.3.4	CCR	The Ludwig visual score is preferred for assessing the degree and distribution of alopecia ❖❖❖❖
1.3.5	CPP	There are no universally accepted visual assessments for evaluating acne
1.3.6	CPP	The prevalence of hirsutism is the same across ethnicities, yet the mFG cut-off scores for defining hirsutism and the severity of hirsutism varies by ethnicity
1.3.7	CPP	As ethnic variation in vellus hair density is notable, overestimation of hirsutism may occur if vellus hair is confused with terminal hair; only terminal hairs need to be considered in pathological hirsutism, with terminal hairs clinically growing > 5 mm in length if untreated, varying in shape and texture and generally being pigmented
1.4		**Ultrasound and polycystic ovarian morphology (PCOM)**
1.4.1	CCR	Ultrasound should not be used for the diagnosis of PCOS in those with a gynecological age of < 8 years (< 8 years after menarche), due to the high incidence of multi-follicular ovaries in this life stage ❖❖❖❖
1.4.2	CCR	The threshold for PCOM should be revised regularly with advancing ultrasound technology, and age-specific cut off values for PCOM should be defined ❖❖❖❖
1.4.3	CCR	The transvaginal ultrasound approach is preferred in the diagnosis of PCOS, if sexually active and if acceptable to the individual being assessed ❖❖❖❖
1.4.4	CCR	Using endovaginal ultrasound transducers with a frequency bandwidth that includes 8 MHz, the threshold for PCOM should be on either ovary, a follicle number per ovary of >20 and/or an ovarian volume ≥ 10 mL, ensuring no corpora lutea, cysts or dominant follicles are present ❖❖❖❖
1.4.5	CPP	If using older technology, the threshold for PCOM could be an ovarian volume ≥ 10 mL on either ovary
1.4.6	CPP	In patients with irregular menstrual cycles and hyperandrogenism, an ovarian ultrasound is not necessary for PCOS diagnosis; however, ultrasound will identify the complete PCOS phenotype
1.4.7	CPP	In transabdominal ultrasound, reporting is best focused on ovarian volume with a threshold of ≥10 mL, given the difficulty of reliably assessing follicle number with this approach
1.4.8	CPP	Clear protocols are recommended for reporting follicle number per ovary and ovarian volume on ultrasound. Recommended minimum reporting standards include: • Last menstrual period • Transducer bandwidth frequency • Approach/route assessed • Total follicle number per ovary measuring 2–9 mm

Contd...

Contd…

- Three dimensions and volume of each ovary
- Reporting of endometrial thickness and appearance is preferred—3-layer endometrial assessment may be useful to screen for endometrial pathology
- Other ovarian and uterine pathology, as well as ovarian cysts, corpus luteum, and dominant follicles ≥equal 10 mm

1.4.9	CPP	There is a need for training in careful and meticulous follicle counting per ovary, to improve reporting	
1.5		Anti-Müllerian hormone (AMH)	
1.5.1	EBR	Serum AMH levels should not yet be used as an alternative for the detection of PCOM or as a single test for the diagnosis of PCOS	❖❖❖ ⊕⊕○○
1.5.2	CPP	There is emerging evidence that with improved standardization of assays and establishedcut off levels or thresholds based on large scale validation in populations of different agesand ethnicities, AMH assays will be more accurate in the detection of PCOM	
1.6		Ethnic variation	
1.6.1	CCR	Health professionals should consider ethnic variation in the presentation and manifestations of PCOS, including: • A relatively mild phenotype in Caucasians • Higher body mass index (BMI) in Caucasian women, especially in North America and Australia • More severe hirsutism in Middle Eastern, Hispanic, and Mediterranean women • Increased central adiposity, insulin resistance, diabetes, metabolic risks, and acanthosis nigricans in South East Asians and Indigenous Australians • Lower BMI and milder hirsutism in East Asians • Higher BMI and metabolic features in Africans	❖❖❖❖
1.7		Menopause life stage	
1.7.1	CCR	Postmenopausal persistence of PCOS could be considered likely with continuing evidence of hyperandrogenism	❖❖❖
1.7.2	CCR	A diagnosis of PCOS postmenopause could be considered if there is a past diagnosis of PCOS, a long-term history of irregular menstrual cycles and hyperandrogenism and/or PCOM, during the reproductive years	❖❖❖
1.7.3	CPP	Postmenopausal women presenting with new-onset, severe or worsening hyperandrogenism including hirsutism, require further investigation to rule out androgen-secreting tumors and ovarian hyperthecosis	
1.8		Cardiovascular disease risk (CVD)	
1.8.1	CCR	All those with PCOS should be offered regular monitoring for weight changes and excess weight, in consultation with and where acceptable to the individual woman. Monitoring could be at each visit or at a minimum 6–12 monthly, with frequency planned and agreed between the health professional and the individual	❖❖❖❖

Contd…

Contd...

1.8.2	CCR	Weight, height, and ideally waist circumference should be measured and BMI calculated with the following considered: • BMI categories and waist circumference should follow World Health Organization guidelines, also noting ethnic and adolescent ranges • Consideration should be given for Asian and high-risk ethnic groups including recommended monitoring of waist circumference	❖❖❖❖ ❖❖❖❖
1.8.3	CCR	All women with PCOS should be assessed for cardiovascular risk factors and global CVD risk	❖❖❖❖
1.8.4	CCR	If screening reveals CVD risk factors including obesity, cigarette smoking, dyslipidemia, hypertension, impaired glucose tolerance, and lack of physical activity, women with PCOS should be considered at increased risk of CVD	
1.8.5	CCR	Overweight and obese women with PCOS, regardless of age, should have a fasting lipid profile (cholesterol, low density lipoprotein cholesterol, high density lipoprotein cholesterol, and triglyceride level at diagnosis). Thereafter, frequency of measurement should be based on the presence of hyperlipidemia and global CVD risk	❖❖❖❖
1.8.6	CCR	All women with PCOS should have blood pressure measured annually, or more frequently based on global CVD risk	❖❖❖❖
1.8.7	CPP	Health professionals need to be aware that CVD risk in women with PCOS remains unclear pending high quality studies, however, prevalence of CVD risk factors is increased, warranting consideration of screening	❖❖❖❖
1.8.8	CPP	Consideration needs to be given to the significant differences in CVD risk across ethnicities (see 1.6.1) when determining frequency of risk assessment	❖❖❖❖
1.9		Gestational diabetes, impaired glucose tolerance and type 2 diabetes	❖❖❖❖
1.9.1	CCR	Health professionals and women with PCOS should be aware that, regardless of age, the prevalence of gestational diabetes, impaired glucose tolerance and type 2 diabetes (fivefold in Asia, fourfold in the Americas, and threefold in Europe) are significantly increased in PCOS, with risk independent of, yet exacerbated by, obesity	
1.9.2	CCR	Glycemic status should be assessed at baseline in all women with PCOS. Thereafter, assessment should be every one to three years, influenced by the presence of other diabetes risk factors	❖❖❖❖
1.9.3	CCR	An oral glucose tolerance test (OGTT), fasting plasma glucose, or HbA1c should be performed to assess glycemic status. In high-risk women with PCOS (including a BMI > 25 kg/m^2 or in Asians >23 kg/m^2, history of impaired fasting glucose, impaired glucose tolerance or gestational diabetes, family history of diabetes mellitus type 2, Hypertension, or high-risk ethnicity), an OGTT is recommended	❖❖❖❖
1.9.4	CCR	A 75-g OGTT should be offered in all women with PCOS preconception when planning pregnancy or seeking fertility treatment, given the high risk of hyperglycemia and the associated comorbidities in pregnancy. If not performed preconception, an OGTT should be offered at < 20 weeks gestation, and all women with PCOS should be offered the test at 24–28 weeks gestation	

Contd...

Contd…

1.10		Obstructive sleep apnea (OSA)	
1.10.1	CCR	Screening should only be considered for OSA in PCOS to identify and alleviate related symptoms, such as snoring, waking unrefreshed from sleep, daytime sleepiness, and the potential for fatigue to contribute to mood disorders. Screening should not be considered with the intention of improving cardiometabolic risk, with inadequate evidence for metabolic benefits of OSA treatment in PCOS and in general populations	
1.10.2	CCR	A simple screening questionnaire, preferably the Berlin tool, could be applied and if positive, referral to a specialist considered	
1.10.3	CPP	A positive screen raises the likelihood of OSA, however it does not quantify symptom burden and alone does not justify treatment. If women with PCOS have OSA symptoms and a positive screen, consideration can be given to be referral to a specialist center for further evaluation	
1.11		Endometrial cancer	❖❖❖❖
1.11.1	CCR	Health professionals and women with PCOS should be aware of a two to sixfold increased risk of endometrial cancer, which often presents before menopause; However, absolute risk of endometrial cancer remains relatively low	
1.11.2	CPP	Health professionals require a low threshold for investigation of endometrial cancer in women with PCOS or a history of PCOS, with investigation by transvaginal ultrasound and/or endometrial biopsy recommended with persistent thickened endometrium and/or risk factors including prolonged amenorrhea, abnormal vaginal bleeding, or excess weight. However, routine ultrasound screening of endometrial thickness in PCOS is not recommended	❖❖❖❖
1.11.3	CPP	Optimal prevention for endometrial hyperplasia and endometrial cancer is not known. A pragmatic approach could include COCP or progestin therapy in those with cycles longer than 90 days	
2		Prevalence, screening, diagnostic assessment, and treatment of emotional wellbeing	
2.1		Quality of life	
2.1.1	CCR	Health professionals and women should be aware of the adverse impact of PCOS on quality of life	
2.1.2	CCR	Health professionals should capture and consider perceptions of symptoms, impact on quality of life and personal priorities for care to improve patient outcomes	
2.1.3	CPP	The PCOS quality of life tool (PCOSQ), or the modified PCOSQ, may be useful clinically to highlight PCOS features causing greatest distress, and to evaluate treatment outcomes on women's subjective PCOS health concerns	❖❖❖❖
2.2		Depressive and anxiety symptoms, screening, and treatment	❖❖❖❖
2.2.1	CCR	Health professionals should be aware that in PCOS, there is a high prevalence of moderate to severe anxiety and depressive symptoms in adults; and a likely increased prevalence in adolescents	❖❖❖❖

Contd…

Contd...

2.2.2	CCR	Anxiety and depressive symptoms should be routinely screened in all adolescents and women with PCOS at diagnosis. If the screen for these symptoms and/or other aspects of emotional wellbeing is positive, further assessment and/or referral for assessment and treatment should be completed by suitably qualified health professionals, informed by regional guidelines	❖❖❖❖
2.2.3	CCR	If treatment is warranted, psychological therapy and/or pharmacological treatment should be offered in PCOS, informed by regional clinical practice guidelines	❖❖❖❖
2.2.4	CPP	The optimal interval for anxiety and depressive symptom screening is not known. A pragmatic approach could include repeat screening using clinical judgment, considering risk factors, comorbidities, and life events	
2.2.5	CPP	Assessment of anxiety and or depressive symptoms involves assessment of risk factors, symptoms, and severity. Symptoms can be screened according to regional guidelines, or by using the following stepped approach: *Step 1*: Initial questions could include: Over the last 2 weeks, how often have you been bothered by the following problems? • Feeling down, depressed, or hopeless? • Little interest or pleasure in doing things? • Feeling nervous, anxious or on edge? • Not being able to stop or control worrying? *Step 2*: If any of the responses are positive, further screening should involve: • Assessment of risk factors and symptoms using age, culturally and regionally appropriate tools, such as the Patient Health Questionnaire (PHQ) or the Generalized Anxiety Disorder Scale (GAD7) and/or refer to an appropriate professional for further assessment	
2.2.6	CPP	Where pharmacological treatment for anxiety and depression is offered in PCOS, the following need consideration: • Caution is needed to avoid inappropriate treatment with antidepressants or anxiolytics. Where mental health disorders are clearly documented and persistent, or if suicidal symptoms are present, treatment of depression or anxiety need to be informed by clinical regional practice guidelines • Use of agents that exacerbate PCOS symptoms, including weight gain, needs careful consideration	
2.2.7	CPP	Factors including obesity, infertility, and hirsutism need consideration along with use of hormonal medications in PCOS, as they may independently exacerbate depressive and anxiety symptoms and other aspects of emotional wellbeing	
2.3		Psychosexual function	
2.3.1	CCR	All health professionals should be aware of the increased prevalence of psychosexual dysfunction and should consider exploring how features of PCOS, including hirsutism and body image, impact on sex life and relationships in PCOS	❖❖❖❖
2.3.2	CCR	If psychosexual dysfunction is suspected, tools such as the Female Sexual Function index can be considered	❖❖❖❖

Contd...

Contd…

2.4		Body image	
2.4.1	CCR	Health professionals and women should be aware that features of PCOS can impact on body image	❖❖❖❖
2.4.2	CPP	Negative body image, can be screened according to regional guidelines or by using the following stepped approach:	

- *Step 1:* Initial questions could include:
  - Do you worry a lot about the way you look and wish you could think about it less?
  - On a typical day, do you spend >1 hour per day worrying about your appearance? (>1 hour a day is considered excessive)
  - What specific concerns do you have about your appearance?
  - What effect does it have on your life?
  - Does it make it hard to do your work or be with your friends and family?
- *Step 2:* If an issue is identified, health professionals could further assess by:
  - Identifying any focus of concern of the patient and respond appropriately
  - Assessing the level of depression and/or anxiety
  - Identifying distortion of body image or disordered eating

2.5		Eating disorders and disordered eating	
2.5.1	CCR	All health professionals and women should be aware of the increased prevalence of eating disorders and disordered eating associated with PCOS	❖❖
2.5.2	CCR	If eating disorders and disordered eating are suspected, further assessment, referral, and treatment, including psychological therapy, could be offered by appropriately trained health professionals, informed by regional clinical practice guidelines	❖❖
2.5.3	CPP	Eating disorders and disordered eating can be screened using the following stepped approach	

Step 1: The SCOFF (Sick, Control, One stone, Fat, Food) screening tool can be used or initial screening questions can include:
- Does your weight affect the way you feel about yourself?
- Are you satisfied with your eating patterns?

Step 2: If the SCOFF tool or any of these questions are positive, further screening should involve:
- Assessment of risk factors and symptoms using age, culturally and regionally appropriate tools;
- Referral to an appropriate health professional for further mental health assessment and diagnostic interview. If this is not the patient's usual healthcare provider, inform the primary care physician

2.6		Information resources, models of care, cultural, and linguistic considerations	
2.6.1	CCR	Information and education resources for women with PCOS should be culturally appropriate, tailored, and high-quality, should use a respectful and empathetic approach, and promote self-care and highlight peer support groups	❖❖❖❖
2.6.2	CCR	Information and education resources for healthcare professionals should promote the recommended diagnostic criteria, appropriate screening for comorbidities and effective lifestyle and pharmacological management	❖❖❖❖

Contd…

Contd...

2.6.3	CCR	PCOS information should be comprehensive, evidence-based and inclusive of the biopsychosocial dimensions of PCOS across the lifespan	✦✦✦✦
2.6.4	CCR	Women's needs, communication preferences, beliefs, and culture should be considered and addressed through provision of culturally and linguistically appropriate code-signed resources and care	✦✦✦✦
2.6.5	CCR	Interdisciplinary care needs to be considered for those with PCOS where appropriate and available. Primary care is generally well placed to diagnose, screen, and coordinate interdisciplinary care	✦✦✦✦
2.6.6	CCR	Care needs to be person centered, address women's priorities and be provided in partnership with those with PCOS and where appropriate, their families	✦✦✦✦
2.6.7	CPP	Guideline dissemination and translation including multimodal education tools and resources is important, with consultation and engagement with stakeholders internationally	
3		Lifestyle	
3.1		Effectiveness of lifestyle interventions	
3.1.1	CCR	Healthy lifestyle behaviors encompassing healthy eating and regular physical activity should be recommended in all those with PCOS to achieve and/or maintain healthy weight and to optimize hormonal outcomes, general health, and quality of life across the life course.	✦✦✦✦
3.1.2	EBR	Lifestyle intervention (preferably multicomponent including diet, exercise, and behavioral strategies) should be recommended in all those with PCOS and excess weight, for reductions in weight, central obesity, and insulin resistance	✦✦✦
3.1.3	CPP	Achievable goals such as 5–10% weight loss in those with excess weight yields significant clinical improvements and are considered successful weight reduction within 6 months. Ongoing assessment and monitoring are important during weight loss and maintenance in all women with PCOS	⊕⊕○○
3.1.4	CPP	SMART (Specific Measurable, Achievable, Realistic, and Timely), goal setting and self-monitoring can enable achievement of realistic lifestyle goals	
3.1.5	CPP	Psychological factors such as anxiety and depressive symptoms, body image concerns and disordered eating, need consideration and management to optimize engagement and adherence to lifestyle interventions	
3.1.6	CPP	Health professional interactions around healthy lifestyle, including diet and exercise, need to be respectful, patient-centered and to value women's individualized healthy lifestyle preferences and cultural, socioeconomic, and ethnic differences. Health professionals need to also consider personal sensitivities, marginalization and potential weight-related stigma	
3.1.7	CPP	Adolescent and ethnic-specific BMI and waist circumference categories need to be considered when optimizing lifestyle and weight	
3.1.8	CPP	Healthy lifestyle may contribute to health and quality of life benefits in the absence of weight loss	
3.1.9	CPP	Healthy lifestyle and optimal weight management appears equally effective in PCOS as in the general population and is the joint responsibility of all health professionals, partnering with women with PCOS. Where complex issues arise, referral to suitably trained allied health professionals needs to be considered	

Contd...

Contd…

3.1.10	CPP	Ethnic groups with PCOS who are at high cardiometabolic risk as per 1.6.1 require greater consideration in terms of healthy lifestyle and lifestyle intervention
3.2		**Behavioral strategies**
3.2.1	CCR	Lifestyle interventions could include behavioral strategies such as goal-setting, self-monitoring, stimulus control, problem solving, assertiveness training, slower eating, reinforcing changes, and relapse prevention, to optimize weight management, healthy lifestyle and emotional wellbeing in women with PCOS
3.2.2	CPP	Comprehensive health behavioral or cognitive behavioral interventions could be considered to increase support, engagement, retention, adherence, and maintenance of healthy lifestyle and improve health outcomes in women with PCOS
3.3		**Dietary intervention**
3.3.1	CCR	A variety of balanced dietary approaches could be recommended to reduce dietary energy intake and induce weight loss in women with PCOS and overweight and obesity, as per general population recommendations
3.3.2	CCR	General healthy eating principles should be followed for all women with PCOS across the life course, as per general population recommendations
3.3.3	CPP	To achieve weight loss in those with excess weight, an energy deficit of 30% or 500–750 kcal/day (1,200–1,500 kcal/day) could be prescribed for women, also considering individual energy requirements, body weight and physical activity levels
3.3.4	CPP	In women with PCOS, there is no or limited evidence that any specific energy equivalent diet type is better than another, or that there is any differential response to weight management intervention, compared to women without PCOS
3.3.5	CPP	Tailoring of dietary changes to food preferences, allowing for a flexible and individual approach to reducing energy intake and avoiding unduly restrictive and nutritionally unbalanced diets, are important, as per general population recommendations
3.4		**Exercise intervention**
3.4.1	CCR	Health professionals should encourage and advise the following for prevention of weight gain and maintenance of health: • In adults from 18–64 years, a minimum of 150 min/week of moderate intensity physical activity or 75 min/week of vigorous intensities or an equivalent combination of both, including muscle strengthening activities on 2 nonconsecutive days/week • In adolescents, at least 60 minutes of moderate to vigorous intensity physical activity/ day, including those that strengthen muscle and bone at least 3 times weekly • Activity be performed in at least 10-minute bouts or around 1,000 steps, aiming to achieve at least 30 minutes daily on most days

Contd…

Contd...

3.4.2	CCR	Health professionals should encourage and advise the following for modest weight-loss, prevention of weight-regain and greater health benefits: • A minimum of 250 min/week of moderate intensity activities or 150 min/week of vigorous intensity or an equivalent combination of both, and muscle strengthening activities involving major muscle groups on 2 nonconsecutive days/week • Minimized sedentary, screen, or sitting time	❖❖❖
3.4.3	CPP	Physical activity includes leisure time physical activity, transportation such as walking or cycling, occupational work, household chores, games, sports or planned exercise, in the context of daily, family, and community activities. Daily, 10,000 steps is ideal, including activities of daily living and 30 minutes of structured physical activity or around 3,000 steps. Structuring of recommended activities need to consider women's and family routines as well as cultural preferences	
3.4.4	CPP	Realistic physical activity SMART goals could include 10-minute bouts, progressively increasing physical activity 5% weekly, up to and above recommendations	
3.4.5	CPP	Self-monitoring including with fitness tracking devices and technologies for step count and exercise intensity could be used as an adjunct to support and promote active lifestyles and minimize sedentary behaviors	
3.5		Obesity and weight assessment	❖❖❖
3.5.1	CCR	Health professionals and women should be aware that women with PCOS have a higher prevalence of weight gain and obesity, presenting significant concerns for women, impacting on health and emotional wellbeing, with a clear need for prevention	❖❖❖❖
3.5.2	CCR	All those with PCOS should be offered regular monitoring for weight changes and excess weight as per 1.8.1 and 1.8.2	
3.5.3	PP	When assessing weight, related stigma, negative body image, and/or low self-esteem need to be considered and assessment needs to be respectful and considerate. Beforehand, explanations on the purpose and how the information will be used and the opportunity for questions and preferences needs to be provided, permission sought and scales and tape measures adequate. Implications of results need to be explained and where this impacts on emotional wellbeing, support provided	
3.5.4	CPP	Prevention of weight gain, monitoring of weight and encouraging evidence-based, and socio-culturally appropriate healthy lifestyle is important in PCOS, particularly from adolescence	
4		Pharmacological treatment for nonfertility indications	
4.1		Pharmacological treatment principles in PCOS	
4.1.1	CPP	Consideration of the individual's personal characteristics, preferences, and values is important in recommending pharmacological treatment	
4.1.2	CPP	When prescribing pharmacological therapy in PCOS, benefits, adverse effects, and contraindications in PCOS and general populations need to be considered and discussed before commencement	

Contd...

Contd...

4.1.3	CPP	COCPs, metformin, and other pharmacological treatments are generally off label in PCOS. However, off label use is predominantly evidence-based and is allowed in many countries. Where is it allowed, health professionals need to inform women and discuss the evidence, possible concerns and side effects of treatment	
4.1.4	CPP	Holistic approaches are required and pharmacological therapy in PCOS needs to be considered alongside education, lifestyle and other options including cosmetic therapy and counseling	
4.2		Combined oral contraceptive pills (COCPs)	
4.2.1	EBR	The COCP alone should be recommended in adult women with PCOS for management of hyperandrogenism and/or irregular menstrual cycles	❖❖❖❖ ⊕⊕○○
4.2.2	EBR	The COCP alone should be considered in adolescents with a clear diagnosis of PCOS for management of clinical hyperandrogenism and/or irregular menstrual cycles	❖❖❖ ⊕⊕○○
4.2.3	EBR	The COCP could be considered in adolescents who are deemed "at risk" but not yet diagnosed with PCOS, for management of clinical hyperandrogenism and irregular menstrual cycles	❖❖❖ ⊕⊕○○
4.2.4	EBR	Specific types or dose of progestins, estrogens, or combinations of COCP cannot currently be recommended in adults and adolescents with PCOS and practice should be informed by general population guidelines	❖❖❖ ⊕⊕○○
4.2.5	CCR	The 35 microgram ethinylestradiol plus cyproterone acetate preparations should not be considered first line in PCOS as per general population guidelines, due to adverse effects including venous thromboembolic risks	❖
4.2.6	CPP	When prescribing COCPs in adults and adolescents with PCOS: • Various COCP preparations have similar efficacy in treating hirsutism • The lowest effective estrogen doses (such as 20–30 micrograms of ethinylestradiol or equivalent), and natural estrogen preparations need consideration, balancing efficacy, metabolic risk profile, side effects, cost, and availability • The generally limited evidence on effects of COCPs in PCOS needs to be appreciated with practice informed by general population guidelines (WHO guidelines) • The relative and absolute contraindications and side effects of COCPs need to be considered and be the subject of individualized discussion • PCOS-specific risk factors such as high BMI, hyperlipidemia and hypertension need to be considered	
4.3		Combined oral contraceptive pills in combination with metformin and/or anti-androgen pharmacological agents	
4.3.1	EBR	In combination with the COCP, metformin should be considered in women with PCOS for management of metabolic features where COCP and lifestyle changes do not achieve desired goals	❖❖❖❖ ⊕⊕○○
4.3.2	EBR	In combination with the COCP, metformin could be considered in adolescents with PCOS and BMI ≥25 kg/m^2 where COCP and lifestyle changes do not achieve desired goals	❖❖❖❖ ⊕⊕○○

Contd...

Contd…

4.3.3	CPP	In combination with the COCP, metformin may be most beneficial in high metabolic risk groups including those with diabetes risk factors, impaired glucose tolerance, or high-risk ethnic groups	❖❖ ⊕⊕OO
4.3.4	EBR	In combination with the COCP, antiandrogens should only be considered in PCOS to treat hirsutism, after 6 months or more of COCP and cosmetic therapy have failed to adequately improve symptoms	
4.3.5	CCR	In combination with the COCP, antiandrogens could be considered for the treatment of androgen-related alopecia in PCOS	❖❖
4.3.6	CPP	In PCOS, antiandrogens must be used with effective contraception, to avoid male fetal undervirilization. Variable availability and regulatory status of these agents are notable and for some agents, potential liver toxicity requires caution	
4.4		**Metformin**	
4.4.1	EBR	Metformin in addition to lifestyle could be recommended in adult women with PCOS, for the treatment of weight, hormonal, and metabolic outcomes	❖❖❖ ⊕⊕OO
4.4.2	EBR	Metformin in addition to lifestyle should be considered in adult women with PCOS with BMI ≥ 25 kg/m² for management of weight and metabolic outcomes	❖❖❖ ⊕⊕OO
4.4.3	EBR	Metformin in additional to lifestyle could be considered in adolescents with a clear diagnosis of PCOS or with symptoms of PCOS before the diagnosis is made	❖❖❖ ⊕⊕OO
4.4.4	CPP	Metformin may offer greater benefit in high metabolic risk groups including those with diabetes risk factors, impaired glucose tolerance or high-risk ethnic groups	
4.4.5	CPP	Where metformin is prescribed the following need to be considered: • Adverse effects, including gastrointestinal side-effects that are generally dose dependent and self-limiting, need to be the subject of individualized discussion • Starting at a low dose, with 500 mg increments 1–2 weekly and extended release preparations may minimize side effects • Metformin use appears safe long-term, based on use in other populations, however, ongoing requirement needs to be considered and use may be associated with low vitamin B12 levels • Use is generally off label and health professionals need to inform women and discuss the evidence, possible concerns, and side effects	
4.5		**Antiobesity pharmacological agents**	
4.5.1	CCR	Antiobesity medications in addition to lifestyle could be considered for the management of obesity in adults with PCOS after lifestyle intervention, as per general population recommendations	❖❖
4.5.2	CPP	For antiobesity medications, cost, contraindications, side effects, variable availability, and regulatory status need to be considered and pregnancy needs to be avoided whilst taking these medications	

Contd…

Contd…

4.6		Antiandrogen pharmacological agents
4.6.1	EBR	Where COCPs are contraindicated or poorly tolerated, in the presence of other effective forms of contraception, antiandrogens could be considered to treat hirsutism and androgen-related alopecia
4.6.2	CPP	Specific types or doses of antiandrogens cannot currently be recommended with inadequate evidence in PCOS
4.7		Inositol
4.7.1	EBR	Inositol (in any form) should currently be considered an experimental therapy in PCOS, with emerging evidence on efficacy highlighting the need for further research
4.7.2	CPP	Women taking inositol and other complementary therapies are encouraged to advise their health professional
5		Assessment and treatment of infertility
5.1		Assessment of factors that may affect fertility, treatment response, or pregnancy outcomes
5.1.1	CPP	Factors such as blood glucose, weight, blood pressure, smoking, alcohol, diet, exercise, sleep and mental, emotional, and sexual health need to be optimized in women with PCOS, to improve reproductive and obstetric outcomes, aligned with recommendations in the general population Refer to lifestyle, emotional wellbeing, and diabetes risk sections
5.1.2	CPP	Monitoring during pregnancy is important in women with PCOS, given increased risk of adverse maternal and offspring outcomes
5.1.3	CCR	In women with PCOS and infertility due to anovulation alone with normal semen analysis, the risks, benefits, costs, and timing of tubal patency testing should be discussed on an individual basis
5.1.4	CCR	Tubal patency testing should be considered prior to ovulation induction in women with PCOS where there is suspected tubal infertility
5.2		Ovulation induction principles
5.2.1	CPP	The use of ovulation induction agents, including letrozole, metformin, and clomiphene citrate is off label in many countries. Where off label use of ovulation induction agents is allowed, health professionals need to inform women and discuss the evidence, possible concerns, and side effects
5.2.2	CPP	Pregnancy needs to be excluded prior to ovulation induction
5.2.3	CPP	Unsuccessful, prolonged use of ovulation induction agents needs to be avoided, due to poor success rates
5.3		Letrozole
5.3.1	EBR	Letrozole should be considered first-line pharmacological treatment for ovulation induction in women with PCOS with anovulatory infertility and no other infertility factors to improve ovulation, pregnancy, and live birth rates
5.3.2	CPP	Where letrozole is not available or use is not permitted or cost is prohibitive, health professionals can use other ovulation induction agents

Contd…

Contd…

5.3.3	CPP	Health professionals and women need to be aware that the risk of multiple pregnancy appears to be less with letrozole, compared to clomiphene citrate	
5.4		**Clomiphene citrate and metformin**	
5.4.1	EBR	Clomiphene citrate could be used alone in women with PCOS with anovulatory infertility and no other infertility factors to improve ovulation and pregnancy rates	❖❖❖ ⊕○○○
5.4.2	EBR	Metformin could be used alone in women with PCOS, with anovulatory infertility and no other infertility factors, to improve ovulation, pregnancy and live birth rates, although women should be informed that there are more effective ovulation induction agents	❖❖❖ ⊕⊕⊕○
5.4.3	EBR	Clomiphene citrate could be used in preference, when considering clomiphene citrate or metformin for ovulation induction in women with PCOS who are obese (BMI is ≥30 kg/m^2) with anovulatory infertility and no other infertility factors	❖❖❖ ⊕⊕○○
5.4.4	EBR	If metformin is being used for ovulation induction in women with PCOS who are obese (BMI ≥30 kg/m^2) with anovulatory infertility and no other infertility factors, clomiphene citrate could be added to improve ovulation, pregnancy, and live birth rates	❖❖❖ ⊕⊕○○
5.4.5	EBR	Clomiphene citrate could be combined with metformin, rather than persisting with clomiphene citrate alone, in women with PCOS who are clomiphene citrate-resistant, with anovulatory infertility and no other infertility factors, to improve ovulation and pregnancy rates	❖❖❖ ⊕⊕○○
5.4.6	CPP	The risk of multiple pregnancy is increased with clomiphene citrate use and therefore monitoring needs to be considered	
5.5		**Gonadotropins**	
5.5.1	EBR	Gonadotropins could be used as second-line pharmacological agents in women with PCOS who have failed first line oral ovulation induction therapy and are anovulatory and infertile, with no other infertility factors	❖❖❖ ⊕⊕○○
5.5.2	EBR	Gonadotropins could be considered as first-line treatment, in the presence of ultrasound monitoring, following counseling on cost and potential risk of multiple pregnancy, in women with PCOS with anovulatory infertility and no other infertility factors	❖❖❖ ⊕⊕○○
5.5.3	EBR	Gonadotropins, where available and affordable, should be used in preference to clomiphene citrate combined with metformin therapy for ovulation induction, in women with PCOS with anovulatory infertility, clomiphene citrate-resistance and no other infertility factors, to improve ovulation, pregnancy, and live birth rates	❖❖❖ ⊕⊕⊕○
5.5.4	EBR	Gonadotropins with the addition of metformin could be used rather than gonadotropin alone, in women with PCOS with anovulatory infertility, clomiphene citrate-resistance and no other infertility factors, to improve ovulation, pregnancy, and live birth rates	❖❖❖ ⊕⊕⊕○
5.5.5	EBR	Either gonadotropins or laparoscopic ovarian surgery could be used in women with PCOS with anovulatory infertility, clomiphene citrate-resistance, and no other infertility factors, following counseling on benefits and risks of each therapy	❖❖❖ ⊕⊕⊕○

Contd…

Contd...

5.5.6	CPP	Where gonadotropins are prescribed, considerations include: • Cost and availability • Expertise required for use in ovulation induction • Degree of intensive ultrasound monitoring required • Lack of difference in clinical efficacy of available gonadotropin preparations • Low dose gonadotropin protocols optimize monofollicular development • Risk and implications of potential multiple pregnancy
5.5.7	CPP	Gonadotropin-induced ovulation is only triggered when there are fewer than three mature follicles and needs to be cancelled if there are more than two mature follicles with the patient advised to avoid unprotected intercourse
5.6		Antiobesity agents
5.6.1	CCR	Pharmacological antiobesity agents should be considered an experimental therapy in women with PCOS for the purpose of improving fertility, with risk to benefit ratios currently too uncertain to advocate this as fertility therapy ❖
5.7		Laparoscopic surgery
5.7.1	EBR	Laparoscopic ovarian surgery could be second-line therapy for women with PCOS, who are clomiphene citrate resistant, with anovulatory infertility, and no other infertility factors ❖❖❖ ⊕⊕○○
5.7.2	CCR	Laparoscopic ovarian surgery could potentially be offered as first-line treatment if laparoscopy is indicated for another reason in women with PCOS with anovulatory infertility and no other infertility factors ❖❖❖
5.7.3	CPP	Risks need to be explained to all women with PCOS considering laparoscopic ovarian surgery
5.7.4	CPP	Where laparoscopic ovarian surgery is to be recommended, the following need to be considered: • Comparative cost • Expertise required for use in ovulation induction • Intraoperative and postoperative risks are higher in women who are overweight and obese • There may be a small associated risk of lower ovarian reserve or loss of ovarian function • Periadnexal adhesion formation may be an associated risk
5.8		Bariatric surgery ❖
5.8.1	CCR	Bariatric surgery should be considered an experimental therapy in women with PCOS, for the purpose of having a healthy baby, with risk to benefit ratios currently too uncertain to advocate this as fertility therapy
5.8.2	CPP	If bariatric surgery is to be prescribed, the following need to be considered: • Comparative cost • The need for a structured weight management program involving diet, physical activity, and interventions to improve psychological, musculoskeletal, and cardiovascular health to continue post-operatively • Perinatal risks such as small for gestational age, premature delivery, possibly increased infant mortality

Contd...

Contd…

- Potential benefits such as reduced incidence of large for gestational age fetus and gestational diabetes
- Recommendations for pregnancy avoidance during periods of rapid weight loss and for at least 12 months after bariatric surgery with appropriate contraception

If pregnancy occurs, the following need to be considered:
- Awareness and preventative management of pre and postoperative nutritional deficiencies is important, ideally in a specialist interdisciplinary care setting
- Monitoring of fetal growth during pregnancy

5.9		In vitro fertilization (IVF)
5.9.1	CCR	In the absence of an absolute indication for IVF ± intracytoplasmic sperm injection (ICSI), women with PCOS and anovulatory infertility could be offered IVF as third-line therapy where first or second-line ovulation induction therapies have failed
5.9.2	CPP	In women with anovulatory PCOS, the use of IVF is effective and when elective single embryo transfer is used multiple pregnancies can be minimized
5.9.3	CPP	Women with PCOS undergoing IVF ± ICSI therapy need to be counseled prior to starting treatment including on: • Availability, cost, and convenience • Increased risk of ovarian hyperstimulation syndrome • Options to reduce the risk of ovarian hyperstimulation
5.9.4	CCR	Urinary or recombinant follicle stimulation hormone can be used in women with PCOS undergoing controlled ovarian hyperstimulation for IVF ± ICSI, with insufficient evidence to recommend specific follicle stimulating hormone (FSH) preparations
5.9.5	CCR	Exogenous recombinant luteinizing hormone treatment should not be routinely used in combination with follicle stimulating hormone therapy in women with PCOS undergoing controlled ovarian hyperstimulation for IVF ± ICSI
5.9.6	EBR	A gonadotropin-releasing hormone (GnRH) antagonist protocol is preferred in women with PCOS undergoing an IVF ± ICSI cycle, over a GnRH agonist long protocol, to reduce the duration of stimulation, total gonadotropin dose and incidence of ovarian hyperstimulation syndrome (OHSS)
5.9.7	CPP	Human chorionic gonadotropins is best used at the lowest doses to trigger final oocyte maturation in women with PCOS undergoing an IVF ± ICSI cycle to reduce the incidence of OHSS
5.9.8	CPP	Triggering final oocyte maturation with a GnRH agonist and freezing all suitable embryos could be considered in women with PCOS having an IVF/ICSI cycle with a GnRH antagonist protocol and at an increased risk of developing OHSS or where fresh embryo transfer is not planned
5.9.9	CPP	In IVF ± ICSI cycles in women with PCOS, consideration needs to be given to an elective freeze of all embryos

Contd…

Contd...

5.9.10	EBR	Adjunct metformin therapy could be used before and/or during follicle stimulating hormone ovarian stimulation in women with PCOS undergoing an IVF ± ICSI therapywith a GnRH agonist protocol, to improve the clinical pregnancy rate and reduce the risk of OHSS	❖❖❖ ⊕⊕○○
5.9.11	CCR	In a GnRH agonist protocol with adjunct metformin therapy, in women with PCOSundergoing IVF ± ICSI treatment, the following could be considered: • Metformin commencement at the start of GnRH agonist treatment • Metformin use at a dose of between 1,000 mg and 2,550 mg daily • Metformin cessation at the time of the pregnancy test or menses (unless the metformin therapy is otherwise indicated) • Metformin side-effects (see above metformin section)	❖❖❖
5.9.12	CPP	In IVF ± ICSI cycles, women with PCOS could be counseled on potential benefitsof adjunct metformin in a GnRH antagonist protocol to reduce risk of ovarian hyperstimulation syndrome (see above for metformin therapy considerations)	
5.9.13	CPP	The term in vitro maturation (IVM) treatment cycle is applied to "the maturationin vitro of immature cumulus oocyte complexes collected from antral follicles" (encompassing both stimulated and unstimulated cycles, but without the use of a human gonadotropin trigger)	❖❖❖
5.9.14	CCR	In units with sufficient expertise, IVM could be offered to achieve pregnancy and live birth rates approaching those of standard IVF ± ICSI treatment without the riskof OHSS for women with PCOS, where an embryo is generated, then vitrified andthawed and transferred in a subsequent cycle	

Off-label prescribing occurs when a drug is prescribed for an indication, a route of administration, or a patient group that is not included in the approved product information document for that drug by the regulatory body. Prescribing off label is often unavoidable and common and does not mean that the regulatory body has rejected the indication, more commonly there has not been a submission to request evaluation of the indication or that patient group for any given drug.

Index

Page numbers followed by *b* refer to box, *f* refer to figure, *fc* refer to flowchart, and *t* refer to table

A

Abnormal glucose tolerance 167
   prevalence of 192
Abortion, spontaneous 155
Acanthosis nigricans 32, 173, 176, 177, 178*f*
   appearance of 35*f*
   formation of 35*f*
Acne 1, 20, 32, 39, 123, 173, 175
   comedonal 34*f*
   distribution 35*t*
   severity, grading of 35*t*
   treatment for 123
   types of 176*f*
Acupuncture 152
Adapalene 176
Adrenal hyperandrogenism, functional 4, 6, 10
Adrenal hyperplasia, congenital 56, 188
Adrenal suppression 62
Adrenarche, premature 189
Adrenocorticotropic hormone 4, 6, 58, 151
   test 6
Advanced glycation end products 11, 84
Alexandrite laser 63
Alistipes 89
Alopecia 20, 32, 39
   Christmas tree pattern of 34*f*
   frontotemporal 34*f*
Alpha-reductase inhibitors 61
Amenorrhea 18
   anovulation 101
   weight-related 142
American Society for Reproductive Medicine 107
Amino acids 87
Androgen 74
   blocker 61
   Excess Society 19, 36
      criteria 101
   hyperproduction of 57
   levels, high 101
   metabolic action of 54
   overproduction of 11
   production 5
   receptor 54
      blockers 61
   secreting tumors 56
   source of 6, 6*t*
   suppression 61
   synthesis 190
      dysregulation of 138
   systemic 129
   types of 56*fc*
Androgenic alopecia 173
Anorexia nervosa 69
Anovulation 23, 54, 101, 136, 147
   chronic 128
Anovulatory cycles 136
Anovulatory infertility 140, 142, 143
   treatment for 124
Antenatal fetal surveillance 163
Anthropometry 119
Antiandrogens 123
   therapy, monitoring of 124
Antifungal lotions 179
Anti-Müllerian hormone 15, 38, 96, 101, 105, 137
   levels 7, 20, 38, 41
   serum 20
Anti-obesity agents 47
Antioxidants 40
Anxiety 68
Arizona sexual experience scale 66
Aromatase inhibitors 125, 131, 142, 143
Assisted reproductive technique 26, 128, 144, 154, 161

B

Bacteroidaceae 88
Bacteroides 88, 89
   fragilis 89
   role of 87*f*
   vulgatus 86
Bariatric surgery 167, 168, 171
   effects of 171
   types of 168
Behavioral strategies 162
Benzoyl peroxide 176
Bicalutamide 124
Bifidobacterium 89
Biliopancreatic diversion 169
Bilophila 89
Binding protein 35
Binge eating disorder 69
Biochemical hyperandrogenism 20, 133
Bisphenol A 92
Blood
   pressure 46, 109, 183
   sugar 96
Body image
   distress 65
   disturbances 65
Body mass index 44, 47, 65, 74, 82, 96, 105, 109, 114, 119, 133, 151, 156, 162, 187
Bodyweight 65
Breast
   cancer 112, 114, 156
   carcinoma 182
Broadband light 63
Bromocriptine 144
Bulimia nervosa 69
Bupropion 126

C

Calcium 171
   deficiency 84
Cancer 45, 182
   endometrial 102, 105, 105*f*, 112, 114, 114*f*, 183, 183*fc*
   gynecologic 114*t*
Carbohydrates 117
   proportion of 117
Carcinoma, endometrial 121
Cardiovascular disease 44, 98, 104, 106, 109, 181
Carotenoids 82

Carotid intima media thickness 109
Central nervous system 55
Cervical mucus, production of 143
Cesarean delivery 171
Cetrorelix 146
Choriogonadotropin receptor 191
Chromium 82, 83
   polynicotinate 149, 150, 152
Chronic anovulation 128
   effects of 138*fc*
Chronic obstructive pulmonary disease 77
Clomiphene 125, 140, 144, 146, 155
   citrate 125, 131, 142, 143, 151
      resistant polycystic ovarian syndrome 131*t*
      role of 142
Clostridium 89
   perfringens 89
Combined oral contraceptive 45
   pill 37, 121
Comedonal acne 34*f*
   formation of 34*f*
Computed tomography 27, 58
Continuous positive airway pressure 74, 109
Contraceptive pills, low-dose 122
Copper 171
Coronary artery calcification 109
Corpus luteum 23
Craniopharyngiomas 142
Cyproterone acetate 61, 124

D

Danish National Patient Register 112
Daytime sleepiness, excessive 75
D-chiro-inositol 40, 99, 155
Dehydroepiandrosterone 6
   sulfate 10, 20, 38, 41, 56, 102, 151, 190
Dendritic cells 130
Depression 68
Depressive disorder, major 68
Dexamethasone androgen suppression test 4, 6
Diabetes mellitus 31*f*, 45, 50, 104, 168, 181, 191
   gestational 161, 163, 167, 171
   noninsulin-dependent 181
   type 2 30, 81, 98, 106, 173, 184

Diet 39, 89, 116, 117
Dietary fiber 116
Diode laser 63
Dominant follicle 23
Doxycycline 176
Dumping syndrome 171
Duodenal switch 170*f*
Duodenum, division of 169
Dysbiosis 11
Dysfunctional steroidogenesis 137
Dyslipidemia 44, 47, 81, 104, 107, 126, 168
   atherogenic 44

E

Eating disorders 69
Elevated luteinizing hormone 155
Ellipsoid, volume of 25*f*
Embryos 152, 155
   implantation 156
Endocrine disorder 121
Endocrine disrupting chemicals 30, 92
   mechanism of action of 93*fc*
Endocrine disturbances 136
Endocrinological disorder 173
Endometrial homeobox gene expression, effects on 132
Endothelial function 181
Enterobacteria 89
Epigenetics 10
Epworth sleepiness scale 73, 76*b*
Erythema, postinflammatory 176
Escherichia coli 11
Esophagogastric junction 168
Estimated glomerular filtration rate 123
Estrogen 143
   component 122
   levels 143
   receptor 11
   sensitive tumors 156
Ethinylestradiol 61, 108, 122
European Society for Human Reproduction and Embryology 65, 107
Exercise 39
Extreme stress 142

F

Facial hair, excessive 34*f*

Faecalibacterium 89
   prausnitzii 11
Fatty acids 87, 117
Fecal microbiota transplantation 90
Female pattern hair loss, scoring systems for 177*f*
Female sexual function index 66
Ferryman-Gallwey score system 32, 33*f*, 124
   modified 20, 58, 59*f*
Fertilization 156
Fibroblast proliferation 177
Finasteride 124*f*
First-line pharmacologic therapy 121
Flutamide 62, 124
Folate 171
Folic acid 96, 171
Follicles 155
   number of 25
   peripheral distribution of 102
   stimulating hormone 5, 6, 38, 41, 58, 82, 95, 96, 101, 106, 107, 122, 136, 143, 152, 188
   serum 104
Follicular somatic cells 140
Free androgen index 20, 38, 41, 102, 105
Free testosterone 20, 98*f*

G

Gastric band 168
   adjustable 169*f*
Gastroesophageal reflux disease 168
Gene
   expression, abnormal 138
   polymorphism 191
      cytokine-related 191
Genome-wide association studies 10, 55
Gestational age
   large for 162, 163
   small for 162, 163
Glucagon-like peptide receptor 48
   agonists 126
Glucocorticoids 62, 144, 149-151
Glucose
   intolerance 74, 180
   metabolism, postprandial abnormalities of 50

transport proteins 138
transporter 51, 52*f*
Glycodeoxycholic acid 86, 87
Glycolic acid 179
Gonadotropin 140, 144, 145
   abnormalities 8
   duration of 145
   exogenous 144
   recombinant 144
   releasing hormone 6, 54, 62, 93, 107, 122, 142, 154, 188
      agonist 4, 6, 62, 145
      antagonists 145
   secretion 188
   therapy 125
   total 155
   use of 140
Granulosa cells 136, 138
   dysfunction 4, 7
Growth hormone 108
Gut
   microbes 86
   microbiome 86
   microbiota, dysbiosis of 86, 87*fc*

H

Hair
   follicular growth, biological modifiers of 62
   growth, severity of 174
   removal 175
Heartbeat, irregular 184
Hematopoietic system 113
Hepatic insulin extraction 54
Hepatobiliary tract 170
High sensitivity C-reactive protein 151
High-density lipoprotein 37*f*, 83, 105
   cholesterol 46, 106, 180
Hirsutism 20, 23, 32, 39, 56, 56*fc*, 57, 60*fc*, 62, 63, 97, 173, 174
   causes of 57
   eflornithine for 124
   first-line antiandrogen for 123
   idiopathic 56
   manifestation of 167
   peripheral 56
   second-line antiandrogen for 124*f*
   treatment for 61, 123
   typical symptoms of 34*f*

Home sleep apnea testing 76, 77
Homeostasis model assessment 105
Hormonal contraceptives 121, 123, 126
Hormone, reproductive 54
Human chorionic gonadotropin 4, 144, 156
Human pregnancy X receptor 92
Hunger hormone 169
Hydrolaparoscopy, transvaginal 133
Hydroxyprogesterone 6, 58, 188
Hyperandrogenemia 23, 30, 65, 136, 139
Hyperandrogenic phenotypes 192
Hyperandrogenism 18, 23, 50, 51, 56, 101, 104, 112, 128, 167, 177, 190*f*
   biochemical signs of 23, 101
   clinical 19, 173
   effects of 173
   in utero 15
   inheritance of 54
   signs of 174
Hyperinsulinemia 8, 52, 54, 81, 133, 136, 177, 189
Hyperkalemia 61
Hyperketonemia 45
Hyperpigmentation, postinflammatory 176
Hyperplasia, endometrial 121, 182
Hyperplastic central stroma 128
Hyperstimulation, risk of 156
Hypertension 44, 104, 122, 126, 167, 168
   gestational 161
Hypertensive spectrum disorder 161
Hypertrichosis 56
Hypogonadism
   eugonadotropic 154
   hypergonadotropic 142
   hypogonadotropic 142, 145
   normogonadotropic 142
Hypopnea 73
Hypothalamic-pituitary-ovarian axis 65, 93, 116, 142
Hypothyroidism, hypophyseal 58

I

Impaired glucose tolerance 44, 50, 106, 151

In vitro
   fertilization 97, 98, 140, 149, 154, 155, 161
   maturation 154, 156
Infertility 1, 161
   factors 134
   stigma of 186
   treatment 128, 156
   unexplained 143, 145
Inflammation 81, 88, 161
Inflammatory bowel disease 89
Innate lymphoid cells 87
Inositols 47
Insulin 54, 140
   like growth factor 7, 31*f*, 35, 52, 106, 183, 190
      binding protein 137
   metabolic actions of 51
   receptor 30
   substrate 30, 55
   resistance 4, 38, 41, 44, 50, 65, 81, 98, 106, 107*f*, 112, 137, 139*fc*, 161, 164, 173, 177, 181, 186*t*, 188, 190*f*
      causes of 137*b*
      diagnosis of 181
      hyperinsulinism 5*f*, 7, 8
      pathogenesis of 87*f*
   secretion 52, 189
   sensitivity 44, 131
   sensitizing
      agents 47, 155
      medications 122
   signaling pathways 139*fc*
Intense pulse light 63
Interleukin 87, 106, 108
International Diabetes Federation 37
Intracytoplasmic sperm injection 154
Intraovarian androgen 7
Intrauterine
   androgen 101
   insemination 97, 98
   origin, theory of 15
Iron 171
Irregular menstrual periods 1, 18
Isotretinoin 176

J

Jejunoileal bypass 169
Jejunum, roux limb of 170

Index

K

Kallmann's syndrome 142
Kaplan-Meier survival estimates 114*f*
Keratinocyte 177

L

Lactobacillus 89
Laparoscopic ovarian drilling 128, 131, 131*t*, 133, 134, 140, 146, 149, 152
 bilateral 131
 effects of 130
 endocrinological aspects of 129
 indications for 129
 technique of 132*f*
 unilateral 131
Laparotomy 128
Laser therapy 175
Lean protein 117
Lesions
 location of 35
 types of 35
Letrozole 125, 140, 144, 146, 154-156
Lipopolysaccharide 87, 88
Lipoprotein
 high-density 37*f*, 83, 105
 low-density 81, 105, 182
 very-low-density 81
Liquid chromatography mass spectrometry 20
Liraglutide 48
Liver disease, end-stage 168
L-methylfolate 40
Low-density lipoprotein 81, 105, 182
 cholesterol 106
Ludwig's classification 173
Ludwig's patterns 177*f*
Luteinization, premature 136
Luteinizing hormone 4, 5, 8, 38, 41, 51, 58, 82, 95, 96, 101, 106, 107, 122, 136, 137, 188-191
 hypersecretion of 182

M

Macrosomia 171
Magnesium 96
Magnetic resonance imaging 27, 58
Male androgenetic alopecia 177*f*
Maternal nutrition, theory of 15
Medical ovulation induction 128
Melatonin 149, 151, 152
Menopause 104, 126
 age of 105
Menstrual cycles 121, 146
 abnormalities 121
Menstrual irregularities 31, 101
 criteria for 31*t*
 treatment for 39
Mental health 103, 108
 disorders 163
 issues 102
Mental well-being 184
Metabolic disorder 173
 causes of 108*fc*
Metabolic dysfunction 86, 137*fc*, 180
Metabolic syndrome 1, 44-46, 46*t*, 104, 106, 106*fc*, 167, 191
 criteria for 180*t*
 diagnosis of 37*f*
 diagnostic criteria for 37, 46
 pathophysiology of 44
 primary intervention for 46
 recommendations for 47*t*
Metformin 40, 47, 84, 122, 123, 131, 144, 149, 150, 155, 164, 175, 176
 monitoring of 123
 role of 144
 therapy 126
Microbiome 11
Micronutrients 81
 role of 81
Mineral deficiency 171
Minocycline 176
M-inositol 96
Miscarriages 164
 rate 161
 lower 140
Mitogen-activated protein kinase 51, 52*f*
Mono-ovulation 147
Mood disorders 68, 180
Multiple pregnancy 155
 rate 146
 risk of 140
Multivitamins 171
Myoinositol 40, 99, 146, 149, 150, 151, 155

N

N-acetyl cysteine 149, 151, 152
Nadifloxacin 176
Naltrexone 126
National Institutes of Health 2, 18, 23, 36, 100
Neodymium-doped yttrium aluminum garnet laser 63
Neoplasm 104
New York Heart Association 77
Nonalcoholic fatty liver disease 45, 107, 126, 162
Non-laparoscopic ovarian drilling 131*t*
Northeast cerebrovascular consortium 105

O

Obesity 2, 9, 32, 36*f*, 41, 44, 65, 81, 102, 104, 107, 107*fc*, 119, 139, 167, 172, 180, 182, 189
 abdominal 106
 atypical polycystic ovarian syndrome of 9, 6*f*
 index 161
 role of 74, 139
Obsessive-compulsive disorder 69
Obstructive sleep apnea 45, 73, 75*fc*, 77, 78*b*, 108, 163, 168
 diagnosis of 75
 management of 75
 pathophysiology 74
 prevalence of 73, 74*f*
 syndrome 73
Oily skin 174
Oligomenorrhea 18, 19, 101
Oligo-ovulation 173
Oocytes 138, 152, 155
 quality 162
Oral contraceptive 156
 effects, monitoring of 122
 pill 21, 61
 selection of 121
Oral glucose tolerance test 38, 41, 45, 163, 192
Oral ovulation induction 142
Oral ovulogen 140
Orlistat 47, 125
Ovarian cancer 106*t*, 112-114, 183
 higher risk of 183

Index

Ovarian dysfunction 23, 140
Ovarian hyperandrogenism,
    functional 4, 5f, 6
Ovarian hyperstimulation
    syndrome 26, 140, 145,
    151, 154, 161
Ovarian malignancy 105
Ovarian stroma,
    hypertrophy of 102
Ovarian surgery,
    laparoscopic 134
Ovary, normal 186
Ovulation 130
    amelioration of 129f
    induction 43, 98, 142, 154, 155
Ovulatory disturbance, causes
    of 136
Ovulatory dysfunction 100, 136
Oxidative stress 81, 152, 191

P

Pancreas 170
Pediatric Endocrine Society
    Criteria 101
Pelvic ultrasonography 58
Peripheral androgen blockade 61
Peritoneal cavity 133
Peroxisome proliferator-activated
    receptor gamma 191
Phenotype 18, 19
Phosphatidylinositol 3-kinase 51,
    52f, 53
Pihydrotestosterone, local 124
Pioglitazone 123
Pittsburgh sleep quality 73
Plasminogen activator
    inhibitor-1 106
Polycystic ovarian
    disease 1, 70, 173
    management of 1
Polycystic ovarian morphology 4,
    5, 18-20, 31, 88, 100-102,
    105, 186
Polycystic ovarian syndrome 1,
    4-6, 8, 14, 18, 23, 31,
    38b, 41, 47, 48f, 50-52,
    54-56, 65, 73, 74f, 78, 82,
    87f, 88, 92, 95, 95f, 97f,
    98, 103-107, 108, 108fc,
    114t, 116-119, 136, 149,
    154, 162f, 163f, 167, 173,
    180, 180t, 181, 186, 187f
    adjuvants in 149, 150t
    association of 106fc
    bariatric surgery in 167
    basic pathophysiology in 192f
    cancer in 112
    clinical
        features of 31, 31f, 140b, 192
        spectrum of 100
    defective oocytes in 138
    development of 15
    diagnosis of 18, 21, 24f, 37, 139
    diagnostic criteria of 36, 36f
    endocrine
        disruptors in 92
        dysfunction in 136
    epidemiology of 1, 186
    etiopathogenesis of 31f
    functional classification of 6t
    genetics of 191
    hyperandrogenism in 56, 190f
    in vitro
        fertilization in 155
        maturation in 156
    incidence of 192
    infertility in 98f, 136
    insulin resistance in 50, 186t,
        190f
    lifestyle interventions in 116
    management of 38, 78b, 121,
        154, 192
    metabolic
        dysfunction in 137fc
        phenotypes 50
    mitogenic action of
        insulin in 52
    neuroendocrine abnormalities
        in 139
    nonhyperandrogenic 19
    nutraceuticals in 95
    ovulation induction in 142
    ovulatory 19
    pathogenesis of 87fc
    pathophysiology of 4, 188
    phenotypes 50, 100t
    pregnancy in 161
    prevalence of 186
    psychological aspects of 65
    questionnaire 66
    Rotterdam's criteria for 24f
    sequelae of 180
    spectrum 149fc
    surgery in 128
    surgical treatment of 129f
    treatment of 38f
Polycystic ovary 1, 18, 19, 23, 27,
    128, 136, 173, 191
Polysomnography 77
Post-letrozole
    supplementation 143
Postpartum androgen 101
Prednisolone 144
Preeclampsia 161, 171
Pregnancy
    disorders of 161
    loss, early 161
    rate 130, 146
Premenstrual flare 175
Preterm births 161
Prevotella 88
Progestin
    component 122
    eluting intrauterine
        device 122
    only pill 122
Propionibacterium acnes 175
Protisol 95
Psychiatric disorders 68

R

Randomized controlled
    trial 84, 89, 131
Reactive oxygen species 81
Renal disease, end-stage 168
Renin-angiotensin-aldosterone
    system 44
Reproductive cycle,
    hypothalamic-pituitary-
    ovarian axis of 116
Rosiglitazone 123, 175
Rotterdam's criteria 18, 19, 24f,
    101, 136
    revised 18
Rotterdam's European Society of
    Human Reproduction
    and Embryology 23
Roux-en-Y gastric bypass 168,
    169, 170f
Ruby laser 62

S

Salicylic acid 179
Scar formation 128
Seborrhea 32, 174, 178
Sebum accumulation
    34f
Selective estrogen receptor
    modulator 125, 142
Selenium 81, 149, 151,
    152, 171
Selenoproteins 81

Index

Sex hormone 88
   binding globulin 11, 31*f*, 38, 41, 51, 53*fc*, 57, 93, 96, 99, 102, 106, 107, 136, 137, 183, 190
Sex steroids, role of 74
Sheehan syndrome 142
Short-chain free fatty acid 89
Single-nucleotide polymorphisms 191
Skin
   issues 97*f*
   tags 174, 178, 178*f*
Sleep apnea 73, 183
   testing 76, 77*fc*
Sleeve gastrectomy 168, 169
Social phobia 68
Spironolactone 61, 123
Stein-Leventhal syndrome 182
Steroid hormone 183
Steroidogenesis 138
Stomach 170
   lesser curvature of 170
STOP-bang
   interpretation 76*t*
   questionnaire 75*t*
Stress 67, 67*fc*
Striae 173, 177
   albae 178
   atrophicans 178
   caerulea 178
   nigrae 178
   rubrae 178
Subfertility 161
   stigma of 186

Surgery, laparoscopic 128, 132

T

Tamoxifen 143
Tauroursodeoxycholic acid 86
T-cell
   counts 130
   regulatory 130
Terminal hair 56*fc*, 174, 174*f*
Testosterone 56, 58, 136
   levels 105, 124
   lower 39
   total 98*f*
Theca cell 44, 136
   steroidogenesis, dysregulation of 5
Thermal injury 130
Thiamine 171
Thiazolidinediones 109, 123, 155
Thyroid
   adenoma 191
   associated gene 10
   stimulating hormone 38, 41, 108
   serum 58
Total antioxidant capacity 82
Transforming growth factor beta 7, 14
Transvaginal sonography 102, 106, 109
Tretinoin 176, 177
Trichoscopy 176
Tumor necrosis factor 106, 108
   alpha 7, 88

U

Ultrasonography 1, 24, 101
United States Environmental Protection Agency 11
Urinary protein 145

V

Vasoactive intestinal peptide 87
Vellus hair 56*fc*, 174*f*
Vertical sleeve gastrectomy 169*f*
Vitamin 96
   A 171
   B12 171
   D 40, 84, 96, 149, 151, 152, 171
      deficiency 84
      supplementation 84
   deficiency 171
   E 171
   K 171

W

Weight 189
   gain 1, 102
      gestational 163
      loss 61, 97*f*, 121, 154

Z

Zinc 83, 96, 171, 176
   deficiency 84
Zygotic genome 138

www.ingramcontent.com/pod-product-compliance
Ingram Content Group UK Ltd.
Pitfield, Milton Keynes, MK11 3LW, UK
UKHW051509150425
457402UK00019B/26